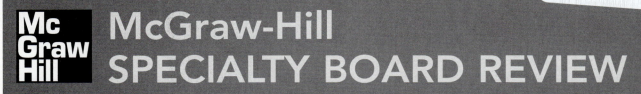

Neurology
Examination & Board Review

Nizar Souayah, MD
Assistant Professor of Neurology
University of Medicine and Dentistry of New Jersey
Director, EMG Laboratory and Peripheral Neuropathy Center
Newark, New Jersey

Sami Khella, MD
Clinical Associate Professor of Neurology
University of Pennsylvania School of Medicine
Philadelphia, Pennsylvania

McGraw-Hill
Medical Publishing Division

New York Chicago San Francisco Lisbon London Madrid Mexico City Milan
New Delhi San Juan Seoul Singapore Sydney Toronto

Neurology Examination & Board Review

Copyright © 2005 by The McGraw-Hill Companies, Inc. All rights reserved. Printed in the United States of America. Except as permitted under the United States Copyright Act of 1976, no part of this publication may be reproduced or distributed in any form or by any means, or stored in a data base or retrieval system, without the prior written permission of the publisher.

3 4 5 6 7 8 9 0   QPD/QPD   0 1 0 9 8 7 6

ISBN: 0-07-137839-1

Notice

Medicine is an ever-changing science. As new research and clinical experience broaden our knowledge, changes in treatment and drug therapy are required. The authors and the publisher of this work have checked with sources believed to be reliable in their efforts to provide information that is complete and generally in accord with the standards accepted at the time of publication. However, in view of the possibility of human error or changes in medical sciences, neither the authors nor the publisher nor any other party who has been involved in the preparation or publication of this work warrants that the information contained herein is in every respect accurate or complete, and they disclaim all responsibility for any errors or omissions or for the results obtained from use of the information contained in this work. Readers are encouraged to confirm the information contained herein with other sources. For example and in particular, readers are advised to check the product information sheet included in the package of each drug they plan to administer to be certain that the information contained in this work is accurate and that changes have not been made in the recommended dose or in the contraindications for administration. This recommendation is of particular importance in connection with new or infrequently used drugs.

This book was set in Palatino by International Typesetting and Composition.
The editor was Catherine A. Johnson.
The production supervisor was Rick Ruzycka.
Project management was provided by International Typesetting and Composition.
Quebecor World Dubuque was printer and binder.

This book is printed on acid-free paper.

Cataloging-in-publication data is on file for this title at the Library of Congress.

To my son Sami—let your dreams be your guide through this life.
To my wife Sonia—without your help and sacrifice this work would not have been possible.
To my parents—for your love, great affection, inspiration, and patience.

Contents

Color Plates appear between pages 280 and 281

Preface

My experience in teaching medical students, neurology residents, and fellows has been that they love multiple-choice questions when combined with didactic teaching. For this reason I developed several board-style questions at the end of most of the lectures I performed in the past few years, encouraging the audience to memorize the provided information.

The idea for this review initially arose when I was studying for the neurology board myself. I was surprised by the lack of review books in a question-and-answer format to help me assess my progress and identify areas of weakness. The few neurology reviews that did have multiple-choice questions were intended for medical students preparing for the USMLE, but lacked the deep and broad coverage needed for the neurology board exam.

Additional impetus for this book came from my years of teaching. Many of my students, residents, fellows, and even colleagues asked whether there was a book in question-and-answer format to use as an exam preparation tool in studying for certification/recertification for the neurology board. This format simulates the board exam and serves as an excellent tool to identify areas of strength and weakness and to sharpen already acquired knowledge.

This book is not designed to substitute for didactic lectures, seminars, and conferences offered during residency or fellowship training but to augment residents' experimental learning, reinforce their self-assessment and self-growth, and better prepare them for the certification examination of the American Board of Psychiatry and Neurology.

The content of this book is divided into 17 chapters, including an entire chapter devoted to psychiatry and another one for localization signs, offering a comprehensive coverage of the neurology board topics.

The best way to go through this book, especially for the "choose the one best response" questions is to follow these steps:

- First read the question without reading the answer choices (A to E) and guess the answer based on the information offered by the question.
- Then read the answer choices (A to E); these may confirm or refute the answer that you have already developed. In the latter case, choose an answer from the different offered choices.
- Go to the answer section of the chapter, check if your answer is correct, and read the answer.

The answers offer a comprehensive review of the different question choices. Whether or not you answered the question correctly, I strongly advise you to go in depth through the incorrect choices to find out why they are incorrect by consulting the answer references or other references. They will enlarge your knowledge provided by the question and will help identify any hidden weakness in your knowledge base.

I am indebted to many people who allowed us the luxury of time for this effort; most importantly, my family carried much of my personal daily workload with understanding. Numerous friends and colleagues deserve credit in helping me with this arduous project; without their support, I could not have completed it.

I am grateful to the many reviewers who made suggestions for improvement in the early stages of manuscript preparation: in particular, Dr. Sami Khella, who reviewed the final version of the book and who provided us with excellent comments and suggestions; Catherine Johnson for her help in contacting and coordinating with the reviewers; and Ben Kolstad, PhD, for providing the final editing.

I hope you have fun studying for the neurology board via the multiple-choice question-and-answer study approach.

Nizar Souayah, MD

CHAPTER 1

Anatomy and Physiology of the Central and Peripheral Nervous System

Questions

1. Which of the following sensory pathways does NOT project to the thalamus?

   (A) Visual sensation pathway
   (B) Auditory sensation pathway
   (C) Vibration sensation pathway
   (D) Olfactory sensation pathway
   (E) Temperature sensation pathway

2. The long thoracic nerve innervates the

   (A) serratus anterior muscle
   (B) rhomboid muscle
   (C) levator scapula
   (D) supraspinatus muscle
   (E) infraspinatus muscle

3. Which of the following is INCORRECT about the axillary nerve?

   (A) It arises from C5-C6.
   (B) It innervates the deltoid and teres minor muscles.
   (C) It is a pure motor nerve.
   (D) Its injury may lead to weakness of arm abduction in the horizontal position.
   (E) In neuralgic amyotrophy, the axillary nerve may be affected in isolation in 10% of cases.

4. A musculocutaneous lesion affects

   (A) hand sensation
   (B) supination with the forearm extended
   (C) supination with the elbow in flexion
   (D) wrist extension
   (E) upper arm abduction

5. Which of the following is a compression site of the radial nerve?

   (A) Suprascapular notch
   (B) Carpal tunnel
   (C) Spinoglenoid notch
   (D) The elbow posterior to the medial epicondyle
   (E) Spiral groove in the posterior aspect of the humerus

6. All of the following muscles are innervated by the medial division of the sciatic nerve EXCEPT the

   (A) semimembranosus
   (B) long head of the biceps femoris
   (C) semitendinosus
   (D) short head of the biceps femoris
   (E) adductor magnus muscle

7. In carpal tunnel syndrome, the median nerve is entrapped

   (A) beneath the flexor retinaculum ligament
   (B) above the flexor retinaculum ligament
   (C) at the hamate bone
   (D) in Guyon's canal
   (E) on the radial side of the wrist at the level of the styloid process

Questions 8 through 12
Link each of the following nerves to its anatomical location.

    (A) Posterior cutaneous nerve of the thigh
    (B) Lateral cutaneous nerve of the thigh
    (C) Genitofemoral nerve
    (D) Femoral nerve
    (E) Obturator nerve

8. The nerve arises from S1-S3. It passes through the greater sciatic notch below the piriform muscle. In the thigh, it branches to the skin of the perineum and scrotum. The nerve descends over the hamstring muscles, supplying fibers to the dorsal side and proximal third of the calf and lower part of the buttock.

9. The nerve arises from L2-L4 roots. It innervates the sartorius and the quadriceps muscles.

10. The nerve arises from L2-L3 roots. It enters the thigh in a fibrous canal within the fascia lata and changes its position from horizontal to vertical. Distal to the inguinal canal, the nerve divides into twigs to innervate the skin of the lateral part of the thigh.

11. This nerve is responsible for the innervation of the adductor muscles of the thigh.

12. The nerve arises from the L1-L2 roots. It runs downward through the psoas muscle. At the level of the inguinal ligament, it divides into branches to innervate the skin of the anterior surface of the thigh and the cremaster muscle.

13. Which of the following structures is involved in vertical saccades?

    (A) Parietal cortex
    (B) Cerebellar vermis
    (C) Caudate nuclei
    (D) Interstitial nucleus of the medial longitudinal fasciculus
    (E) Fastigial nucleus

14. Eye position information reaches the abducens nucleus from neuronal integrator neurons coming from the

    (A) rostral interstitial nucleus of the medial longitudinal fasciculus
    (B) interstitial nucleus of Cajal
    (C) parapontine reticular formation
    (D) red nucleus
    (E) nucleus prepositus hypoglossi

15. The gaze-holding neural integrator for vertical gaze is located in the

    (A) interstitial nucleus of Cajal
    (B) medial vestibular nucleus
    (C) nucleus prepositus hypoglossi
    (D) red nucleus
    (E) rostral interstitial nucleus of the medial longitudinal fasciculus

16. Which of the following cranial nerves exits the brainstem from its dorsal aspect?

    (A) Oculomotor nerve
    (B) Facial nerve
    (C) Trigeminal nerve
    (D) Glossopharyngeal nerve
    (E) Trochlear nerve

17. Which of the following neurological structures does NOT travel through the cavernous sinus?

    (A) Sympathetic carotid plexus
    (B) Oculomotor nerve
    (C) Mandibular branch of the trigeminal nerve
    (D) Trochlear nerve
    (E) Abducens nerve

18. Which of the following is TRUE about the trigeminal nerve?

    (A) The spinal nucleus of the trigeminal nerve subserves light touch in the ipsilateral side of the face.
    (B) The motor nucleus of the trigeminal nerve lies in the pons medial to the sensory nucleus and sends axons to the

maxillary division of the trigeminal nerve.

(C) The three divisions of the trigeminal nerve converge at the Gasserian ganglion.

(D) The mesencephalic nucleus of the trigeminal nerve subserves pain and temperature in the ipsilateral side of the face.

(E) The mandibular division of the trigeminal nerve subserves sensation to the ipsilateral angle of the mandible.

19. Which of the following pairs of cranial nerves travel through the internal auditory canal?

(A) Vestibulocochlear and trigeminal
(B) Facial and trigeminal
(C) Facial and optic
(D) Facial and vestibulocochlear
(E) Vestibulocochlear and vagus

20. The origin of the nervus intermedius of Wrisberg is the

(A) sensory nucleus of the trigeminal nerve
(B) motor facial nucleus
(C) superior salivary nucleus
(D) inferior salivary nucleus
(E) nucleus of the vestibulocochlear nerve

21. A 40-year-old man developed chronic pain in the right forearm that lasted hours each day. Neurological examination demonstrated normal sensory examination, mild right forearm pronation weakness, and weak flexion of terminal phalanges of right thumb, index, and middle fingers. An attempt to make a full circle by applying the end phalanx of the thumb to that of the index finger with firm pressure showed consistent weakness. Which of the following structures is affected?

(A) Right anterior interosseous nerve
(B) Right median nerve at the upper axilla

(C) Right ulnar nerve
(D) Right radial nerve
(E) Right musculocutaneous nerve

22. The substantia gelatinosa of the spinal cord is located in

(A) lamina I
(B) lamina II
(C) lamina IV
(D) lamina VII
(E) lamina IX

23. The striatum is formed by all of the following structures EXCEPT the

(A) caudate nucleus
(B) globus pallidus
(C) olfactory tubercles
(D) nucleus accumbens
(E) substantia innominata

24. The direct circuit loop between the basal ganglia and the cortex is

(A) cerebral cortex → striatum → internal globus pallidus → substantia nigra pars reticulata → dorsal thalamus → cerebral cortex

(B) cerebral cortex → striatum → external globus pallidus → substantia nigra pars reticulata → dorsal thalamus → cerebral cortex

(C) cerebral cortex → striatum → internal globus pallidus → dorsal thalamus → cerebral cortex

(D) cerebral cortex → striatum → external globus pallidus → substantia nigra pars compacta → dorsal thalamus → cerebral cortex

(E) cerebral cortex → striatum → internal globus pallidus → subthalamic nucleus → internal globus pallidus → dorsal thalamus → cerebral cortex

25. The indirect circuit loop between the basal ganglia and the cerebral cortex is

    (A) cortical fibers → striatum → external globus pallidus → subthalamic nucleus → internal globus pallidus → dorsal thalamus → cerebral cortex
    (B) cortical fibers → striatum → external globus pallidus → internal globus pallidus → dorsal thalamus → cerebral cortex
    (C) cortical fibers → striatum → external globus pallidus → substantia nigra pars reticulata → dorsal thalamus → cerebral cortex
    (D) cortical fibers → striatum → external globus pallidus → subthalamic nucleus → substantia nigra pars compacta → dorsal thalamus → cerebral cortex
    (E) cortical fibers → striatum → external globus pallidus → subthalamic nucleus → internal globus pallidus → substantia nigra pars compacta → dorsal thalamus → cerebral cortex

26. The superior cerebellar peduncle contains one cerebellar afferent, which is the

    (A) ventral spinocerebellar tract
    (B) pontocerebellar tract
    (C) dorsal spinocerebellar tract
    (D) olivocerebellar fibers
    (E) reticulocerebellar fibers

Questions 27 through 29
Link each of the following cerebellar nuclei to the structure to which it sends efferent projections.

    (A) Fastigial nucleus
    (B) Dentate nucleus
    (C) Emboliform nucleus

27. Red nucleus

28. Posterior division of the ventrolateral nucleus of the thalamus

29. Vestibular nucleus

30. The cerebellar cortex contains all of the following types of cells EXCEPT

    (A) pyramidal cells
    (B) Purkinje cells
    (C) granule cells
    (D) Golgi cells
    (E) basket cells

31. The source of noradrenergic projection to the cerebellum is the

    (A) dorsomedial nucleus of the hypothalamus
    (B) locus ceruleus
    (C) raphe nucleus
    (D) thalamus
    (E) inferior olivary nucleus

32. The learning of complex motor tasks and motor plasticity are two functions that mainly involve the

    (A) olivocerebellar climbing fibers
    (B) mossy fibers
    (C) emboliform nuclei
    (D) motor cortical area
    (E) parallel fibers from granular cell axons

33. The tuberoinfandibular hypothalamic tract arises from the

    (A) arcuate nuclei
    (B) mammillary nuclei
    (C) fornix
    (D) paraventricular nucleus
    (E) supraoptic nucleus

34. The most likely neurotransmitter for cerebellar climbing fibers is

    (A) acetylcholine
    (B) glutamate
    (C) aspartate
    (D) dopamine
    (E) glycine

35. The only efferent fibers from the cerebellar cortex come from

    (A) axons of Purkinje cells
    (B) mossy fiber projections
    (C) parallel fibers
    (D) climbing fibers
    (E) axons of Golgi cells

36. Hyperphagia is caused by a lesion in the

    (A) ventromedial nucleus
    (B) supraoptic nucleus
    (C) anterior nucleus
    (D) arcuate nucleus
    (E) mammillary nucleus

37. Which of the following extraocular muscles is innervated by a nucleus located on the contralateral side?

    (A) Superior rectus
    (B) Inferior rectus
    (C) Medial rectus
    (D) Lateral rectus
    (E) Inferior oblique

38. All of the following cranial nerve nuclei are sources of general somatic efferents EXCEPT the

    (A) oculomotor nucleus
    (B) trochlear nucleus
    (C) abducens nucleus
    (D) motor nucleus of the facial nerve
    (E) hypoglossal nucleus

39. The parasympathetic innervation of the parotid gland is provided by the

    (A) facial nerve
    (B) vestibulocochlear nerve
    (C) glossopharyngeal nerve
    (D) vagus nerve
    (E) spinal accessory nerve

40. Which of the following is true about the trigeminal nerve nuclei?

    (A) The trigeminal nerve has two sensory nuclei.
    (B) Pain and temperature are carried predominantly by the spinal nucleus of the trigeminal nerve.
    (C) Most small fibers afferent of the spinal tract of the trigeminal nerve end in the main sensory nucleus of that nerve.
    (D) The motor nucleus of the trigeminal nerve innervates the muscles of mastication via its maxillary division.
    (E) The motor nucleus of the trigeminal nerve contains only alpha motor neurons.

41. Which of the following neurons are NOT found in the cerebral cortex?

    (A) Pyramidal cells
    (B) Granular cells
    (C) Purkinje cells
    (D) Horizontal cells
    (E) Fusiform cells

42. The principal efferent neuron layer of the cerebral neocortex is

    (A) II
    (B) III
    (C) IV
    (D) V
    (E) VI

43. Thalamocortical afferents have their main terminals in the cerebral cortex layer number

    (A) I
    (B) II
    (C) III
    (D) IV
    (E) V

44. The extrathalamic cortical modulatory system, using acetylcholine as a neurotransmitter, arises from the

(A) midbrain raphe

(B) locus ceruleus

(C) ventral midbrain

(D) nucleus basalis of Meynert of the basal forebrain

(E) hypothalamic nuclei

Questions 45 through 47

Link each of the following association areas of the cerebral cortex to the appropriate clinical signs and symptoms.

(A) Posterior parietal association cortex lesion

(B) Temporal association cortex lesion

(C) Prefrontal association cortex lesion

45. Affected patient displays bizarre, socially unacceptable behavior, with labile and unpredictable emotion.

46. Prosopagnosia

47. Neglect of the contralateral body

48. Which of the following arteries supplies the medial part of the lateral geniculate body?

(A) Ophthalmic artery

(B) Anterior communicating artery

(C) Anterior choroidal artery

(D) Posterior choroidal artery

(E) Middle cerebral artery

49. Which of the following cranial nerves is responsible for eye closure?

(A) Oculomotor nerve

(B) Trochlear nerve

(C) Abducens nerve

(D) Facial nerve

(E) Spinal accessory nerve

50. Which of the following structures receives afferents responsible for taste sensation in the anterior two-thirds of the tongue?

(A) Submaxillary ganglion

(B) Pterygopalatine ganglion

(C) Superior salivary nucleus

(D) Geniculate ganglion

(E) Submandibular ganglion

51. Which of the following arteries supplies the intracranial part of the facial nerve?

(A) Middle meningeal artery

(B) Superior cerebellar artery

(C) Posterior inferior cerebellar artery

(D) Anterior inferior cerebellar artery

(E) Posterior auricular artery

52. The third-order neurons of the auditory pathway terminate at the

(A) inferior colliculus

(B) auditory radiation

(C) medial geniculate body

(D) lateral geniculate body

(E) dorsal portion of the cochlear nucleus

53. The glossopharyngeal nerve crosses the jugular foramen with the

(A) facial and vestibulocochlear nerves

(B) vestibulocochlear and vagus nerves

(C) vagus and spinal accessory nerves

(D) vestibulocochlear and spinal accessory nerves

(E) facial and spinal accessory nerves

54. Jugular foramen syndrome includes all the following signs EXCEPT

(A) ipsilateral trapezoid weakness

(B) dysphonia

(C) dysphagia

(D) ipsilateral tongue deviation

(E) depressed gag reflex

55. All of the following arteries supply the mid-brain EXCEPT the

    (A) posterior cerebral artery
    (B) superior cerebellar artery
    (C) anterior inferior cerebellar artery
    (D) posterior choroidal artery
    (E) anterior choroidal artery

56. Which of the following is true about ion channel sequestration in central nervous system axons?

    (A) Sodium and potassium channel clustering causes an inhibition of proper electrical signal generation in the central nervous system.
    (B) Sodium channel clustering is located within the juxtaparanodal axonal region.
    (C) Sodium channel clustering is initiated by Schwann cells in the peripheral nervous system.
    (D) Shaker-type potassium channels are clustered in the node of Ranvier and may serve to inhibit sodium channel clustering.
    (E) Axonal sodium channel expression decreases in multiple sclerosis.

57. Which of the following proteins is found in noncompact myelin of the peripheral nervous system?

    (A) Connexin 32
    (B) Myelin basic protein
    (C) Proteolipid protein (PLP)
    (D) Peripheral myelin protein 22 (PMP22)
    (E) Myelin-oligodendrocyte-specific protein

Questions 58 through 64
Link the following.

    (A) Oligodendrocyte
    (B) Schwann
    (C) Both
    (D) Neither

58. The cell ensheathes multiple axons.

59. The cell makes multiple myelin sheaths for different axons.

60. The cell has a basal lamina.

61. The cell synthesizes myelin basic protein.

62. The cell expresses connexin 32.

63. The cell expresses myelin-oligodendrocyte glycoprotein.

64. The cell is responsible for myelin synthesis in the central nervous system.

Questions 65 through 69
Link the following.

    (A) Astrocyte
    (B) Oligodendrocyte
    (C) Both
    (D) Neither

65. Class I MHC expression

66. Class II MHC expression

67. Expression of adhesion molecules

68. Expression of costimulatory molecules

69. Expression of complement components

70. The resting membrane potential in a typical neuron is

    (A) −50 mV
    (B) −70 mV
    (C) −80 mV
    (D) −30 mV
    (E) −40 mV

71. Which of the following types of axons has the fastest conduction velocity?

    (A) Ia
    (B) Ib
    (C) II
    (D) III
    (E) IV

72. Neurulation does not occur when the embryo is exposed to colchicine because

    (A) it inhibits induction
    (B) it inhibits anterior neuropore closure
    (C) it inhibits posterior neuropore closure
    (D) it induces microfilament-based contraction
    (E) it induces the depolymerization of microtubules

73. After fertilization, the anterior neuropore closes at

    (A) 14 days
    (B) 20 days
    (C) 18 days
    (D) 24 days
    (E) 28 days

74. Failure of the anterior neuropore to close causes

    (A) anencephaly
    (B) spina bifida
    (C) meningocele
    (D) meningomyelocele
    (E) tethered cord syndrome

75. Failure of the forebrain to undergo cleavage results in

    (A) anencephaly
    (B) holoprosencephaly
    (C) myelodysplasia
    (D) meningoencephalocele
    (E) spina bifida

Questions 76 through 79
Link each of the following secondary brain vesicles to the corresponding brain structure that derives from each vesicle.

    (A) Diencephalon
    (B) Telencephalon
    (C) Rhombencephalon
    (D) Mesencephalon

76. Internal capsule

77. Cerebral aqueductus of Sylvius

78. Thalamus

79. Fourth ventricle

80. All of the following cells and structures derive from the neural crest EXCEPT

    (A) melanocytes
    (B) neuroblasts
    (C) Schwann cells
    (D) cartilage of pharyngeal arches
    (E) chromaffin cells of the adrenal medulla

Questions 81 through 87
Link the following.

    (A) Basal plate
    (B) Alar plate

81. General somatic efferent

82. General visceral afferent

83. General visceral efferent

84. General somatic afferent

85. Special visceral efferent

86. Special visceral afferent

87. Special somatic afferent

88. Which of the following structures sends afferents to the mammillary body?

    (A) Medial temporal cortex
    (B) Retinal pregeniculate nucleus
    (C) Nucleus of locus coeruleus
    (D) Arcuate nucleus
    (E) Supraoptic nucleus

Questions 89 through 99
Link each of the following thalamic nuclei to the corresponding afferent connection.

    (A) Anterior nucleus
    (B) Dorsomedial nucleus
    (C) Midline nucleus
    (D) Lateral dorsal nucleus
    (E) Ventral anterior nucleus
    (F) Ventral lateral nucleus
    (G) Ventral posterolateral nucleus
    (H) Ventral posteromedial nucleus
    (I) Lateral posterior nucleus
    (J) Medial geniculate body
    (K) Lateral geniculate body

89. Substantia nigra

90. Medial lemniscus

91. Trigeminal nucleus

92. Mammillary body

93. Cerebellum

94. Hypothalamus

95. Fornix

96. Frontal lobe

97. Optic tract

98. Pulvinar

99. Brachium of the inferior colliculus

100. Which of the following arteries does (do) NOT supply the thalamus?

    (A) Polar arteries
    (B) Anterior choroidal arteries
    (C) Posterior choroidal artery
    (D) Posterior cerebral artery
    (E) Posterior communicating arteries

101. The Papez circuit involves all of the following structures EXCEPT the

    (A) hippocampus
    (B) fornix
    (C) hypothalamus
    (D) anterior thalamic nuclei
    (E) cingulate gyrus

Answers and Explanations

1. **(D)** The olfactory pathway is the only sensory pathway that does not project to the thalamus. The olfactory nerve penetrates the cribriform plate of the ethmoid bone and enters the olfactory bulb to synapse with the second-order neurons: mitral and tufted cells. The axons of the second-order neurons course posteriorly as the olfactory tract in the orbital surfaces of the frontal lobe and project to the primary olfactory cortex in the temporal lobe. *(Parent, 748–754)*

2. **(A)** The long thoracic nerve arises from the motor roots of C5, C6, and C7. It courses downward through and in front of the medial scalenus muscle and further descends dorsal to the brachial plexus along the medial axillary wall to innervate the serratus anterior muscle. The suprascapular nerve innervates the supraspinatus and infraspinatus. The dorsal scapular nerve innervates the rhomboid and levator scapulae. *(Parent, 276; Staal 19)*

3. **(C)** The axillary nerve originates from the posterior fascicle of the brachial plexus and carries fibers from C5 and C6. It innervates the deltoid muscle and teres minor muscle. The axillary nerve sends a sensory branch, the lateral brachial cutaneous nerve, to the skin of the upper outer surface of the arm mainly in the deltoid region. An axillary nerve lesion results in weakness of arm abduction in the horizontal position against resistance. The first 30 degrees of abduction of the upper arm from the trunk is performed by the supraspinatus muscle, which is innervated by the suprascapular nerve, not by the axillary nerve. There is also weakness of the horizontal upper arm retraction against resistance with sensory loss in the skin area overlying the deltoid muscle. The axillary nerve is often involved in neuralgic amyotrophy, and in about ten percent of cases it is affected in isolation. *(Parent, 275–277; Staal, 27–29)*

4. **(C)** The musculocutaneous nerve arises from the lateral cord of the brachial plexus and carries fibers from the root of C5, C6, and C7. The nerve proceeds obliquely downward between the axillary artery and the median nerve. The nerve pierces the coracobrachialis muscle while giving off branches to it, and it descends further between the biceps and brachialis muscles to supply both of them. The lateral cutaneous nerve of the forearm is the sensory continuation of the musculocutaneous nerve. It innervates the skin from the elbow to the wrist and covers the entire forearm from the dorsal to the ventral midline. The coracobrachialis muscle is a forward elevator of the arm. The biceps is a forearm supinator, especially if the elbow is flexed at 90 degrees. Isolated lesions of the musculocutaneous nerve are rare. Such lesions would cause weakness of elbow flexion against resistance in a fully supinated hand, possible arm elevation weakness, arm pain, and radial forearm parasthesia. *(Brazis, 9–10; Staal, 31–33)*

5. **(E)** The radial nerve arises from the posterior cord of the brachial plexus and comprises fibers from spinal levels C5 to C8. After descending posterior to the axillary artery, the nerve courses posterior to the humerus in the spiral groove. It is at this site that the nerve is most often damaged by compression. *(Staal, 35)*

6. **(D)** The sciatic nerve is a mixed nerve that carries fibers from L4 to S3 and leaves the pelvis

through the sciatic foramen below the piriform muscle. The nerve then curves laterally and downward beneath the gluteus maximus muscle and runs on the dorsal side of the femoral bone to terminate at the proximal part of the popliteal fossa to divide into the tibial nerve medially and the peroneal nerve laterally. Within the sciatic nerve, as proximal as the gluteal region, the fibers of the tibial and peroneal nerves are arranged into two separate divisions: the medial and the lateral trunks, respectively. The medial part of the nerve innervates the adductor magnus and the hamstring muscles, except for the short head of the biceps femoris (it is the only thigh muscle supplied by the lateral peroneal division). The hamstring muscles are flexors of the knee joint and include the semimembranosus muscle, the semitendinous muscle, and the short and long heads of the biceps femoris. *(Staal, 117–118)*

7. **(A)** The point of entrapment of the median nerve in carpal tunnel syndrome lies under the flexor retinaculum. The flexor retinaculum forms the roof of the carpal tunnel, whereas the carpal bones and their connective tissue components form the floor of the carpal tunnel. In Guyon's canal, the hamate, and the pisiform bones are sites of compression of the ulnar nerve at the wrist. Rarely, radial nerve compression occurs at the level of the styloid process, just proximal to the wrist. *(Staal, 56–66)*

8. **(A)**

9. **(D)**

10. **(B)**

11. **(E)**

12. **(C)**

Explanations 8 through 12

The posterior femoral cutaneous nerve is a purely sensory nerve that arises from the anterior primary rami of the first through third sacral segments. It supplies the skin of the posterior thigh and popliteal fossa. The lateral femoral cutaneous nerve is also a purely sensory nerve that derives from the second and third lumbar segments within the substance of the psoas muscle. It supplies the skin of the anterior thigh to the knee and the upper half of the lateral aspect of the thigh. The genitofemoral nerve is predominantly a sensory nerve. It divides near the inguinal ligament into the external genital branch (responsible for the innervation of the cremaster muscle) and the medial femoral branch (responsible for the innervation of the skin of the upper thigh over the femoral triangle). The femoral nerve supplies the sartorius muscle (a flexor and evertor of the thigh) and the quadriceps (an extensor of the leg). The obturator nerve supplies the adductor muscles of the thigh. *(Brazis, Masdeu, and Biller, 27–32)*

13. **(D)** Vertical saccades are controlled by cortical pathways descending to the rostral interstitial nucleus of the medial longitudinal fasciculus at the junction between the midbrain and the thalamus. *(Kline and Bajandas, 54–55)*

14. **(E)** The abducens nucleus is the site of horizontal versional control. The nucleus of the abducens nerve contains two types of neurons: those that innervate the ipsilateral lateral rectus, and those that project via the contralateral medial longitudinal fasciculus to the contralateral oculomotor nucleus. The parapontine reticular formation contains cells that project to the abducens nucleus and activate it. The parapontine reticular formation contains excitatory burst neurons that discharge just prior to a horizontal saccade to stimulate cells in the abducens nucleus. Once the eye reaches a new eccentric position at the end of the saccade, stimulation of the abducens nucleus by the parapontine reticular formation burst neurons is substituted by a tonic gaze-holding mechanism to maintain the eccentric position. This requires a neuronal network that integrates a velocity-coded signal into a position-coded signal. This is referred to as the neural integrator, which includes the horizontal gaze center, the medial vestibular nucleus, and the nucleus prepositus hypoglossi. *(Kline and Bajandas, 61)*

15. **(A)** The rostral interstitial nucleus of the medial longitudinal fasciculus contains excitatory burst neurons for vertical and torsional saccade. It projects bilaterally to the oculomotor nuclei in the case of upward gaze and mainly ipsilaterally in the case of downward gaze. The gaze-holding neural integrator for vertical gaze is located in the interstitial nucleus of Cajal. *(Kline and Bajandas, 62)*

16. **(E)** The trochlear nerve is purely a motor nerve and is the only cranial nerve to exit the brain dorsally. The trochlear nerve supplies one muscle: the superior oblique. The cell bodies that originate in the trochlear nerve are located in the ventral part of the brain stem in the trochlear nucleus. The trochlear nucleus gives rise to fibers that cross to the other side of the brain stem just prior to exiting the pons. Thus, each superior oblique muscle is supplied by nerve fibers from the trochlear nucleus of the opposite side. The nerve travels in the lateral wall of the cavernous sinus and then enters the orbit via the superior orbital fissure. It passes medially and diagonally across the levator palpebral superioris and superior rectus muscles to innervate the superior oblique. *(Parent, 531)*

17. **(C)** The medial wall of the cavernous sinus contains the abducens nerve, the internal carotid artery and the sympathetic fibers of the carotid plexus. The lateral wall contains the oculomotor and trochlear nerves, and the ophthalmic and maxillary divisions of the trigeminal nerve. *(Afifi and Bergman, 240)*

18. **(C)** The trigeminal nerve is a mixed nerve. It subserves the sensory innervation of the ipsilateral side of the face and the ipsilateral muscles of mastication (masseter, temporalis, and pterygoids). The sensory nucleus of the trigeminal nerve extends from the midbrain to the upper cervical cord: (a) The mesencephalic nucleus subserves proprioception and deep sensation from the tendons and muscles of mastication. (b) The main sensory nucleus (located in the pons) subserves light touch. (c) The spinal nucleus (which extends from the pons to the upper cervical cord and is divided into segments that correspond to concentric

dermatomes around the mouth) subserves pain and temperature. The trigeminal nerve supplies sensation to the ipsilateral side of the face via three branches: the ophthalmic division (which innervates the frontal, lacrimal, and nasociliary areas), the maxillary division (which innervates the cheek and lower eyelid), and the mandibular division (which innervates the lower lip, the tongue, the mandible, except for the angle of the mandible). The motor nucleus lies medially to the main sensory nucleus and sends axons to the mandibular division of the trigeminal nerve. All divisions of the trigeminal nerve converge at the Gasserian ganglion, which lies in Meckel's cave of the temporal bone. *(Afifi and Bergman, 173–175)*

19. **(D)** The facial nerve leaves the pons and travels with the vestibulocochlear nerve through the internal auditory canal. *(Parent, 154–168)*

20. **(C)** The nervus intermedius is the sensory and parasympathetic division of the facial nerve. Its preganglionic parasympathetic fibers arise from the superior salivary nucleus and synapse in the pterygopalatine and submandibular, which then send postganglionic fibers to submandibular, sublingual, lacrimal, palatal, and nasal glands. The sensory fibers of the nervus intermedius arrive at the nerve intermedius via the geniculate ganglion. They provide taste sensation to the anterior two-thirds of the tongue. *(Afifi and Bergman, 163)*

21. **(A)** The patient described in this vignette has a pure motor deficit. The right pronator quadratus is weak because of paresis of forearm pronation. Also there is paresis of the flexor digitorum profundus I & II and the flexor pollicis longus because of loss of flexion of the terminal phalanges of the second and third fingers, and the thumb, respectively. All of these muscles are innervated by an anterior interosseous nerve. The characteristic feature of a lesion of this nerve is the inability to make a circle with the thumb and index finger. *(Staal, 55–56)*

22. **(B)** The gray matter of the spinal cord is divided into the 10 laminae of Rexed, which

form a cytoarchitectonic map of the spinal cord that correlates well with synaptic connections and neurophysiological data. Laminae I, II, III, and IV encompass most of the dorsal horn, which receives primary sensory fibers. Lamina I corresponds to the nucleus postmarginalis, lamina II corresponds to the substantia gelatinosa, and laminae III and IV correspond to the nucleus proprius dorsalis. All these nuclei integrate and modulate sensory information. They relay sensory information to higher centers like the cerebellum, thalamus, and brain stem. *(Afifi and Bergman, 66)*

23. **(B)** The striatum is the main receiving station for the basal ganglia. It receives massive projections from all areas of the cerebral cortex and from certain thalamic nuclei, the substantia nigra, and other brain stem nuclei. The caudate nucleus and the putamen are the largest of the nuclei composing the striatum. The ventral striatum consists of the ventral portion of the caudate nucleus, the putamen, the deep layers of the olfactory tubercle, the nucleus accumbens, and the substantia innominata. Although the nucleus accumbens and the substantia innominata are frequently referred to as parts of the olfactory system, they play an important functional role in the basal ganglia. *(Afifi and Bergman, 275–294)*

24. **(C)** In the direct loop, cortical fibers project to the striatum, and striatal efferent neurons project to the internal globus pallidus and the substantia nigra pars reticulata. Efferents from the internal globus pallidus and the substantia nigra pars reticulata project to the dorsal thalamus, and the thalamic neurons project to specific areas of the cerebral cortex. Both the glutaminergic corticostriate projections and the thalamocortical projections are excitatory. However, the efferents from the striatum to the internal globus pallidus and the substantia nigra pars reticulata, and their projections to the thalamus, are all GABAergic inhibitory. The glutaminergic corticostriate fibers excite a select population of striatal efferent neurons that project to the internal globus pallidus and the substantia nigra pars reticulata. These striatal efferents, using GABA and substance P as a neurotransmitter, inhibit the spontaneous firing of internal globus pallidus and substantia nigra pars reticulata efferents to the thalamus. These latter projections inhibit cortical relay neurons in the dorsal thalamus. Inhibition of these inhibitory neurons in the internal globus pallidus and substantia nigra pars reticulata leads to a disinhibition of the thalamocortical projections and an increase in cortical activity. *(Afifi and Bergman, 279–281; Brazis, Masdeu, and Biller 427–430)*

25. **(A)** In the indirect loop, linking the cerebral cortex to the basal ganglia, cortical fibers project to the striatum, and striatal efferent neurons project to the external globus pallidus. Efferents from the external part of the globus pallidus project to the subthalamic nucleus. Neurons in the subthalamic nucleus project to both the internal globus pallidus and the substantia nigra pars reticulata. The internal globus pallidus and the substantia nigra pars reticulata project to the dorsal thalamus. The dorsal thalamus projects to the cerebral cortex. The glutaminergic corticostriate fibers excite a specific population of striatal efferent neurons that project to the external globus pallidus. These striatal efferent neurons are GABAergic, with enkephalin as a co-transmitter. They inhibit neurons on the external globus pallidus. The external globus pallidus projection to the subthalamic nucleus has a high rate of spontaneous firing and is inhibitory. Subthalamic nucleus neurons are excitatory glutaminergic and project to both the internal globus pallidus and the substantia nigra pars reticulata.

Because of the high spontaneous firing rate of the inhibitory neurons in the external globus pallidus, the excitatory effects of the subthalamic nucleus on neurons in the internal globus pallidus and substantia nigra pars reticulata normally are minimal. However, when the activity of the indirect loop increases, there is a disinhibition of the subthalamic nucleus. The increased rate of firing of the subthalamic nucleus neurons in the internal globus pallidus and substantia nigra pars reticulata results in inhibition of the thalamic relay neurons. A corresponding decrease in the level of cortical activity occurs. *(Afifi and Bergman, 270–281; Brazis, Masdeu, and Biller 427–430)*

26. (A) The cerebellum communicates with the brain stem through three pairs of masses of projection fibers called cerebellar peduncles: the superior cerebellar peduncle, the middle cerebellar peduncle, and the inferior cerebellar peduncle. The superior cerebellar peduncle contains most of the cerebellar efferent fibers and all those arising from the dentate nucleus, the emboliform nucleus, and the globose nucleus. In addition, the superior cerebellar peduncle contains one cerebellar afferent pathway, the ventral spinocerebellar tract, which carries proprioceptive information to the cerebellum from the lower extremities and the trunk. *(Burt, 352)*

27. (C)

28. (B)

29. (A)

Explanations 27 through 29

Cerebellar nuclei are the principal source of efferent fibers from the cerebellum projecting to the dorsal thalamus, vestibular nuclei, red nucleus, and other brain stem nuclei. The dentate nucleus receives projections from Purkinje cells in the cerebro-cerebellum, and collaterals from some of the pontocerebellar fibers. Fibers from the dentate nucleus enter the brachium conjunctivum in the superior cerebellar peduncle, cross at the level of the inferior colliculus, and terminate in the contralateral ventral nucleus of the thalamus. The emboliform nucleus receives projections from the Purkinje cells in the spinocerebellum and collaterals from the fibers entering the restiform body and ventral spinocerebellar tract. Fibers from the emboliform nucleus enter the brachium conjunctivum, decussate to the contralateral side, and terminate in both the contralateral ventral nucleus of the thalamus and the red nucleus. The fastigial nucleus receives axons of the Purkinje cells in the vestibulocerebellum. It projects primarily to the lateral and inferior vestibular nuclei and to the pontine and medullary reticular formation. *(Burt, 352–354)*

30. (A) The cerebellar cortex contains three laminated cellular layers: the outermost molecular cell layer, a sheet of single large neurons; the Purkinje cell layer; and a deeper granular cell layer. These layers contain six types of neurons: basket, satellite, Purkinje, Golgi, granule cells, and the relatively rare Legato cells. Pyramidal cells are the most abundant cells of the cerebral cortex neuron types, are not found in the cerebellum, and are the most characteristic of the cerebral cortex. *(Afifi and Bergman, 308–310)*

31. (B) The monoaminergic projections to the cerebellum originate from the pontine raphe nuclei, the locus ceruleus, and the hypothalamus. The raphe nuclei are the source of serotoninergic projections to both the granular and molecular layers. The locus ceruleus is the source of noradrenergic projection to the three layers of the cerebellar cortex. The dorsomedial, dorsal, and lateral areas of the hypothalamus are the sources of histaminergic projections to all three layers of the cerebellar cortex. *(Afifi and Bergman, 322)*

32. (A) Learning complex motor tasks requires modifying motor responses or sequences in order to adapt the responses to a new situation or changes in the surrounding conditions. A major component of this learning ability resides in the cerebellum and in the olivocerebellar climbing fiber system. Selective damage to this system results in a loss of the ability to modify a motor response and the ability to maintain or store a modified response. *(Burt, 363)*

33. (A) The tuberoinfundibular tract is an efferent hypothalamic pathway. It arises from the arcuate nuclei and periventricular nuclei. Axons from these neurons extend into the infundibular stalk of the neurohypophysis, where they end. *(Afifi and Bergman, 408)*

34. (C) Climbing fibers are axons of neurons originating from the contralateral inferior olivary nucleus that project to all areas of the cerebellar cortex. Climbing fibers are excitatory. Aspartate is the most likely transmitter for these fibers. Each single climbing fiber establishes 1000 to 2000 synaptic contacts with its Purkinje cell. When the climbing fibers fire, there is a massive synchronous depolarization of Purkinje cells, which activates Ca^{++} channels in the dendritic membrane. The major source of climbing fibers in the cerebellum is the inferior olive. Degeneration of the inferior olive (seen in olivocerebellar atrophy) induces a drop in aspartate level in the cerebrospinal fluid. *(Afifi and Bergman, 313–314)*

35. **(A)** Purkinje cells are the largest cells in the central nervous system. Their cell bodies form a single cell layer. Their axons project primarily to the cerebellar nuclei, although a few exit the cerebellum and terminate directly into the vestibular nuclei. The Purkinje cell axon is the primary route for information leaving the cerebellar cortex. Each Purkinje cell axon courses through the granule cell layer and deep white matter to project onto deep cerebellar nuclei. However, some Purkinje cell axons from the vermis bypass the deep cerebellar nuclei to reach the lateral vestibular nucleus. Mossy fibers, climbing fibers, parallel fibers, and monoaminergic fibers are afferent projections to the cerebellum. Golgi cells are inhibitory interneurons in which the cell axons branch profusely in the granular layer and synapse with dendrites of a large number of granule cells, forming a negative feedback loop. *(Burt, 450–451)*

36. **(A)** The hypothalamus plays a major role in regulating eating behavior. The ventromedial nucleus is located in the tuberal region of the hypothalamus. Animal studies have demonstrated that bilateral lesions of the ventromedial nuclei of the hypothalamus cause hyperphagia, obesity, and savage behavior, whereas lesions of the lateral hypothalamus produce loss of appetite. The supraoptic nucleus belongs to the suprachiasmatic region and is located above the optic tract. With the paraventricular nucleus, the supraoptic nucleus is responsible for vasopressin and oxytocin secretion. Lesions of the paraventricular nucleus or the supraoptic nucleus cause diabetes insipidus. The anterior nucleus is located in the suprachiasmatic region. Stimulation of this nucleus may cause

excessive water intake. The arcuate nucleus is located in the tuberal region. The nucleus contains dopamine, which is responsible for control of prolactin and growth hormone secretion. The mammillary nucleus plays a role in memory. *(Afifi and Bergman, 403–406)*

37. **(A)** General somatic efferent fibers of the oculomotor nerve arise from the oculomotor nucleus situated near the midline of the midbrain at the level of the superior colliculus. This nucleus is formed by subnuclei for each of the extraocular muscles. The superior rectus muscle receives innervation from neurons in the contralateral subnucleus. The levator palpebral superioris muscle receives innervation from a medial subnucleus. The inferior rectus, medial rectus, and inferior oblique muscles receive innervation from ipsilateral subnuclei. *(Burt, 403–406)*

38. **(D)** General somatic efferents provide the motor innervation of somatic structures developed from the embryonic ectoderm and somatic mesoderm. The oculomotor nucleus provides general somatic efferent innervation to all extraocular muscles except the lateral rectus (which is innervated by the abducens nerve) and the superior oblique (which is innervated by the trochlear nerve). The hypoglossal nucleus provides general somatic efferents to tongue musculature. The facial motor nucleus provides special visceral efferents to the muscles of facial expression and the stapedius muscle. *(Burt, 404)*

39. **(C)** The glossopharyngeal nerve provides parasympathetic innervation to the parotid gland via the otic ganglion. *(Afifi and Bergman, 131–132)*

40. **(B)** The trigeminal nerve has three sensory nuclei: the spinal nucleus, the main sensory nucleus, and the mesencephalic nucleus. The spinal nucleus of the trigeminal nerve is a long column of neurons extending from the point of entry of the trigeminal nerve to the upper cervical spinal cord. It is divided into three parts: the oral part, responsible for tactile sensation from the oral mucosa; the interpolar part, receiving afferents for dental pain; and the

caudal part, receiving pain and temperature sensations from the face. Most of the small afferent fibers of the spinal tract of the trigeminal nerve terminate in the spinal nucleus. Most of the afferent large fibers that originate from the trigeminal ganglion end in the main sensory nucleus and are responsible for the transmission of discriminative touch. The mesencephalic nucleus is located at the rostral pons. It receives afferent fibers conveying kinesthesia and pressure from the teeth, periodontium, hard palate, joint capsules, and stretch receptors from the muscles of mastication. It sends efferent fibers to the cerebellum, the thalamus, the motor nuclei of the brain stem, and the reticular formation. The motor nucleus of the trigeminal nerve provides somatic visceral efferents that innervate the muscles of mastication via the mandibular division and contains α and γ motor neurons. (*Afifi and Bergman, 171–175*)

41. **(C)** Purkinje cells are found in the cerebellum. They constitute the sole output neurons of the cerebellar cortex. Their cell bodies are arranged in a single sheet at the border zone between the molecular and the granule cell layers. Their axons project primarily to cerebellar nuclei, although some axons from the vermis bypass the deep cerebellar nuclei to reach the vestibular nuclei directly. (*Afifi and Bergman, 317–320*)

42. **(D)** The cerebral neocortex has a laminar pattern of organization because of the distribution and size of neuronal cells and the horizontal pattern of incoming afferents. It is divided into six layers: Layer I, primarily a synaptic area, is the molecular layer. It is the most superficial layer of the cerebral cortex; its most characteristic cells are horizontal cells. Layer II, the external granular layer, is characterized by an abundance of small, densely packed neurons and a paucity of myelinated fibers. The dendrites of neurons in this layer project to layer I, while their axons project to deeper layers. Layer III, the external pyramidal layer, contains medium-large pyramidal cells and granule cells. Axons of most pyramidal cells descend through the cortex, forming cortical association fibers, both callosal and intrahemispherical. Layer IV, the internal granular layer, is the principal receiving station of the cerebral cortex. Layer V, the internal pyramidal layer, is the principal efferent layer of the cortex. This layer contains pyramidal cells that send their axons through the cortical white matter to the internal capsule and all subcortical sites except the thalamus, which receives fibers from layer VI. Layer VI, the fusiform layer, contains fusiform and pyramidal cells, which are the principal source of corticothalamic fibers and contribute to the intrahemispheric cortical association fibers. (*Afifi and Bergman, 340–343; Burt, 451–452*)

43. **(D)** Layer IV of the cerebral cortex, the internal granular layer, is the principal receiving station of the cortex. The input from the modality-specific thalamic nuclei projects mainly onto neurons in lamina IV, with some projections on laminae III and IV. The nonspecific thalamocortical input originating from nonspecific thalamic nuclei projects diffusely on all laminae and establishes mostly axodendritic types of synapses. (*Afifi and Bergman, 340–343; Burt, 451–452*)

44. **(D)** There are at least six neurochemically distinct extrathalamic projection systems that reach the cerebrum monosynaptically, without a relay in the thalamus: three arise from the brain stem reticular formation, two from the hypothalamus, and one from the basal forebrain. The first system arises from the locus ceruleus of the pontine reticular formation using norepinephrine. The second system arises from the midbrain raphe nuclei using serotonin. The third system arises from the ventral midbrain using dopamine. The fourth and fifth systems arise from two hypothalamic nuclei using histamine and GABA, respectively, as a neurotransmitter. From the nucleus basalis, located in the basal forebrain, arises a cholinergic extrathalamic modulatory system. The basal forebrain contains four populations of cholinergic neurons with projection to the cerebral cortex, with the nucleus basalis of Meynert as the principal source of cholinergic neurons. (*Burt, 459–463*)

45. (C)

46. (B)

47. (A)

Explanations 45 through 47

Damage to the right posterior parietal lobe causes neglect of the left side of the body. This neglect may have several dimensions: sensory, motor, cognitive, and attentional. In addition to the primary auditory function, the whole temporal cortex is involved in associative function. Temporal lobe damage may lead to difficulties in the performance of visually cued tasks requiring a high degree of visual discrimination. Temporal lobe lesions may also cause prosopagnosia, an inability to recognize familiar faces. This disorder is caused by impairment of some of the pathways responsible for visual processing. The patient is still able to recognize family and friends from the sound of their voices. Prefrontal association cortex lesions may cause problem-solving and emotional deficits. A problem-solving deficit is characterized by the inability of the patient to make an informed decision. The emotional deficit is characterized by bizarre and socially unacceptable behavior. The patient has a labile and unpredictable emotional status. *(Burt, 466–468)*

48. (D) The lateral geniculate body receives a dual arterial supply: the anterior choroidal artery laterally and the lateral posterior choroidal artery medially. *(Brazis, Masdeu, and Biller, 127)*

49. (D) The orbicularis oculi controls eye closure and is innervated by the facial nerve. Eye opening is controlled by the levator of the lid, which is innervated by the oculomotor nerve. *(Brazis, Masdeu, and Biller, 271–272)*

50. (D) The nervus intermedius is the sensory and parasympathetic division of the facial nerve. It carries preganglionic parasympathetic fibers to the submaxillary ganglion and to the pterygopalatine ganglion. It receives sensory fibers from the geniculate ganglion. This ganglion receives fibers that carry taste sensation from the anterior two-thirds of the tongue and afferents from the mucosae of the pharynx, nose, and palate. *(Afifi and Bergman, 166–167)*

51. (D) The intracranial portion of the facial nerve is supplied by the anterior inferior cerebellar artery. The intrapetrosal portion is supplied by the superficial branch of the middle meningeal artery and the stylomastoid branch of the posterior auricular artery. The extracranial part of the facial nerve is supplied by the stylomastoid, posterior auricular, superficial temporal, and transverse facial arteries. *(Brazis, Masdeu, and Biller, 275)*

52. (C) The first-order neurons of the auditory pathway have their cell bodies in the spiral ganglion of the cochlear nerve and enter the brain stem at the level of the ventral cochlear nuclei, as the cochlear nerve. The second-order neurons arise from the ventral and dorsal cochlear nuclei and send several projections to the contralateral brain stem that ascend as the lateral lemniscus. Fibers in the lateral lemniscus project on the nucleus of the lateral lemniscus and then to the inferior colliculus. The inferior colliculus contains the third-order neurons of the auditory pathway. These neurons project to the medial geniculate body. Geniculotemporal fibers, the fourth-order neurons of the auditory pathway, project to the primary auditory cortex. *(Brazis, Masdeu, and Biller, 293–295)*

53. (C) The glossopharyngeal nerves travel through the jugular foramen with the vagus nerve and the bulbar fibers of the spinal accessory nerve. *(Burt, 420–423)*

54. (D) Glomus jugulare tumors or basal skull fractures may cause jugular foramen syndrome. The glossopharyngeal nerve, the vagus nerve, and the spinal accessory nerve may be injured in this syndrome. Clinical signs include ipsilateral trapezius and sternocleidomastoid weakness, dysphonia, dysphagia, depressed gag reflex, ipsilateral loss of taste in the ipsilateral posterior third of the tongue, ipsilateral vocal cord paresis, and anesthesia of the posterior third of the tongue. There is no tongue deviation, since the twelfth cranial nerve is not affected. *(Brazis, Masdeu, and Biller, 318)*

55. **(C)** Paramedian and circumferential vessels supply the midbrain. The paramedian vessels arise from the posterior cerebral arteries and include the thalamoperforating and the peduncular arteries, which supply the medial peduncles and midbrain tegmentum. The circumferential arteries include the quadrigeminal arteries (which supply the superior and inferior colliculi), the superior cerebellar arteries (which supply the cerebral peduncles and brachium conjunctivum), and the posterior and anterior choroidal arteries. *(Brazis, Masdeu, and Biller, 357–358)*

56. **(C)** Na^+ and K^+ channel localization and clustering are essential for proper electrical signal generation and transmission in CNS myelinated nerve fibers. In particular, Na^+ channels are clustered at high density at nodes of Ranvier, and Shaker-type K^+ channels are sequestered in juxtaparanodal zones, just beyond the paranodal axoglial junctions. There is strong evidence that Schwann cells initiate sodium channel clustering in the peripheral nervous system just after the latter become committed to myelination. In the peripheral nervous system, conduction is invariably blocked when the myelin is stripped from the entire internode, but it can be restored by just minimal glial ensheathment. This conduction restoration is likely related to the early sodium channel clustering that accompanies initial steps in remyelination. As myelination proceeds, Na^+ channels are initially found in broad zones within gaps between neighboring oligodendroglial processes, and then are condensed into focal clusters. This process appears to depend on the formation of axoglial junctions. It has been suggested that juxtaparanodal potassium channels may serve to inhibit repetitive activation of nodal sodium channels. Sodium channel expression is increased in demyelinated lesions in multiple sclerosis. *(Rasband and Shrager, 63–73)*

57. **(A)** Central and peripheral nervous system myelin sheaths contain distinct sets of proteins. In the peripheral nervous system, the noncompact myelin contains E-cadherin, myelin-associated glycoprotein (MAG), and connexin 32 (Cx32). The compact myelin in the peripheral nervous system contains protein 0 (P0), peripheral myelin protein 22 (PMP22), and myelin basic protein (MBP). In the central nervous system, the compact myelin contains proteolipid protein (PLP), oligodendrocyte-specific protein (OSP), myelin-oligodendrocyte basic protein, and myelin basic protein. *(Arroyo and Scherer, 1–18)*

58. **(C)**

59. **(A)**

60. **(B)**

61. **(C)**

62. **(B)**

63. **(A)**

64. **(A)**

Explanations 58 through 64

Myelination in the central nervous system differs from that in the peripheral nervous system in several ways. Oligodendrocytes are responsible for myelination in the central nervous system, whereas Schwann cells are responsible for myelination in the peripheral nervous system. Both oligodendrocytes and Schwann cells ensheathe multiple axons; however, each Schwann cell is responsible for the myelination of only one axon. Each oligodendrocyte makes multiple myelin sheaths. The number varies from tract to tract and appears to relate to the caliber of the axons. Oligodendrocytes make fewer sheaths in tracts containing large myelinated fibers, the result of axooligodendrocyte interactions rather than an intrinsic trait of the oligodendrocytes themselves. Oligodendrocytes do not have a basal lamina or microvilli, and their incisures do not have distinguishing molecular markers such as connexin 32 (Cx32), myelin-associated glycoprotein (MAG), or E-cadherin. The molecular components of the central nervous system myelin sheaths partially overlap with those of the peripheral nervous system. Both contain high amounts of lipids, especially cholesterol and sphingolipids, including galactocerebroside and sulfatide. Similarly, in both systems, the central nervous system and the peripheral nervous system, compact myelin contains myelin basic protein (MBP), and the adaxonal surface contains MAG. Like myelinating Schwann cells, oligodendrocytes also express Cx32, but mainly on their cell bodies and proximal processes. Oligodendrocytes express two proteins that are not expressed by Schwann cells: myelin-oligodendrocyte glycoprotein (MOG) on their outer cell membrane, and myelin-oligodendrocyte basic protein (MOBP) in the major dense line of compact myelin. (*Arroyo and Scherer, 1–18*)

65. **(C)**

66. **(A)**

67. **(C)**

68. **(A)**

69. **(A)**

Explanations 65 through 69

All glial cells express class I MHC, but only astrocytes and microglia express class II MHC. All glial cells express adhesion molecules and synthesize cytokines. Astrocytes, as well as microglia cells, express co-stimulatory molecules (B7) and complement components. They may play the role of antigen-presenting cells. (*Antel, Birnbaum, and Hartung, 29–31*)

70. **(B)** The plasma membrane of a nerve controls ion transport, so that sodium and chloride are more concentrated outside the cell than inside it, whereas potassium and organic anions are relatively more concentrated inside the cell. The interior of the cell ends up with a relative excess of negative charges, so a voltage difference exists across the cell membrane. This voltage difference is called the resting potential; in a typical neuron it has a value of about –70 mV. (*Haines, 23*)

71. **(A)** Sensory axons are grouped on the basis of their diameters and myelin thickness into groups

I, II, III, and IV. The thicker the diameter of the axon and its myelin, the faster the conduction velocity. Class I axons are large and heavily myelinated. Classes II and III are progressively smaller and less myelinated. Class IV axons are smallest and unmyelinated. Class I is divided into subclasses Ia and Ib; the faster Ia fibers supply muscle spindles and the slower Ib fibers supply Golgi tendon organs. (*Haines, 251*)

72. **(E)** Neurulation is brought about by morphologic changes in the neuroblasts, the immature and dividing future neurons. Microfilaments in each cell form a circular bundle parallel to the future lamina surface, whereas microtubules extend along the length of the cell. Colchicine may stop neurulation by inhibiting microfilament-based contraction or by depolymerizing microtubules. (*Haines, 73–76*)

73. **(D)** Secondary neurulation induces the formation of the neural canal, which is open to the amniotic cavity both rostrally and caudally. In the rostral opening, the anterior neuropore closes at about 24 days; in the caudal opening, the posterior neuropore closes about 2 days later. (*Haines, 75–76*)

74. **(A)** Congenital malformations associated with defective neurulation are called dysraphic defects. There is an intimate relationship between the neural tissue and the surrounding bone, meninges, muscle, and skin. They are interdependent via inductive factors, so failure of neurulation also impairs the formation of these surrounding structures. Most dysraphic disorders occur either at the anterior or posterior neuropores. Failure of the anterior neuropore to close causes anencephaly. In this disorder, the brain is not formed, the surrounding meninges and skull may be absent, and there may be associated facial abnormalities. Failure in the closure of the posterior neuropore causes a range of malformations known collectively as myeloschisis. These defects always involve a failure of the vertebral arches at the affected levels to form completely and fuse to cover the spinal cord. This defect is called spina bifida. Spina bifida may be accompanied by a saccular structure that contains

only meninges and cerebrospinal fluid. The defect is called a meningocele. If the saccular structure contains meninges, cerebrospinal fluid, and spinal neural tissue, it is called a meningomyelocele. Myelodysplasia refers to malformation of the neural tube during secondary neurulation, such as a tethered cord syndrome, in which the conus medullaris and filum terminale are abnormally fixed to a defective vertebral column. *(Haines, 73–76)*

75. **(B)** Prosencephalization is the process in which the forebrain vesicle differentiates into diencephalon and telencephalon. Failure of this process results in a holoprosencephaly. *(Haines, 75–77)*

76. **(B)**

77. **(D)**

78. **(A)**

79. **(C)**

Explanations 76 through 79

The process of forebrain development into diencephalon and telencephalon is referred to as central induction and occurs mainly in the second month of gestation. The adult telencephalon derivatives include the cerebral cortex, the subcortical white matter (including the internal capsule), the olfactory bulb and tract, the basal ganglia, the amygdala, and the hippocampus. The diencephalon develops into the thalamic nuclei and associated structures. The ventricular system is an elaboration of the lumen of the cephalic portions of the neural tube. The cavities of the telencephalon become the lateral ventricles, the diencephalic cavity becomes the third ventricle, the rhombencephalic cavity becomes the fourth ventricle, and the mesencephalic cavity becomes the narrow cerebral aqueduct of Sylvius. *(Haines, 75–77)*

80. **(B)** Neuroblasts arise from the ventricular surface of the developing brain, which is the luminal surface of the neural tube. *(Haines, 81)*

81. **(A)**

82. **(B)**

83. **(A)**

84. **(B)**

85. **(A)**

86. **(B)**

87. **(B)**

Explanations 81 through 87

In the brainstem, the dorsal portion of the neural tube rotates dorsolaterally as the developing cerebellum invades it. The central canal of the mesencephalon invaginates into the fourth ventricle. This results in a lateral-to-medial orientation of the sensory area, which is the alar plate, versus the motor areas of the developing brainstem which is the basal plate. The basal plates in the brainstem give rise to cranial nerve motor nuclei, whereas the alar plates give rise to cranial nerve sensory nuclei. *(Haines, 81–82)*

88. **(A)** The mammillary body is located in the posterolateral part of the hypothalamus. The mammillary body receives afferents from the medial temporal lobe through the fornix, from the midbrain tegmental nuclei through the mammillary peduncle, and from the septal nuclei through the medial forebrain bundle. *(Burt, 384–386)*

89. **(E)**

90. **(G)**

91. **(H)**

92. **(A)**

93. **(F)**

94. **(C)**

95. **(D)**

96. **(B)**

97. **(K)**

98. (I)

99. (J)

Explanations 89 through 99

The thalamus is the largest component of the diencephalon. It is divided by a band of myelinated fibers, the internal medullary lamina, into the rostrocaudal and the mediolateral group of nuclei. *(Martin, 40, Figure 2-10)*

(1) The first group includes the midline, the intralaminar, the reticular, and the ventral anterior nuclei. They mediate general cortical alerting responses and are termed nonspecific thalamic nuclei, but recent studies suggest they may have a specific role in various aspects of awareness. The midline nuclei have reciprocal connection with the hypothalamus and receive efferents from the dorsal medial thalamic nucleus. The intralaminar nuclei (centromedian and parafascicular nuclei) send efferents to the striatum and ventrolateral thalamic nuclei and receive afferents from the pallidum and areas 4 and 6 of the frontal lobe. The ventral anterior nucleus has a reciprocal connection with the dorsomedial thalamic nucleus, sends efferents to the orbitofrontal cortex (as well as the intralaminar thalamic nuclei), and receives afferents from the pallidum and the substantia nigra. The reticular nucleus sends efferents to thalamic nuclei and receives thalamocortical afferents.

(2) The second group includes the dorsomedial and anterior thalamic nuclear groups. They play an important role in memory and emotion. The dorsomedial nucleus has efferent connections to the frontal lobe, lateral hypothalamus, and ventral anterior thalamus. It receives afferent connections from the frontal lobe, amygdala, inferior temporal cortex, and centromedian thalamic cortex.

(3) The third group includes the ventral lateral and basal nuclear groups, which are concerned with processing and relaying sensory information to the cortex. The ventral posterolateral nucleus receives afferents from the medial lemniscus, responsible for conveying proprioceptive sensation, and the spinothalamic tract, responsible for conveying pain and temperature sensation. It receives afferents also from the dorsomedial nucleus, the septal region, the frontal lobe, and the somatosensory cortex. It sends efferents to the postcentral gyrus areas 3b, 1, and 2. The ventral posteromedial nucleus receives afferents from the contralateral sensory trigeminal nuclei, located in the brain stem and spinal cord, and sends efferents to the cortical postcentral gyrus.

The medial geniculate body carries auditory information from the brachium of the inferior colliculus and sends efferents to the transverse temporal gyrus of Heschl. The lateral geniculate body is a relay station for the visual pathway, which receives afferents from the retinal ganglion cells the axons that form the optic tract, and from which originates the axons that project to the calcarine cortex through the optic radiation.

The ventrolateral nucleus receives afferents from the pallidum and contralateral cerebellum and sends efferents to the paracentral cortex areas 4 and 3a. It integrates input from the cerebellum, basal ganglia, and mechanoreceptors from the musculoskeletal system. It contributes to the coordination of fine distal motor movements and the proximal axial movements that support them.

The ventral anterior nucleus has a reciprocal connection with the dorsomedial thalamic nucleus. It receives input from the pallidum and substantia nigra and sends output to the orbitofrontal cortex. It may play a role in voluntary attention. The lateral dorsal nucleus receives afferents from the fornix.

(4) The fourth group corresponds to the dorsolateral and posterior nuclear group. The pulvinar receives afferents from the medial and lateral geniculate body as well as from the ventrolateral thalamic nucleus. It sends efferents to the cortex to modulate the attention needed for the accurate production of language-related tasks in the left hemisphere and visuospatial tasks in the right. The lateral posterior nucleus receives afferents from the pulvinar and sends efferents to the parietal lobe. *(Brazis, Masdeu, and Biller, 401–406; Martin, 40; Van der Werf et al, 107–140)*

100. **(B)** The thalamic arteries arise from the posterior communicating arteries and from the perimesencephalic segment of the posterior cerebral arteries. The polar arteries arise from the posterior communicating arteries and supply the reticular, ventral, and medial anterior nuclei. The posteromedian and posterolateral choroidal arteries, as well as the thalamogeniculate and thalamomesencephalic arteries, come from the posterior cerebral artery and are responsible for the vascular supply of the thalamus. The anterior choroidal artery does not participate in the vascular supply of the thalamus. *(Afifi, 255)*

101. **(C)** The Papez circuit is a closed circuit starting and ending in the hippocampus. It is thought to play a role in emotional reactions. The circuit consists of outflow of impulses from the hippocampus, fornix, mammillary body, mammillothalamic tract, anterior and dorsomedial thalamic nuclei, cingulate gyrus, and cingulum. *(Haines, 499)*

REFERENCES

Afifi AK, Bergman RA, ed. *Functional Neuroanatomy: Text and Atlas*. New York, NY: McGraw-Hill; 1998.

Antel JP, Birnbaum G, Hartung HP, ed. *Clinical Neuroimmunology*. Oxford, UK: Blackwell Science; 1998.

Arroyo EJ, Scherer SS. On the molecular architecture of myelinated fibers. *Histochem & Cell Biol* 2000; 113(1): 1–18.

Brazis PW, Joseph, Masdeu C, Biller J, ed. *Localization in Clinical Neurology*. 3rd ed. London, UK: Little, Brown; 1996.

Burt AM, ed. *Textbook of Neuroanatomy*. Philadelphia, Pa: W.B. Saunders; 1993.

Haines DE, ed. *Fundamental Neuroscience*. 2nd ed. New York, NY: Churchill Livingstone; 2002.

Kline LB, Bajandas, FJ, ed. *Neuroophthalmology Review Manual*. 5th ed. Thorofare, NJ: Slack; 2001.

Martin JH, ed. *Neuroanatomy. Text and Atlas*. New York, NY: McGraw-Hill; 2003.

Parent A, ed. *Carpenter's Human Neuroanatomy*. 9th ed. Media, PA: Williams & Wilkins; 1996.

Rasband MN, Shrager P. Ion channel sequestration in central nervous system axons. *J Physiol* 2000; 525 (1):63–73.

Staal A, Van Gijn J, Spaams F, ed. *Mononeuropathies. Examination, Diagnosis and Treatment*. London, UK: W.B. Saunders; 1999.

Van der Werf YD, Witter MP, Groenewegen HJ. The intralaminar and midline nuclei of the thalamus. Anatomical and functional evidence for participation in processes of arousal and awareness. *Brain Res Brain Res Rev* 2002; 39: 107–140.

CHAPTER 2

Localization Signs in Neurology
Questions

1. Which of the following statements about the Marcus-Gunn pupil is correct?

    (A) When each eye is stimulated by a rapid alternating light, each constricts.
    (B) When both eyes are stimulated by a rapid alternating light, the normal eye constricts, whereas the affected eye dilates as the light falls on it.
    (C) When both eyes are stimulated by a rapid alternating light, the normal and the affected eye constrict as the light falls on each one.
    (D) When both eyes are stimulated by a rapid alternating light, the normal eye dilates, whereas the affected eye constricts as the light falls on each one.
    (E) When both eyes are stimulated by a rapid alternating light, the normal and the affected eye dilate as the light falls on each one.

Questions 2 through 5
Match the following.

    (A) Holmes-Adie's pupil
    (B) Argyll-Robertson pupil
    (C) Epidemic encephalitis
    (D) Parinaud syndrome

2. Small irregular pupils fixed to light but reactive to accommodation

3. Pupils reactive to light but not to accommodation

4. Widely dilated pupils poorly reactive to light; associated with impaired sweating and loss of knee and ankle jerks

5. Dilated pupils fixed to light with loss of upward gaze

Questions 6 through 10
Match each of the following neurological symptoms and/or signs to the most likely root lesion.

    (A) First thoracic root lesion (T1)
    (B) Fifth cervical root lesion (C5)
    (C) Sixth cervical root lesion (C6)
    (D) Seventh cervical root lesion (C7)
    (E) Eighth cervical root lesion (C8)

6. Pain radiating into the arm and shoulder with weakness of shoulder abduction

7. Weakness of elbow flexion in its fully supine and half-pronated positions, associated with deep aching pain spreading down the lateral forearm to the thumb and index finger, affecting both the palmar and dorsal aspects of the hand

8. Weakness of shoulder adduction, elbow extension, and flexion and extension of the wrist with pain in the forearm, radiating into the middle, index, and ring fingers

9. Weakness of the long extensor and flexor muscles of the hand with pain in the olecranon, radiating into the little and ring fingers

10. Weakness of all intrinsic hand muscles with pain in the shoulder joint, axilla, and medial side of the upper arm down to the olecranon

Questions 11 through 14
Link each of the following clinical features to the most likely injured nerve.

  (A) Radial nerve lesion at the spiral groove
  (B) Ulnar nerve entrapment at the wrist
  (C) Musculocutaneous nerve
  (D) Median nerve lesion in the upper arm

11. Proximal forearm pain exacerbated by elbow extension with muscle wasting in the ventral arm, weakness of elbow flexion, and loss of the biceps reflex

12. Saturday night palsy

13. Pain in the little and medial half of the ring finger with weakness of all intrinsic hand muscles except for thumb abduction

14. Pain from the thumb to the middle finger and forearm with weakness of wrist flexion, thumb abduction, and the inability to form an O with the thumb and index fingers (pinch sign).

Questions 15 through 23
Link the following clinical signs and symptoms to the most likely anatomic location.

  (A) A 65-year-old woman developed a pain located diagonally across the thigh, with weakness on hip flexion, knee extension, and thigh adduction.
  (B) A 23-year-old pregnant woman developed pain in the medial right thigh and weakness of thigh adduction.
  (C) A 50-year-old man developed a progressive loss of sensation to all modalities in the sole and lateral border of the foot with weakness on plantar flexion and inversion of the foot.
  (D) A 56-year-old man developed a left flail foot, weakness of left knee flexion, decreased left Achilles reflex, and loss of sensation in the lateral left leg and dorsum of the foot after an intramuscular injection in his left buttock.

  (E) A 22-year-old female began, late in her pregnancy, to complain of tingling and burning sensations from her left lateral thigh spreading to the popliteal fossa.
  (F) A 66-year-old woman with a past medical history of breast cancer developed loss of sensation in her left posterior thigh, lateral calf, and dorsum of the foot, including all toes. Motor examination demonstrated weakness of left hip extension, left thigh abduction, and all left foot movements.
  (G) A 71-year-old man on warfarin for severe cardiomyopathy developed, after a fall on his back, severe pain in his anterior left thigh and medial leg down to his ankle. Neurological assessment was significant for the absence of left knee jerk and weakness of knee extension.
  (H) A 78-year-old woman developed loss of sensation in the dorsum of her foot and a dull ache in the anterolateral leg after a left knee arthroplasty. Neurological examination demonstrated weakness on dorsiflexion and eversion of her left foot.
  (I) A 22-year-old woman developed pain in her perineum and clitoris with fecal incontinence.

15. Lumbar plexus

16. Sacral plexus

17. Obturator nerve

18. Femoral nerve

19. Tibial nerve

20. Peroneal nerve

21. Sciatic nerve

22. Pudendal nerve

23. Lateral femoral cutaneous nerve

Questions 24 through 31
Match the following.

(A) Cecocentral scotoma
(B) Binasal hemianopia
(C) Optic neuritis
(D) Optic nerve compression at the junction with the optic chiasm
(E) Compression of the optic chiasm
(F) Anton syndrome
(G) Anterior visual cortex infarction

24. B_{12} deficiency

25. Ethanol abuse

26. Hydrocephalus

27. A 23-year-old male treated with ethambutol for tuberculosis

28. Ipsilateral central scotoma with contralateral temporal visual field defect

29. Bitemporal hemianopia

30. Cortical blindness

31. Hemianopia with macula sparing

32. Which of the following is true about Bell's phenomenon in Bell's palsy?

(A) Eyeball deviation up and slightly outward on the affected side when the patient attempts to close both eyes
(B) Eyeball deviation down and slightly inward on the affected side when the patient attempts to close both eyes
(C) Eyeball deviation down and slightly inward on the normal side when the patient attempts to close both eyes
(D) Eyeball deviation up and slightly inward on the normal side when the patient attempts to close both eyes
(E) Eyeball deviation in Bell's phenomenon is not a physiologic phenomenon and it

is only seen in peripheral facial nerve disease.

33. Tolosa-Hunt syndrome is characterized by all of the following EXCEPT

(A) recurrent unilateral orbital pain
(B) transient extraocular nerve palsies
(C) high sedimentation rate
(D) insensitivity to corticosteroids
(E) equal prevalence in both sexes

34. A 28-year-old right-handed volleyball player noticed, for the last three weeks, mild right arm weakness on elevation, especially when shaving or combing his hair. The weakness has been accompanied by a dull aching in the shoulder. On neurological examination, there was winging of the right scapula when the patient was asked to push against the wall with both arms. The lesion is most likely located in the

(A) C7-C8 cervical root
(B) long thoracic nerve
(C) suprascapular nerve
(D) dorsal scapular nerve
(E) trapezius muscle

Questions 35 through 38
For each of the following clinical cases, identify the location of the radial nerve damage.

(A) Radial nerve lesion at the upper arm
(B) Radial nerve lesion at the axilla
(C) Radial nerve lesion at the forearm
(D) Radial nerve lesion at the wrist

35. A 45-year-old right-handed porter used to keep his arms outstretched and forearms in maximum supination when carrying heavy bags on his back. He consulted a neurologist because of weakness on extension of his right elbow, wrist, and fingers with slightly decreased sensation to all modalities in his lateral arm and posterior forearm and the web between the index finger and thumb.

36. A 56-year-old alcoholic man awoke in the morning after a heavy alcoholic binge complaining of inability to extend his right wrist and fingers, including the thumb. Neurological examination demonstrated weakness of wrist and metacarpophalangeal extension. Right arm extension was normal. Elbow flexion was weak with the thumb pointing to the ceiling.

37. A 60-year-old man described progressive difficulty in extending his right little finger. This symptom progressed over several weeks to total inability to extend the fingers and thumb. Neurological examination demonstrated dropped fingers without wrist drop.

38. A 30-year-old man developed a shooting pain on the radial side of his right wrist and paresthesias radiating into the thumb and index finger after he had been handcuffed by a police officer.

Questions 39 through 41
For each of the following clinical cases, identify the location of the median nerve damage.

(A) Median nerve lesion at the upper arm
(B) Median nerve lesion at the elbow
(C) Median nerve lesion at the wrist

39. A 40-year-old woman, recently diagnosed with non-Hodgkin's lymphoma, noticed difficulty in holding a glass with her right hand and numbness of the palmar side of the thumb, index, and middle fingers of her right hand. Neurological examination of the right hand demonstrated weak pronation and abduction of the wrist against resistance, weak flexion of the proximal and distal interphalangeal joint against resistance of the second and third fingers, and inability to form an O with the thumb and index finger.

40. A 60-year-old African American man, a few days after reduction of a dislocated left elbow, developed dull pain in his left forearm over several days. The pain spread to his index finger and thumb. Neurological examination demonstrated normal sensation and wrist flexion. There was weakness in pronation of the

forearm when the elbow was flexed but not in extension.

41. A 45-year-old woman with a history of rheumatoid arthritis has noticed for the past 4 months intermittent sensation of pins and needles in both hands. The pain worsens when just awakening from sleep. She has also noticed hand clumsiness with fine finger movements. Neurological examination demonstrated abnormal pinprick sensation on the palmar surface of both hands; with hypesthesia in the distal aspect of the first three digits bilaterally, there was mild thenar atrophy, weakness of thumb abduction, and weakness on opposing the thumb against the little finger.

Questions 42 through 43
For each of the following clinical cases, identify the location of the ulnar nerve damage.

(A) Ulnar nerve lesion at the elbow
(B) Ulnar nerve lesion at the wrist

42. A 40-year-old woman noticed pins-and-needles sensation in her right ring and little finger. After a few weeks, she noticed atrophy of her nails in the two last fingers as her hand became claw-like. Neurological examination demonstrated weakness on right wrist abduction and adduction, decreased pinprick sensation in the palmar surface of the right hand, diminished dorsal sensation of the little and medial aspect of the ring fingers. There was weakness on flexion of the little finger.

43. A 37-year-old man developed a history of right hand weakness, mostly in the ring and little fingers, over the last 6 weeks. Neurological examination demonstrated weakness on thumb adduction, little finger abduction, and flexion. There was mild hypothenar muscle atrophy. The right palmaris brevis was spared on clinical examination.

44. A 45-year-old woman had been recently started on warfarin for atrial fibrillation. She developed severe pain in her anterior right thigh and difficulty walking and rising from a chair.

Neurological examination demonstrated weakness on right thigh, hip flexion, and weakness on extension of the leg against resistance. The most likely diagnosis is

(A) right lower extremity embolism

(B) obturator nerve neuropathy

(C) femoral nerve neuropathy

(D) sciatic nerve neuropathy

(E) tibial nerve neuropathy

45. Papillomacular bundle lesions cause which of the following visual field defects?

(A) Paracentral scotoma

(B) Wedge-shaped temporal scotoma

(C) Comma-shaped extension of the blind spot

(D) Bjerrum arcuate scotoma

(E) Nasal step of Ronne

46. Optic tract lesions result in

(A) congruous hemianopia

(B) unilateral retinal nerve fiber atrophy

(C) normal pupillary reflex

(D) Wernicke's pupil

(E) decreased visual acuity

47. Left homonymous superior quadranopsia (pie in the sky) field defect is caused by a

(A) left geniculate body lesion

(B) left optic tract lesion

(C) right parietal lobe lesion

(D) left parietal lobe lesion

(E) right anterior temporal lobe lesion

Questions 48 through 54
Link each of the following syndromes to the corresponding clinical case.

(A) Millard-Gubler syndrome (lesion of the ventrocaudal pons)

(B) Foville syndrome (lesion of the dorsal pons)

(C) Raymond-Cestan syndrome (lesion of the ventral medial pons)

(D) Subarachnoid syndrome of the abducens cranial nerve

(E) Gradenigo syndrome (lesion of the apex of the temporal bone)

(F) Petrous bone fracture

(G) Cavernous sinus syndrome

48. A 50-year-old woman with a history of pituitary adenoma developed pain and paresthesias in the right periorbital area. The neurological examination demonstrated right ophthalmoplegia with loss of sensation in the distribution of the ophthalmic branch of the trigeminal nerve.

49. Following an otitis media, a 36-year-old man developed diplopia, left facial pain, and left eye closure weakness. Neurological examination demonstrated a left abducens and facial nerve palsy associated with left sensorineural deafness.

50. A 70-year-old woman with a history of hypertension developed the sudden onset of left side weakness with facial involvement. Neurological examination demonstrated right abducens nerve paresis, right facial paresis, and a left hemiplegia.

51. A 20-year-old woman with a history of pseudotumor cerebri developed an acute headache and blurred vision. Neurological examination demonstrated bilateral papilledema and bilateral abducens nerve palsy.

52. A 75-year-old woman with a history of hypertension consulted a neurologist because of acute left side weakness. Neurological examination demonstrated horizontal conjugate gaze palsy with right trigeminal, facial, and cochleovestibular nerve palsies and right Horner syndrome.

53. A 26-year-old male was brought to the Emergency Room because of a car accident with head trauma. Physical examination demonstrated mastoid ecchymosis, otorrhea, hemotympanum and left trigeminal, abducens, and facial nerve palsy.

54. A 70-year-old man with a history of diabetes developed a left hemiparesis with right abducens palsy.

55. Which of the following is the most suggestive of a lesion in the nucleus of the oculomotor nerve?

(A) Ipsilateral superior rectus palsy

(B) Bilateral ptosis

(C) Contralateral inferior oblique paresis

(D) Contralateral ptosis

(E) Contralateral medial rectus palsy

56. A 52-year-old woman with a history of migraine and HTN developed a left ptosis. Neurological examination demonstrated left oculomotor nerve palsy without pupillary abnormality. The symptoms improved over the next 2 months. A follow-up visit in the third month showed an Argyll Robertson pupil on the left side during convergence. The LEAST likely cause of the pupillary abnormality is

(A) an intracavernous meningioma

(B) ischemic mononeuropathy of the oculomotor nerve

(C) an aneurysm of the posterior communicating artery

(D) trauma

(E) neurinoma

57. A 40-year-old man developed a new onset of diplopia. Neurological examination demonstrated eye misalignment on vertical gaze (the right eye higher than the left eye). The misalignment worsened on left gaze deviation and when the head was tilted to the right. Which of the following ocular muscles was affected?

(A) Right superior oblique

(B) Left superior oblique

(C) Right inferior rectus

(D) Left inferior rectus

(E) Right inferior oblique

58. A lesion at which of the following spinal cord segments causes inversion of the brachioradialis reflex?

(A) C8

(B) C4

(C) C7

(D) C6

(E) T1

Questions 59 through 64

Link each of the following clinical syndromes to the corresponding anatomical location.

(A) Brown-Séquard syndrome

(B) Syringomyelia

(C) B_{12} deficiency

(D) Anterior spinal artery occlusion

(E) Amyotrophic lateral sclerosis

(F) Tabes dorsalis

59. A 35-year-old man developed progressive lower extremity weakness and gait ataxia over 6 months. Neurological examination demonstrated bilateral lower extremity spasticity, increased deep tendon reflexes throughout, and bilateral Babinski sign. Sensory examination showed no sensory level but loss of proprioception and vibratory sensation in both legs with preservation of temperature and pinprick sensations.

60. A 50-year-old man had chronic lancinating leg pain, urinary incontinence, and gait ataxia progressing over 3 months. Neurological examination demonstrated impaired vibratory and joint position sense in the lower extremities, decreased tactile localization, and the presence of the Romberg sign. Examination of the feet showed chronic trophic changes.

61. A 30-year-old man consulted because of generalized weakness and muscle atrophy in the right hand and foot. These symptoms had been progressing over the last 2 years and were associated with painful cramps. Neurological examination demonstrated explosive dysarthria, generalized spasticity, increased deep tendon reflexes throughout, and bilateral Babinski sign. There was prominent muscle atrophy in the right hand and both feet with fasciculations. Sensory examination was normal. Bladder and rectal sphincters were not affected.

62. A 45-year-old female developed thermoanesthesia in a cape-like distribution involving both upper extremities with preservation of light touch sensation and proprioception.

63. A 40-year-old man developed a sudden onset of back pain, followed by flaccid areflexic paraplegia with urinary incontinence. Neurological examination showed loss of sensation to pain and temperature at the T4 level with preservation of vibration and proprioception.

64. A 60-year-old woman developed right lower extremity weakness with urinary incontinence following back trauma. Neurological examination demonstrated spastic right lower extremity monoplegia, loss of vibration, proprioception in the right side below the T6 level, loss of pain and temperature sensation on the left side below the T6 level.

65. Funnel vision is seen in all of the following conditions EXCEPT

(A) glaucoma
(B) hysteria
(C) retinitis pigmentosa
(D) postpapilledema optic atrophy
(E) bilateral occipital infarct with macular sparing

66. Which of the following retrochiasmatic lesions may cause a strictly unilateral visual field defect?

(A) The most anterior aspect of the calcarine cortex
(B) Lateral geniculate body
(C) Optic radiation
(D) Medial occipital lesion
(E) Optic tract

Questions 67 through 72
Link the following syndromes to the appropriate lesion.

(A) Fascicular lesion of the facial nerve
(B) Facial nerve lesion in the meatal canal

(C) Geniculate ganglion lesion
(D) Facial nerve lesion between the departure of the nerve to the stapedius and the departure of the chorda tympani
(E) Facial nerve lesion at the stylomastoid foramen

67. Ipsilateral facial nerve palsy with normal auditory and taste function

68. Foville syndrome (lesion of the dorsal pons)

69. Ramsay Hunt syndrome

70. Ipsilateral facial palsy with loss of taste in the anterior two-thirds of the tongue and normal hearing.

71. Millard-Gubler syndrome (lesion of the ventrocaudal pons)

72. Ipsilateral facial palsy with deafness and loss of taste in the anterior two-thirds of the tongue

Questions 73 through 76
Link the following brain stem syndromes to the appropriate clinical description.

(A) Medial medullary syndrome
(B) Wallenberg syndrome (lateral medullary syndrome)
(C) Locked-in syndrome
(D) Foville syndrome (dorsal pontine tegmentum lesion)

73. A 70-year-old man with a history of atrial fibrillation developed sudden onset of vertigo, nausea, vomiting, diplopia, and dysarthria. He also had pain in the right face and left arm and leg. Neurological examination demonstrated right Horner syndrome, decreased temperature, sensation in the painful areas. The right palate and vocal cord were paralyzed. The right arm and leg were ataxic.

74. A 50-year-old woman with a history of diabetes developed left side weakness and dysarthria. Neurological examination demonstrated tongue deviation to the right side, left hemiplegia, as well as loss of vibratory and position sensation in the left arm and leg with preservation of temperature and pain sensation.

75. The neurological assessment of a 65-year-old comatose patient demonstrated a right facial weakness, left gaze deviation, left hemiplegia, and left Babinski sign.

76. A 65-year-old female with a history of diabetes and hypertension developed severe headache, followed by a dysarthria that progressed to total aphonia and generalized weakness. Neurological examination found an awake and alert patient, quadriparesis, and ophthalmoplegia bilaterally with sparing of vertical eye movement and blinking.

Questions 77 through 80
Link the following.

(A) Marie-Foix syndrome (lateral pontine lesion)
(B) Weber syndrome (medial cerebral peduncle lesion)
(C) Benedict syndrome (mesencephalic tegmentum lesion)
(D) Sylvian aqueduct syndrome

77. A 30-year-old man with a history of cocaine abuse developed sudden onset of ataxia and left-sided weakness. Neurological examination demonstrated right arm ataxia, left hemiparesis, and loss of temperature and pain sensation in the left arm.

78. A 40-year-old woman with a history of diabetes developed sudden onset of diplopia and left-sided tremor. Neurological examination demonstrated right ophthalmoplegia and left intention tremor.

79. An 80-year-old man with a history of hypertension consulted because of new onset of double vision and left-sided weakness. Examination demonstrated right oculomotor paresis with a dilated pupil and left hemiplegia.

80. A 20-year-old man consulted because of chronic headache and blurred vision. Neurological examination demonstrated paralysis of upward gaze and convergence retraction nystagmus on upward gaze. MRI of the head showed pineal tumor with hydrocephalus.

Questions 81 through 85
Link each of the following cerebellar syndromes to the appropriate clinical case.

(A) Rostral vermis syndrome
(B) Caudal vermis syndrome
(C) Posterior inferior cerebellar artery occlusion syndrome
(D) Anterior inferior cerebellar artery occlusion syndrome
(E) Superior cerebellar artery occlusion syndrome

81. A 5-year-old boy was brought to the neurology clinic because of the insidious onset of a staggering gait. Neurological examination demonstrated axial ataxia without limb ataxia and spontaneous nystagmus. MRI of the head showed a cerebellar mass suggesting medulloblastoma.

82. A 70-year-old diabetic woman developed sudden onset of dizziness, nausea, vomiting, right-sided ataxia, and right hearing loss. Cranial nerve examination revealed on the right sensorineural deafness, peripheral facial palsy, and loss of facial pain and temperature sensation. The rest of the neurological examination demonstrated left trunk, arm, and leg, sensory loss to pain and temperature and right Horner syndrome.

83. A 50-year-old man with a history of ethanol abuse consulted because of progressive exacerbation of gait ataxia and slurred speech. Neurological examination demonstrated mild dysarthria, axial ataxia with minimal ataxia on the heel-to-shin maneuver, and normal arm coordination.

84. A 60-year-old man with a history of hypertension developed sudden onset of vertigo and gait disturbance. Neurological examination demonstrated right Horner syndrome with horizontal nystagmus, left sensorineural deafness, right limb ataxia, and intention tremor. Sensory examination was significant for left-sided pain and temperature loss.

85. A 75-year-old woman with a history of hypertension and atrial fibrillation developed acute vertigo, headache, dysarthria, and gait disturbance. Neurological examination was significant for left limb ataxia, facial loss of temperature sensation, vocal cord palsy, Horner syndrome, and on the right temperature and pain loss in the trunk and right arm and leg.

86. The most common location of neurogenic gastrointestinal ulceration after an acute hypothalamic lesion is in the

    (A) upper esophagus
    (B) lower esophagus
    (C) fundus of the stomach
    (D) ileum
    (E) colon

87. The lesion most consistently associated with memory disturbance in patients with Wernicke-Korsakoff syndrome has been found in the

    (A) mammillary bodies
    (B) pulvinar
    (C) medial dorsal nucleus of the thalamus
    (D) fornix
    (E) ventromedial region of the hypothalamus

88. Hemiballismus occurs with damage to each of the following anatomical structures EXCEPT the

    (A) globus pallidus
    (B) subthalamic nucleus
    (C) caudate nucleus
    (D) substantia nigra
    (E) thalamic nuclei

89. Sensory inattention occurs most commonly with a lesion of the

    (A) inferior parietal lobe
    (B) thalamus
    (C) mesencephalic reticular formation
    (D) dorsolateral frontal lobe
    (E) cingulate gyrus

Questions 90 through 97

Link each of the following abnormal behavioral patterns to the appropriate anatomical structure responsible for it.

    (A) Sensory aprosodia
    (B) Indifference to pain
    (C) Blunt affect
    (D) Rage reaction
    (E) Depression
    (F) Hostility
    (G) Paranoid behavior
    (H) Denial

90. Lesion of the septal region

91. Right orbitofrontal lesion

92. Right parietotemporal lesion

93. Bilateral anterior temporal lesion

94. Bilateral anterior cingulate lesion

95. Left dorsofrontal lesion

96. Left temporal lobe lesion

97. Right temporal lesion

98. The association of mutism, gait disturbance, and urinary incontinence may be seen in lesions affecting the

    (A) temporal lobe
    (B) occipital lobe
    (C) medial frontal lobe
    (D) parietal lobe
    (E) lateral frontal lobe

Questions 99 through 103
Link each of the following types of hallucinations to the most likely corresponding anatomical area.

(A) Nocturnal bright-colored people with a cartoon-like appearance

(B) Predominantly black-and-white-colored zigzag linear visual hallucination

(C) Predominantly multicolored patterned hallucination

(D) Pleasant dream-like visual hallucination

(E) "Déjà vécu" illusion

99. Neocortex of the temporal lobe

100. Occipital seizure

101. Midbrain lesion

102. Charles Bonnet syndrome

103. Migraine

104. Which of the following is NOT true about Balint syndrome?

(A) Gaze apraxia

(B) Optic ataxia

(C) Decreased visual attention

(D) Color agnosia

(E) Possible occurrence of bilateral posterior watershed lesion in the hemispheric convexities

105. A 67-year-old White man with a history of diabetes and hypertension developed sudden onset of severe headache and blurred vision on the left. Neurological examination demonstrated a left homonymous hemianopia, normal response to threat, normal optokinetic nystagmus, and normal drawing and copying. Imaging studies showed an acute ischemic stroke. Where is the most likely anatomical location of the lesion?

(A) Right occipitoparietal lesion

(B) Right temporoparietal lesion

(C) Bilateral occipital lesion

(D) Bilateral lesions of the banks of the calcarine fissure

(E) Bilateral lesions of the superior banks of the calcarine fissure

106. Which of the following is NOT characteristic of the frontal hand alien limb syndrome?

(A) Occurrence in the dominant hand

(B) Presence of reflex grasping

(C) Compulsive manipulation of tools

(D) Intermanual conflict

(E) Presence of groping

107. Limb-kinetic apraxia is caused by a lesion in the

(A) peri-rolandic cortex

(B) mesial frontal cortex

(C) supplementary motor cortex

(D) parietal cortex

(E) corpus callosum

Questions 108 through 118
Link each of the following cortical locations to the appropriate clinical manifestation.

(A) Mesial occipital lobe

(B) Lateral occipital lobe

(C) Bilateral anterior tip of the temporal lobe

(D) Lateroinferior aspect of the nondominant temporal lobe

(E) Parietal postcentral gyrus

(F) Mesial parietal lobe lesion

(G) Lateral parietal lesion in the dominant hemisphere

(H) Mesiofrontal lesion

(I) Lateral frontal premotor lesion

(J) Orbitofrontal lesion

(K) Callosal frontal lesion

108. Contralateral somatosensory disturbance

109. Impaired contralateral saccade with pure agraphia

110. Lack of kinesthetic transfer

111. Visual field defect with visual field agnosia and hallucination

112. Amnesia with storage impairment of geometric pattern

113. Blunt affect with impaired association of social nuance

114. Alexia with agraphia, impaired ipsilateral scanning, and nystagmus

115. Klüver-Bucy syndrome

116. Transcortical sensory aphasia

117. Akinesia with perseveration and alien hand syndrome

118. Alexia with agraphia, finger agnosia, and acalculia

Questions 119 through 124
Link each of the following syndromes to the appropriate clinical description.

    (A) Erb-Duchenne palsy
    (B) Dejerine-Klumpke palsy
    (C) Cervical plexus lesion
    (D) Thoracic outlet syndrome
    (E) Lumbar segment plexopathy
    (F) Sacral plexopathy

119. A 74-year-old man developed loss of sensation to all modalities in the right mandible and lower external ear after a right endarterectomy. Motor examination showed weakness of right lateral and anterior head flexion and rotation as well as weakness on external rotation of the scapula.

120. A 33-year-old woman with a history of cervical cancer developed insidious onset of lower back pain and right proximal thigh and buttock pain. Sensory examination demonstrated loss of sensation in the lateral right leg and dorsum of the foot. Motor examination demonstrated a flail right foot, weakness of right knee flexion abduction, internal rotation of the right thigh, and paresis of hip extension.

121. A 40-year-old woman consulted because of recurrent left upper extremity coldness and cyanosis with pain of the ulnar border of the right hand. Right hand examination demonstrated thenar wasting.

122. A 22-year-old football player consulted because of an acute transient episode of intense burning and weakness of his left upper extremity following a sudden depression of his left shoulder during a football game. A few weeks later, neurological examination showed weakness of internal rotation and adduction of the left limb. The forearm was held in extension and pronation because of elbow flexion weakness.

123. A 52-year-old man with a history of colorectal cancer consulted because of new onset of back and right lower extremity pain. Neurological assessment demonstrated sensory loss to pin prick over the lateral and medial right thigh and weakness of hip flexion, leg extension, and thigh adduction.

124. A 65-year-old man with a history of thoracotomy for a left lung cancer consulted because he developed paresthesias of the left medial arm and forearm and a left hand claw deformity.

Answers and Explanations

1. **(B)** The pupil size is under the dual control of sympathetic and parasympathetic systems that innervate a ring of radially arranged dilator fibers and a circle of constrictor fibers, respectively. The resting size of the pupil depends on the intensity of light falling on the retina and the integrity of the parasympathetic nerves. A light stimulus is conveyed from the retina to the optic nerve, optic chiasm, and lateral geniculate body. Ten percent of the afferent fibers subserve the light reflex and are related, in the periaqueductal gray, to both Edinger-Westphal nuclei (which induce papillary constriction) and the consensual light reflex. The parasympathetic fibers are then carried by the third cranial nerve to the ciliary ganglion and to the pupil constrictor fibers.

   The sympathetic system starts from the hypothalamus; its fibers pass to the cervicothoracic spinal cord at levels C8 and T1. The second-order neurons pass from the spinal cord to the superior cervical ganglion. The third-order neurons supply the pupillodilator fibers and the blood vessels of the eye, passing over the carotid artery. Any lesion affecting the afferent pathways—the retina, optic chiasm, optic tract, and particularly the optic nerve—will cause Marcus-Gunn pupil. When the abnormal eye is stimulated by light, it will slowly and briefly constrict and may start to dilate while it is still illuminated. This is also illustrated in the swinging flashlight test: the abnormal eye dilates instead of constricting when the light is rapidly alternated from one eye to another, whereas, the normal eye constricts and stays small. *(Patten, 7–9)*

2. **(B)**

3. **(C)**

4. **(A)**

5. **(D)**

Explanations 2 through 5

Holmes-Adie or tonic pupil syndrome is a condition of unknown cause related to degeneration of nerve cells in the ciliary ganglion. The degeneration of short ciliary nerves, with subsequent collateral sprouting, results in predominance of accommodation elements in the innervation of the iris. It is more frequent in females and can be unilateral at first. Typically, the patient presents with blurred near vision, loss of knee and ankle jerks, and impaired sweating. The pupil is round and widely dilated; it reacts poorly to light but better to accommodation. The minimal reaction to accommodation or to light is probably related to partial reinnervation of parasympathetic fibers and slow inhibition of sympathetic fibers. The confirmation of the diagnosis is made by pupillary reaction to pilocarpine drops. Pilocarpine is rapidly hydrolyzed by acetylcholine esterase and has no effect on the normal pupil. In Holmes-Adie syndrome, the denervated pupil with enzyme depletion allows the piloloconstrictor effect to occur.

Argyll-Robertson pupil is classically seen in patients with neurosyphilis. The site of the lesion is thought to be in the rostral midbrain, injuring the supranuclear inhibitory fibers that affect the visceral oculomotor nuclei. The pupils are usually affected bilaterally and are irregularly miotic with variable iris atrophy. There is a decrease or absence of the pupillary light reaction with conservation of the near response in the presence of normal visual acuity. Epidemic encephalitis lethargica causes loss of convergence with parkinsonism. The patient's pupils react to light but not to accommodation. Parinaud syndrome results from a lesion in the dorsal rostral midbrain that interferes with the decussating light reflex fibers in the periaqueductal area. The syndrome is characterized by dilated fixed pupils to light, loss of upward gaze, defective convergence, skew deviation, light near dissociation (reaction to accommodation but not to light) and lid retraction. *(Brazis, Masdeu, and Biller, 181–188; Thompson and Miller, 961–1040)*

6. **(B)**

7. **(C)**

8. **(D)**

9. **(E)**

10. **(A)**

Explanations 6 through 10

A C5 root lesion induces neck, shoulder, and anterior upper arm pain. Muscle weakness occurs predominantly but variably in the following muscles: the supraspinatus and deltoid, resulting in weakness of shoulder abduction, and the rhomboid, serratus anterior, infraspinatus, biceps, and brachioradialis. Biceps and brachioradialis reflexes may be depressed.

A C6 root lesion is often caused by compression from disc herniation at the C5-C6 vertebral level. It results in pain in the lateral arm and dorsal forearm. Paresthesia and hypesthesia occur in the lateral forearm, lateral hand, and first and second digits. Muscle weakness occurs in the biceps, pronator teres,

and brachioradialis, inducing weakness of elbow flexion in both fully supine position and half-pronated position. The extensor carpi radialis longus, flexor carpi radialis brevis, supinator, and serratus anterior are also affected by C6 root damage. The biceps and brachioradialis reflexes may be depressed.

Monoradiculopathy affecting the C7 nerve root is the most commonly affected level of the cervical roots, followed by the C6 nerve root. In C7 radiculopathy, pain is located in the dorsal forearm and middle and ring fingers. Paresis occurs variably in the pectoralis major and latissimus dorsi (inducing weakness of shoulder adduction), the triceps (inducing weakness of elbow extension), and the flexor carpi radialis, extensor carpi radialis longus, extensor carpi radialis brevis, and extensor digitorum (inducing weakness of wrist extension). The triceps reflex may be affected.

A C8 nerve root lesion causes pain in the medial arm, the forearm, and the fifth digit. Paresis occurs predominantly in the long forearm extensors and flexors of the fingers.

A T1 nerve root lesion causes a deep aching sensation in the shoulder joint, axilla, and me-dial side of the upper arm down to the olecranon. There is a loss of intrinsic hand muscles, including the abductor pollicis brevis muscle, which differentiates T1 nerve root lesions from ulnar nerve lesions (in ulnar nerve lesions all intrinsic muscles of the hand are affected except the abductor pollicis brevis). *(Brazis, Masdeu, and Biller, 67–72; Patten, 288–291)*

11. **(C)**

12. **(A)**

13. **(B)**

14. **(D)**

Explanations 11 through 14

A median nerve lesion at the upper arm may cause pain in the thumb, index, and middle fingers that spreads up from the forearm to the elbow. Motor signs may include paresis of forearm pronation, radial wrist flexion, distal flexion of the thumb, palmar abduction, opposition of the thumb, and flexion of the second and, to a lesser extent, the third finger. Weakness of the pinch sign results from paresis of the flexor digitorum profundus of the index finger and of the flexor pollicis longus.

Saturday night palsy corresponds to compression of the radial nerve within the spiral groove of the humerus. Clinical signs may include paralysis of extension of the wrist and elbow flexion and weakness of supination. Elbow extension is preserved because the radial nerve branches to the triceps muscle originate proximal to the spiral groove.

Musculocutaneous dysfunction causes atrophy of the biceps and brachialis, resulting in wasting of the ventral aspect of the upper arm and absence of the biceps reflex.

An ulnar nerve lesion at the wrist may cause paralysis of all intrinsic hand muscles, except the abductor pollicis brevis, which is innervated by the median nerve. Since the ulnar nerve lesion is proximal to the origin of the superficial terminal cutaneous branch of the ulnar nerve, there is sensory loss on the distal part and the palmar surfaces of the fifth and medial half of the fourth fingers. (Brazis, Masdeu, and Biller, 4–26; Patten, 292–296)

15. (A)

16. (F)

17. (B)

18. (G)

19. (C)

20. (H)

21. (D)

22. (I)

23. (E)

Explanations 15 through 23

A lumbar plexus lesion causes pain across the thigh. Sensation may be lost in the inguinal region and over the genitalia innervated by the iliohypogastric, ilioinguinal, and genitofemoral nerves. The sensation of the anterior and medial parts of the thigh may be affected. Motor signs include paresis and atrophy of muscles innervated by the femoral and obturator nerves. Thus, there is weakness of thigh flexion because of paresis of the iliopsoas, leg extension because of paresis of the quadriceps, thigh eversion because of paresis of the sartorius, and thigh adduction weakness because of paresis of the adductor muscles. The patellar and cremasteric reflexes may be decreased or absent.

The patient described in case F developed loss of sensation in the territory of the left posterior femoral cutaneous and sciatic nerves. There is weakness of all movement of the foot. This includes foot plantar flexion (due to weakness of the gastrocnemius and soleus), toe dorsiflexion and plantar flexion, foot eversion and inversion (due to weakness of the peronei and tibialis anterior and to posterior calf muscles, respectively). All of these muscles are in the sciatic distribution. Paresis of hip extension results from weakness of the gluteus maximus, innervated by the inferior gluteal nerve. Paresis of abduction and internal rotation of the thigh results from weakness of the gluteus medius and minimus, innervated by the superior gluteal nerve. Thus, the patient described in case F has symptoms and signs in the distribution of the sciatic nerve, superior gluteal nerve, and inferior gluteal nerve. Compression of the left sacral plexus by metastasis from the breast may explain the patient's clinical picture.

In case B, the patient developed sensory and motor disturbance in the territory of the obturator nerve: disturbance of sensation in the medial aspect of the thigh and weakness of the adductor muscles. Pregnancy may cause compression of the obturator nerve in the obturator canal.

In case G, the patient developed weakness of left knee extension, presumably by quadriceps weakness, and pain in the anterior thigh and medial leg, caused by injury to the medial cutaneous nerve of the thigh and the saphenous nerves (both are branches of the femoral nerve). These symptoms suggest left femoral nerve dysfunction. As the patient in this case has a history of falling and warfarin use, a retroperitoneal hematoma with femoral nerve compression is the most likely etiology. However, retroperitoneal hematoma is more commonly associated with diffuse weakness because multiple portions of the lumbosacral plexus are involved.

In case C, the patient has sensory loss in the territory of the tibial nerve. Weakness of plantar flexion and inversion of the foot is caused by weakness of the gastrocnemius muscle and the tibialis posterior muscle (both are innervated by the tibial nerve).

The patient in case H has sensory and motor deficits of the left peroneal nerve. Weakness of foot dorsiflexion and eversion may be caused by paralysis of the tibialis anterior, peroneus longus, and brevis muscles, respectively.

In case D, the patient has a flail foot because of paralysis of flexors and extensors of the left foot, and knee flexion weakness due to paresis of the hamstring muscles. A single lesion in the sciatic nerve would result in these and in loss of sensation in the lateral leg. Decreased Achilles reflex can occur in sciatic lesions because the tibial nerve subserves this reflex. Sciatic nerve injury may be caused by fracture dislocation of the hip, pelvic cancer surgery, infection, and buttock intramuscular injection, as illustrated in this case.

The patient in case I has disturbance of sensation in the territory of the pudendal nerve, whereas in case E, sensory disturbance is located in the region of the lateral femoral cutaneous nerve. (Brazis, Masdeu, and Biller, 27–49, 62–66; Patten, 299–314)

24. **(A)**

25. **(A)**

26. **(B)**

27. **(C)**

28. **(D)**

29. **(E)**

30. **(F)**

31. **(G)**

Explanations 24 through 31

B_{12} deficiency and ethanol abuse may cause a cecocentral scotoma that extends to the blind spot. Bilateral compression of the lateral optic chiasm is rare. It may be caused by the intracavernous part of an arteriosclerotic carotid artery pushing the chiasm against the opposite carotid artery. It may be caused also by dilatation of the third ventricle secondary to chronic aqueductal stenosis. The chiasm is splayed laterally by the dilated third ventricle and is damaged by the pulsatile carotid arteries pressing against its lateral edge. Bilateral compression of the lateral chiasm may cause binasal hemianopia.

Ethambutol is a drug used in the treatment of tuberculosis that sometimes causes dose-related optic neuritis. These patients may complain of central vision deficit and often claim that if they could see around it, vision would be normal.

At the chiasm, fibers from the inferior part of the nasal retina are ventral in the chiasm and loop into the proximal part of the contralateral optic nerve before turning back to join uncrossed inferotemporal fibers in the optic tract. Compres-sion of the junction between the optic nerve and optic chiasm may cause an ipsilateral central scotoma with contralateral superior temporal visual defect. Compression of the chiasm by a growing tumor such as a pituitary adenoma causes bitemporal field defect.

Anton syndrome may be caused by a bilateral medial occipital lesion. Affected patients may deny their blindness and confabulate about what they see. The anterior visual cortex is supplied by the posterior cerebral artery. Infarction of this area causes a macular sparing hemianopia because the macular cortex has a dual vascular supply from the middle cerebral and the posterior cerebral arteries. *(Brazis, Masdeu, and Biller, 147–150; Patten, 323–331)*

32. **(A)** With eyelid closure, reflex innervation of the extraocular muscles results in an upward and slightly outward rotation of the globe. This reflex eye movement is Bell's phenomenon, a physiological mechanism that protects the cornea from exposure, ulceration. In patients who have reduced or absent Bell's phenomenon, a tarsorrhaphy or placement of a gold weight in the upper eyelid is sometimes needed to protect the affected eye. *(Brazis, Masdeu, and Biller, 232)*

33. **(D)** The Tolosa-Hunt syndrome, a painful ophthalmoplegia, is characterized by steady, unremitting retro- and supraorbital pain in the trigeminal nerve ophthalmic division distribution in association with paresis of the oculomotor, trochlear, and abducens nerves as well as a diminished corneal reflex. Sensory loss and pain in the mandibular trigeminal distribution may also occur. Less frequently, the optic nerve and oculosympathetic fibers may be affected. Symptoms may persist for weeks to months. Both sexes are equally affected. The sedimentation rate may be elevated. Pathologically, a low-grade, noninfectious granulomatous process adjacent to the cavernous sinus or within the superior orbital fissure has been identified. The granulomas consist of lymphocytes and plasma cells. The Tolosa-Hunt syndrome typically responds dramatically to systemic corticosteroids, although symptoms may recur months to years later. Spontaneous remissions have also been reported. *(Goetz and Pappert, 167)*

34. **(B)** The patient described in the vignette has weakness on right arm elevation associated with winging of the scapula. These signs point toward weakness of the serratus anterior muscle. This muscle fixes and stabilizes the scapula against the chest wall. It is tested by observing for scapula winging (the vertebral border of the scapula stands away from the thorax, forming a wing, while the patient pushes the extended arm against a fixed object). The serratus anterior muscle is innervated by the long thoracic nerve, which may be affected by a variety of athletic activities, like volleyball. A C7 cervical root lesion may cause weakness of the serratus anterior muscle, but in combination with weakness of the extensors of the arm, wrist, or fingers. Volleyball players are also prone to suprascapular nerve injuries. However, a lesion of the suprascapular nerve results in weakness of arm abduction and external rotation without scapula winging. A dorsal scapular nerve lesion causes weakness of the rhomboid and levator scapulae muscles, resulting in weakness of elevation and adduction of the medial border of the shoulder blade. Weakness of the trapezius muscle may cause winging of the scapula on abduction of the arm; the shoulder is lower on the affected side, because there is weakness on elevation and retraction. *(Brazis, Masdeu, and Biller, 5; Staal, 19–21)*

35. **(B)**

36. **(A)**

37. **(C)**

38. **(D)**

Explanations 35 through 38

The radial nerve derives from the posterior cord of the brachial plexus and comprises fibers from spinal levels C5 to C8. In the axilla, the nerve gives rise to the posterior cutaneous nerve of the arm, which supplies the skin over the posterior aspect of the arm as far down as the olecranon. A secondary sensory branch, the posterior cutaneous nerve of the forearm, innervates the skin on the distal extensor aspect of the arm and the extensor aspect of the forearm up to the wrist.

Within or proximal to the spiral groove, the radial nerve supplies the triceps and the anconeus; both are forearm extensors. At the level of the lateral condyle of the humerus, the radial nerve gives off branches to the brachialis muscle (an elbow flexor that is also innervated by the musculocutaneous), the brachioradialis muscle (a forearm flexor midway between pronation and supination), and the extensor carpi radialis longus (radial extensor of the hand). The radial nerve then bifurcates into superficial and deep branches. The superficial branch emerges in the distal forearm and supplies the skin of the medial aspect of the back of the hand and the dorsum of the first four fingers. The deep branch is a purely motor nerve and is referred to as the posterior interosseous nerve. It supplies the supinator muscle (a forearm supinator), the extensor carpi radialis brevis (a radial extensor of the hand), the extensor digitorum (an extensor of the metacarpophalangeal joint of the second through the fifth fingers), the extensor digiti minimi (an extensor of the metacarpophalangeal joint of the fifth finger), the extensor carpi ulnaris (an ulnar extensor of the hand), the abductor pollicis longus (an abductor of the metacarpal of the thumb), the extensor pollicis longus and brevis (extensors of the thumb), and the extensor indicis (an extensor of the second finger).

A lesion of the radial nerve at the axilla causes weakness of elbow extension, loss of the triceps reflex (triceps muscle), wrist drop, fingers drop and sensory loss on the entire extensor surface of the arm, the forearm, the web between the index finger and the thumb, and the radial side of the dorsum of the hand. There is also weakness of forearm flexion and a depressed radial reflex (brachioradialis muscle). A lesion of the radial nerve in the upper arm causes the same symptoms as described above, with sparing of the triceps and the posterior cutaneous nerve of the skin of the arm. A radial nerve lesion in the upper arm may by seen in alcohol-induced sleep, where acute retrohumeral nerve compression occurs. The tingling and pain that normally wake up normal individuals do not occur in the inebriated. A lesion of the radial nerve at the forearm will spare the triceps, brachioradialis, and extensor carpi radialis muscles. Typically, the patient has finger but not wrist

drop. There is a radial deviation of the extended hand when the patient is asked to make a fist, illustrating the weakness of the extensor carpi ulnaris compared to the extensor carpi radialis muscles. The patient described in question 38 has purely sensory symptoms that correspond to a wrist compression of the dorsal digital nerve. (*Brazis, Masdeu, and Biller,* 21–26; *Staal,* 35–48)

39. **(A)**

40. **(B)**

41. **(C)**

Explanations 39 through 41

The median nerve carries fibers from C5 to T1 roots. It is a mixed nerve formed in the axilla by the joining of the lateral cord of the brachial plexus with the medial cord. The nerve descends on the medial side of the arm and enters the forearm, between the two heads of the pronator teres, to supply the pronator teres (C6-C7), the flexor carpi radialis (C6-C7) (a radial flexor of the hand), the palmaris longus (C7-T1) (a flexor of the wrist), and the flexor digitorum superficialis (C7-T1) (a flexor of the middle phalange of the second to the fifth fingers). After it passes between the two heads of the pronator teres, it gives off the anterior interosseous nerve. It then courses deep to the flexor retinaculum at the wrist to reach the hand. The palmar cutaneous branch takes off to the flexor retinaculum either subcutaneously or through the superficial ligament fibers to supply the skin over the thenar eminence and the proximal palm on the radial aspect of the hand.

The purely motor anterior interosseous nerve innervates the flexor pollicis longus (a flexor of the terminal phalanx of the thumb), the flexor digitorum profundus I and II (a flexor of the terminal phalanges of the second and third digit), and the pronator quadratus (a forearm pronator). At the distal end of the carpal tunnel, the median nerve divides into its terminal branches. The motor branches innervate the first and second lumbricals (which are flexors of the proximal phalanges and extensors of the two distal phalanges of the second and third fingers), the thenar muscles (which include the abductor pollicis brevis, an abductor of the thumb, the opponens pollicis, and the superficial head of the flexor pollicis brevis).

Soft tissue tumors, such as lymphomas, may cause a compression of the median nerve in the upper arm. Signs of a lesion at this level include sensory loss in the territory of the palmar cutaneous and palmar digital branches, atrophy of the thenar eminence muscles, paresis of forearm pronation, radial wrist flexion, distal flexion of the thumb, palmar abduction, opposition of the thumb, and flexion of the second and, to a lesser extent, the third fingers. Dislocation of the elbow may expose the patient to median nerve injury in its anterior interosseous branch. Neurological signs in this case are purely motor. They include the inability of the patient to form a small circle by pinching the end of the phalanx of the thumb and index finger together, resulting from a weakness of the flexor digitorum profundus of the index finger and the flexor pollicis longus, and weakness of forearm pronation on flexion because of the pronator quadratus muscle. Elbow pronation on extension is conserved because of the integrity of the pronator teres. The patient described in question 41 has the clinical features of carpal tunnel syndrome. There is sensory loss in the palmar aspect of the hand, weakness, and atrophy of the abductor pollicis brevis and opponens pollicis muscles. *(Brazis, Masdeu, and Biller, 10–16; Staal, 52–60)*

42. **(A)**

43. **(B)**

Explanations 42 through 43

The ulnar nerve carries fibers from C7-T1 roots. Immediately distal to the elbow joint, the ulnar nerve innervates the flexor carpi ulnaris, an ulnar flexor of the wrist, and the flexor digitorum profundus, a flexor of the terminal phalanges of the fourth and fifth fingers. In the middle of the forearm, the ulnar nerve gives off the palmar cutaneous branch, which supplies the skin over the hypothenar eminence. It then gives off a dorsal cutaneous branch, which supplies the dorsal aspect of the hand and dorsal aspect of the fifth and fourth finger. In the hand, it gives off the superficial terminal branch, a sensory branch to the skin of the distal part of the ulnar aspect of the palm and the palmar aspect of the fifth and half of the fourth finger. It then passes between the pisiform and hamate bones to give off superficial terminal branches, which are mainly sensory and deep motor terminal branches. The superficial terminal branch innervates the palmaris brevis muscle. The deep branch innervates the abductor digiti minimi (an abductor of the fifth finger), the opponens digiti minimi, the flexor digiti minimi (a flexor of the fifth finger), and the lumbricals III and IV (flexors of the metacarpophalangeal joints and extensors of the proximal interphalangeal joints). The deep muscle branch also innervates the interosseous muscles (flexors of the metacarpophalangeal joints and extensors of the proximal interphalangeal joints; the dorsal interosseous muscles are finger abductors, whereas the palmar interosseous muscles are finger adductors) and the adductor pollicis.

The patient described in question 42 has a clawlike hand, which is characteristic of ulnar nerve injury. It is caused by the unopposed action of long finger extensors from the paralyzed interossei and ulnar lumbrical muscles. Weakness of hand adduction and flexion associated with weakness of flexion of the little finger in the distal interphalangeal joint suggests involvement of the flexor carpi ulnaris and the flexor digitorum III and IV, respectively. These findings localize the lesion of the ulnar nerve at the elbow in the cubital tunnel. In question 43, the absence of a sensory defect and the preservation of the palmaris brevis with atrophy of the hypothenar muscles localize the nerve injury to the wrist at the level of the pisiform bone. *(Brazis, Masdeu, and Biller, 16–21; Staal, 71–82)*

44. **(C)** The patient described in this vignette shows a weakness of the right quadriceps and

psoas muscles, both of which are innervated by the femoral nerve. In the context of recent anti-coagulation, compression of the femoral nerve by a hematoma of the psoas muscle is the most likely diagnosis. *(Staal, 104–107)*

45. **(A)** Retinal nerve fibers enter the optic disc via the temporal aspect of the disc, the temporal aspect of the superior and inferior poles of the disc, and the nasal aspect of the disc. The papillomacular bundle is formed by macular fibers that enter the temporal aspect of the disc. A lesion in these fibers may cause a central scotoma (a defect covering central fixation), centrocecal scotoma (a central scotoma connected to the blind spot), or a paracentral scotoma. The arcuate bundle is formed by fibers from the retina temporal to the disc that enter the superior or inferior poles of the disc. A lesion of the arcuate fibers may cause Bjerrum arcuate scotoma, Seidel scotoma (a defect in the proximal portion of the nerve fibers that causes a comma-shaped extension of the blind spot), or nasal step of Ronne scotoma respecting the horizontal meridian. A nasal nerve fiber bundle defect results in a wedge-shaped temporal scotoma arising from the blind spot. *(Kline and Bajandas, 5–7)*

46. **(D)** An optic tract lesion causes a contralateral hemianopia. The defect is incongruous (not identical in shape, location, and size in both eyes), since the lesion is located anterior to the occipital lobe, and nerve fibers of corresponding points do not lie adjacent to one another. An optic tract syndrome also includes bilateral nerve fiber atrophy and relative afferent defect on the side opposite to the lesion. Wernicke's pupil consists of absence of pupillary reaction to light stimulation of a blind retina, while stimulation of an intact retina causes normal pupillary response. *(Kline and Bajandas, 10–12)*

47. **(E)** Ipsilateral inferotemporal fibers and contralateral inferonasal fibers course anteriorly from the lateral geniculate body into the temporal lobe, forming Meyer's loop. A right anterior temporal lobe lesion tends to produce left mid-peripheral and peripheral, pie-in-the-sky,

homonymous superior quadrantanopia. *(Kline and Bajandas, 12.)*

48. **(G)**

49. **(E)**

50. **(A)**

51. **(D)**

52. **(B)**

53. **(F)**

54. **(C)**

Explanations 48 through 54

The abducens nucleus is located in the dorsal caudal portion of the pons, separated from the fourth ventricle by the genu of the facial nerve. The abducens nuclear complex coordinates the action of both eyes to produce horizontal gaze by sending axons to the medial longitudinal fasciculus that end in the contralateral nucleus of the third nerve. Axons of the abducens motoneurons ascend along the base of the pons in the prepontine cistern and enter Dorello's canal beneath the petroclinoid ligament. In the lateral wall of the cavernous sinus, the abducens nerve lies between the ophthalmic artery medially and the ophthalmic branch of the trigeminal nerve laterally. After passing through the orbital fissure, the abducens nerve innervates the lateral rectus muscle.

A pituitary tumor may compress the cavernous sinus, which may cause total ophthalmoplegia, Horner syndrome, and pain in the area innervated by the ophthalmic division of the trigeminal nerve. Gradenigo syndrome may be caused by a localized inflammation of the petrous apex following complicated otitis media. Contact with the tip of the petrous pyramid makes the portion of the abducens nerve within Dorello's canal susceptible to injury when the petrous bone is inflamed. Clinical findings include abducens nerve palsy, ipsilateral decreased hearing, facial pain, and ipsilateral facial palsy. Millard-Gubler syndrome is caused by a lesion located in the ventral pons that destroys the fascicles of the abducens and facial nerves and the corticospinal tract. It is characterized by ipsilateral abducens nerve palsy, ipsilateral peripheral-type facial paralysis, and contralateral hemiplegia. Foville syndrome is caused by a lesion located in the pontine tegmentum that destroys the fascicles of the facial nerve, the paramedian pontine reticular formation, and the corticospinal tract. It is characterized by horizontal gaze palsy, dysfunction of the facial and vestibulocochlear nerves, ipsilateral Horner syndrome, and contralateral hemiplegia. In Raymond-Cestan syndrome, the lesion is located in the basal pons but is less extensive than the lesion in Millard-Gubler syndrome: there is only ipsilateral abducens nerve palsy with contralateral hemiplegia. Elevation of intracranial pressure may result in downward displacement of the brain stem, with stretching of the abducens nerve as it exits from the pons and Dorello's canal. Pseudotumor cerebri may cause papilledema, and in 30% of cases it also causes abducens nerve palsy. Petrous bone fracture may follow head trauma. The trigeminal, abducens, facial, and cochleovestibular nerves may be affected. Associated signs may include otorrhea, hemotympanum, and mastoid ecchymosis. *(Brazis, Masdeu, and Biller, 176–180; Kline and Bajandas, 93–101)*

55. **(B)** Oculomotor nerve palsy secondary to a nuclear lesion is extremely rare. Each superior rectus is innervated by the contralateral oculomotor nerve nucleus; therefore, a nuclear oculomotor nerve lesion results in contralateral superior rectus palsy. Both levator muscles are innervated by one subnuclear structure, the central caudal nucleus. Hence, a nuclear oculomotor nerve lesion results in bilateral ptosis. *(Kline and Bajandas, 105)*

56. **(B)** The pupillomotor fibers of the oculomotor nerve travel in the outer layers of the nerve and therefore are closer to the nutrient blood supply. This may explain their susceptibility to compressive lesions of the oculomotor nerve rather than to ischemic causes. The patient described in the vignette developed a pupil-sparing, isolated oculomotor nerve palsy. This may suggest an ischemic oculomotor mononeuropathy. A follow-up examination revealed an Argyll Robertson pupil in the affected eye, which is most likely a pseudo Argyll Robertson sign caused by aberrant regeneration of the oculomotor nerve. Some of the medial rectus fibers may end up innervating the pupillary sphincter muscle so that there is more pupillary constriction during convergence than response to light. Secondary aberrant regeneration does not occur after ischemic oculomotor nerve palsy. The diagnosis of ischemic oculomotor nerve palsy is unlikely in this case. Other diagnoses, such as neoplasm, aneurysm, and trauma, should be considered. *(Kline and Bajandas, 111–112)*

57. **(A)** If a patient has vertical misalignment due to recently acquired weakness of a single vertically acting muscle, then the determination of the weak muscle follows the three steps of the Parks-Bielschowsky test. The median and lateral rectus muscles do not have vertical action. Therefore, vertical misalignment of paretic etiology is caused by weakness of one or more of the following eight vertically acting muscles: right inferior oblique, left inferior oblique, right superior oblique, left superior oblique, right inferior rectus, left inferior rectus, right superior rectus, and left superior rectus.

The first step is to find which is the higher eye. In the vignette, the right eye is higher than the left eye. The weak muscle is then a depressor of the right eye (right inferior rectus or right superior oblique) or an elevator of the left eye (left superior rectus or left inferior oblique).

The second step is to find if the misalignment is worse on right or left gaze. The vertical rectus muscles have their greatest vertical action and least torsional action when the eye is abducted. The oblique muscles have their greatest vertical and least torsional action when the eye is adducted. In the vignette, the patient's hypertropia is getting worse on left abduction of the left eye and adduction of the right eye (left gaze deviation). Therefore, the possible causes of right hypertropia are narrowed from four muscles to two: worsening of the right hypertropia on right eye adduction and left eye abduction is caused by right superior oblique weakness or left superior rectus weakness, respectively.

The third step is to find out if the hypertropia is worse on left or right head tilt (by moving the ear near the ipsilateral shoulder). The superior muscles intort the eyes (superior rectus and superior oblique) and the inferior muscles extort the eyes (inferior rectus and inferior oblique). When the head is tilted downward to the right shoulder, the eyes undergo corrective torsion: the right eye is intorted and the left eye is extorted. Therefore, when the head is tilted to the right, the right eye is intorted by contraction of the right superior rectus or right superior oblique. These two muscles work together in affecting the intorsion and neutralize each other's vertical action. If one of these muscles is weak and thus responsible for the misalignment, then the vertical action is not neutralized, and the hypertropia will become worse, as in this case. From steps one and two, weakness of only two muscles is left: right superior oblique or left superior rectus. So the muscle responsible for the misalignment in this case is the right superior oblique. *(Kline and Bajandas, 118–121)*

58. **(D)** In a C6 radiculopathy, the biceps and the brachioradialis reflexes are absent or diminished, whereas the triceps reflex, mediated by C7 nerve root and spinal cord segments and the finger flexor reflex, mediated by the C8 nerve root and spinal cord segments, are exaggerated as a result of injury of the corticospinal tract below the C6 spinal cord level. Thus, C5-C6 segmental lesions result in an inversion of the brachioradialis reflex. Tapping of the radius elicits exaggerated finger and hand flexion without flexion and supination of the forearm. *(Brazis, Masdeu, and Biller, 71)*

59. **(C)**

60. **(F)**

61. **(E)**

62. **(B)**

63. **(D)**

64. **(A)**

Explanations 59 through 64

The patient in vignette 59 developed signs of dorsal column dysfunction: loss of proprioception and vibration sense in both legs as well as sensory ataxia. He also has bilateral corticospinal tract dysfunction resulting in spasticity, hyperreflexia, and bilateral Babinski sign. The spinothalamic tract seems intact because temperature and pain are conserved. This is selective damage of the posterior and lateral columns that may occur in subacute combined degeneration of the spinal cord due to vitamin B_{12} deficiency (Figs. 2.1 and 2.2).

The patient described in vignette 60 shows pure posterior column dysfunction with loss of proprioception and vibratory sensation and presence of the Romberg sign. Tabes dorsalis affects the posterior columns selectively (see again Fig. 2.1).

The patient described in case 61 has pure chronic motor syndrome, including signs of upper motor neuron dysfunction (paresis, spasticity, increased deep tendon reflexes, and the Babinski sign) and lower motor neuron dysfunction (progressive muscular atrophy and fasciculations). The most likely diagnosis is amyotrophic lateral sclerosis. The disease is characterized by degenerative changes in the anterior horn cells of the spinal cord, the motor nuclei of the brain stem, and the corticospinal tract. Clinically, the onset of the disease is usually focal or in one limb. Sensation is usually preserved. Bulbar or pseudobulbar impairment is often superimposed resulting in explosive dysarthria, dysphagia, emotional incontinence, tongue spasticity, and atrophy. Virtually any striated muscle can be affected. However, the urinary and rectal sphincters are unaffected early in the illness due to the sparing of Onuf's nucleus, located in the ventral margin of the anterior sacral horns (Fig. 2.3). These, as well as the extraocular muscles, are affected late in the illness.

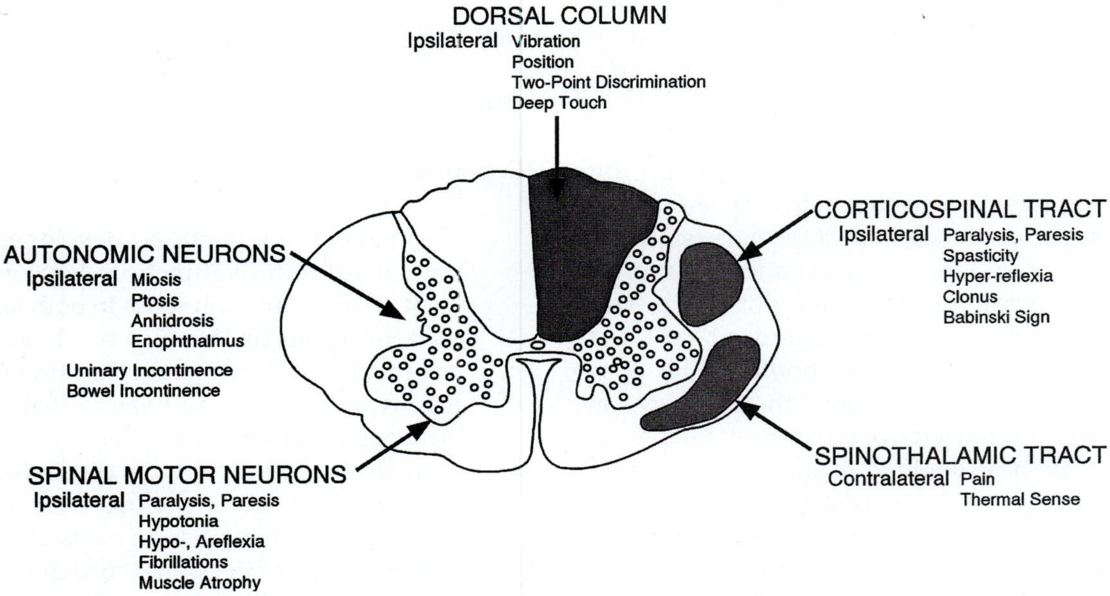

DORSAL COLUMN
Ipsilateral   Vibration
Position
Two-Point Discrimination
Deep Touch

CORTICOSPINAL TRACT
Ipsilateral   Paralysis, Paresis
Spasticity
Hyper-reflexia
Clonus
Babinski Sign

AUTONOMIC NEURONS
Ipsilateral   Miosis
Ptosis
Anhidrosis
Enophthalmus

Uninary Incontinence
Bowel Incontinence

SPINAL MOTOR NEURONS
Ipsilateral   Paralysis, Paresis
Hypotonia
Hypo-, Areflexia
Fibrillations
Muscle Atrophy

SPINOTHALAMIC TRACT
Contralateral   Pain
Thermal Sense

FIG. 2-1

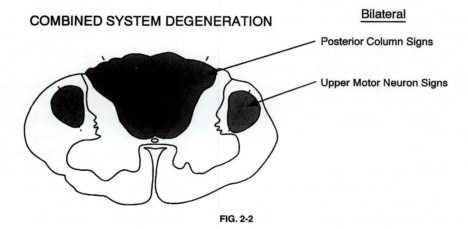

COMBINED SYSTEM DEGENERATION

<u>Bilateral</u>

Posterior Column Signs

Upper Motor Neuron Signs

FIG. 2-2

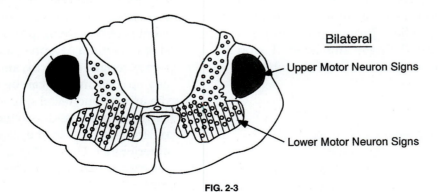

MOTOR NEURON DISEASE

<u>Bilateral</u>

Upper Motor Neuron Signs

Lower Motor Neuron Signs

FIG. 2-3

SYRINGOMYELIA

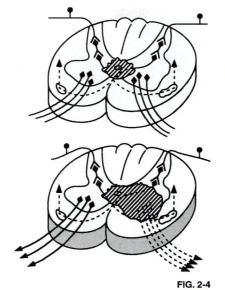

EARLY LESION
(Crossing spinothalamic fibers involved)

LATE LESION
(Crossing spinothalamic fibers and motor neurons involved)

FIG. 2-4

The patient in case 62 shows a central spinal cord syndrome with dissociation of sensory loss that is best exemplified by syringomyelia. Cord damage starts centrally and spreads centrifugally to involve other spinal cord structures. Characteristically, the decussating fibers of the spinothalamic tract, conveying pain and temperature sensation, are affected first. This results in thermoanesthesia and analgesia with suspended bilateral distribution and preservation of sensation to light touch as well as proprioception (Fig. 2.4).

The patient described in question 63 developed a neurological deficit involving the territory of the anterior spinal artery. Spinal cord infarction is rare. The syndrome is characterized the abrupt onset of leg weakness and urinary incontinence associated with loss of thermoanesthesia and analgesia below the level of the lesion. Position sense, vibration, and light touch remain intact due to preservation of the dorsal columns (Fig. 2.5).

The patient described in question 64 developed right lower extremity weakness and loss of proprioceptive function below the T6 spinal cord level with contralateral loss of pain and temperature. This is highly suggestive of right hemisection of the spinal cord at the T6 level. The weakness is caused by a lesion in the ipsilateral corticospinal tract, and the loss of proprioception is related to interruption of the ipsilateral ascending fibers of the posterior columns. The loss of pain and temperature sensation in the contralateral side is related to a lesion of the decussating spinothalamic tract (Fig. 2.6). *(Afifi, 98–100; Brazis, Masdeu, and Biller 88–93)*

65. **(B)** The patient has funnel vision only when the central vision is intact. Funnel vision should not be confused with tunnel vision, a field defect characteristic of hysteria or malingering. This latter field can be easily mapped onto a tangent screen by plotting the fields with the patient seated one and two meters from the screen. In the case of organic defect, the field projected at two meters is larger than the field plotted at one meter. Constricted visual field with retained acuity may be seen in the case of glaucoma, retinitis pigmentosa, cancer-associated retinopathy, postpapilledema optic atrophy, and bilateral occipital infarct with macular sparing. *(Brazis, Masdeu, and Biller, 133)*

66. **(A)** Disease of the choroid, retinal pigment epithelium, retina, optic disc, or optic nerve

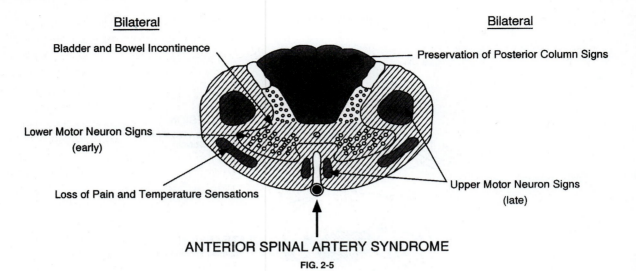

<u>Bilateral</u>   <u>Bilateral</u>

Bladder and Bowel Incontinence   Preservation of Posterior Column Signs

Lower Motor Neuron Signs
(early)

Loss of Pain and Temperature Sensations   Upper Motor Neuron Signs
(late)

ANTERIOR SPINAL ARTERY SYNDROME

FIG. 2-5

almost always causes monocular visual defects. The early stage of a chiasmatic lesion may cause monocular loss of vision in the temporal field of the ipsilateral eye when the defect is located most anterior in the chiasm to affect the nasal retinal fibers crossing from the contralateral eye. A lesion located in the most anterior aspect of the calcarine cortex causes a crescent-shaped defect restricted to the temporal field of the contralateral eye. This is the only retrochiasmatic lesion that may cause a unilateral visual defect. *(Brazis, Masdeu, and Biller, 104)*

67.   (E)

68.   (A)

HEMISECTION
BROWN-SEQUARD SYNDROME

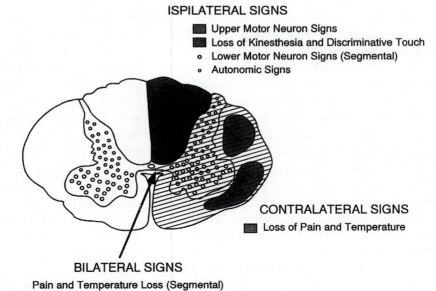

ISPILATERAL SIGNS

    ■ Upper Motor Neuron Signs
    ■ Loss of Kinesthesia and Discriminative Touch
    ○ Lower Motor Neuron Signs (Segmental)
    ○ Autonomic Signs

CONTRALATERAL SIGNS

    ▨ Loss of Pain and Temperature

BILATERAL SIGNS

Pain and Temperature Loss (Segmental)

FIG. 2-6

69. (C)

70. (D)

71. (A)

72. (B)

Explanations 67 through 72

A fascicular lesion of the facial nerve results in a peripheral type of facial nerve palsy (Fig. 2.7). A lesion located in the ventral pons, destroying the fascicles of the facial and abducens nerves, and corticospinal tract, causes the Millard-Gubler syndrome. This syndrome is characterized by an ipsilateral peripheral facial nerve palsy, ipsilateral lateral rectus palsy, and contralateral hemiplegia. A lesion located in the pontine tegmentum that destroys the fascicle of the facial nerve, the paramedian pontine reticular formation, and the corticospinal tract causes Foville's syndrome. It is characterized by an ipsilateral peripheral-type facial palsy, paralysis of the conjugate gaze to the side of the lesion, and contralateral hemiplegia. A lesion of the facial nerve in the meatal canal affects the facial and cochleovestibular nerves: there is ipsilateral facial nerve palsy, impaired taste sensation in the anterior two-thirds of the tongue, impaired lacrimation, and deafness. A lesion of the facial nerve within the facial canal, distal to the meatal segment but proximal to the departure of the nerve to the stapedius muscle, results in ipsilateral facial motor paralysis, loss of taste over the anterior two-thirds of the tongue, and hyperacusis. Lacrimation is preserved if the lesion is distal to the greater superficial petrosal nerve. Ramsay Hunt syndrome results from a herpes zoster infection of the geniculate ganglion. Clinical features may include hyperacusis, loss of taste in the anterior two-thirds of the tongue, geniculate neuralgia, and herpetic vesicles of the external auditory meatus. A lesion affecting the facial nerve, between the departure of the nerve to the stapedius and the departure of the chorda tympani, results in ipsilateral facial palsy and loss of taste sensation in the anterior two-thirds of the tongue. Hearing is spared. A lesion of the facial nerve at the stylomastoid foramen produces isolated ipsilateral motor palsy without hearing or taste loss. (*Brazis, Masdeu, and Biller, 276–281*)

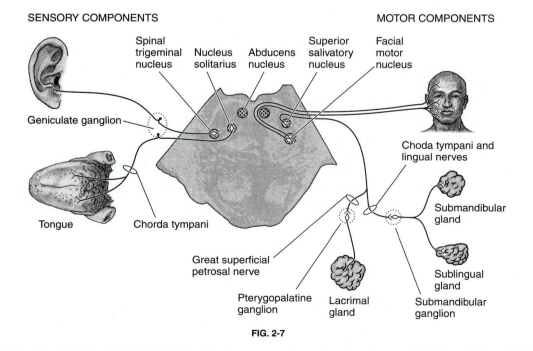

SENSORY COMPONENTS

MOTOR COMPONENTS

Spinal trigeminal nucleus

Nucleus solitarius

Abducens nucleus

Superior salivatory nucleus

Facial motor nucleus

Geniculate ganglion

Tongue

Chorda tympani

Great superficial petrosal nerve

Pterygopalatine ganglion

Lacrimal gland

Choda tympani and lingual nerves

Submandibular gland

Sublingual gland

Submandibular ganglion

FIG. 2-7

73. (B)

74. (A)

75. (D)

76. (C)

Explanations 73 through 76

The patient described in question 73 has decreased pain and temperature in the right face and left side of the trunk and extremities. This results from a lesion affecting the right trigeminal spinal nucleus/tractus and the right spinothalamic tract, respectively. A right nucleus ambiguus lesion causes weakness of the right palate and vocal cord paralysis resulting in hoarseness. Right limb ataxia may be explained by a right cerebellar lesion. All these clinical findings are highly suggestive of a lateral medullary lesion, also known as Wallenberg syndrome. It is most often related to obstruction of the intracranial vertebral artery or the posterior inferior cerebellar artery. The syndrome has been reported with cocaine abuse, medullary metastasis, trauma, abscess, and demyelination. The clinical features of this syndrome may include Horner syndrome (due to injury to the descending sympathetic fibers), vertigo, and vomiting from the involvement of the vestibular nuclei. A lateral lesion of the rostral medulla is associated with more severe dysphagia and dysphonia, whereas a caudal lesion is associated with more marked vertigo, nystagmus, and gait ataxia.

The patient described in question 74 has symptoms consistent with a lesion located in the right pyramidal system, right medial lemniscus, and right hypoglossal nerve, which explain the protrusion of the tongue away from the hemiplegia towards the side of the lesion. These symptoms are consistent with the diagnosis of right medial medullary syndrome. It may be caused by occlusion of the right anterior spinal artery or its parent, the vertebral artery.

In case 75, the neurological examination demonstrates right facial palsy and contralateral hemiplegia. These findings point to a lesion affecting the right pons. The presence of gaze deviation to the left side may suggest a lesion of the paramedian pontine reticular formation or a right abducens lesion. The association of these findings puts the lesion in the right dorsal pontine tegmentum in the caudal third of the pons. This is consistent with a diagnosis of Foville syndrome.

In case 76, the patient's neurological assessment shows the association of quadriparesis, aphonia, impairment of horizontal eye movement with preservation of vertical gaze and maintenance of consciousness. These signs are highly suggestive of the locked-in syndrome. It results from a ventral pontine lesion. It may be caused by a vertebral artery thrombosis, ventral pontine tumor, hemorrhage, trauma, or central pontine myelinolysis from rapid correction of hyponatremia. The quadriplegia is caused by bilateral corticospinal tract lesion, the aphonia is caused by a lesion in the corticobulbar fibers that innervate the lower cranial nerves, and the ophthalmoplegia with impairment of horizontal eye movement results from a lesion of the abducens nerve fascicles. The patient is fully awake because the reticular formation is spared. The supranuclear ocular motor pathways, as well as the blinking pathways, are also spared because they lie more dorsally. Thus, the patient is only able to blink and to look up and down. *(Brazis, Masdeu, and Biller, 345–356)*

77. (A)

78. (C)

79. (B)

80. (D)

Explanations 77 through 80

In question 77 the patient has a right cerebellar syndrome, and right spinothalamic and corticospinal tracts impairment. A lesion of the lateral pons would explain these signs, which correspond to Marie-Foix syndrome. The 40-year-old diabetic woman described in question 78 has signs highly suggestive of a lesion affecting the mesencephalic tegmentum (Benedict syndrome). Ophthalmoplegia is caused by fascicular third cranial nerve damage on the ipsilateral side of the lesion on the right side in this case. The left side tremor is caused by destruction of the right red nucleus, causing a rubral tremor.

In question 79, the patient developed right oculomotor paresis and left hemiplegia. This is compatible with a lesion in the right cerebral peduncle that affects the right oculomotor nerve fascicles and right corticospinal tract, causing left hemiplegia. These signs are consistent with the diagnosis of Weber syndrome. The patient described in question 80 has signs highly suggestive of Sylvian aqueduct syndrome. It results from a dorsal rostral mesencephalic lesion. This is most often seen with pineal gland tumors that cause hydrocephalus. The syndrome may include a paralysis of the conjugate upward gaze and convergence retraction nystagmus on upward gaze. *(Brazis, Masdeu, and Biller, 357–360)*

81. **(B)**

82. **(D)**

83. **(A)**

84. **(E)**

85. **(C)**

Explanations 81 through 85

The clinical case described in question 81 shows a 5-year-old boy complaining of axial ataxia without limb ataxia and spontaneous nystagmus. These symptoms are consistent with damage to the flocculonodular lobe in the caudal part of the vermis, caused in this case by a medulloblastoma. The neurological abnormalities reported in case 82 suggest right anterior inferior cerebellar artery occlusion. The vertigo is caused by ischemia of the vestibular nuclei. The right facial palsy and the loss of sensation are caused by ipsilateral ischemia of the lateral-pontomedullary tegmentum and the trigeminal nuclei and tract, respectively. The right Horner syndrome is caused by a compromise of the descending oculosympathetic fibers. The patient described

in question 83 has a predominant axial ataxia. With the history of ethanol abuse, the most likely diagnosis is cerebellar degeneration from chronic ethanol abuse. Ethanol results in atrophy of the anterior and superior vermis. The patient described in question 84 has symptoms consistent with superior cerebellar artery occlusion. The vertigo and nystagmus are caused by ischemia of the vestibular nuclei. The Horner syndrome is caused by a compromise of the descending oculosympathetic fibers; the left deafness results from a lesion in the crossed right lateral lemniscus; and the right tremor is caused by a lesion of the dentate nucleus and the superior cerebellar peduncle. The left side pain and temperature loss is caused by involvement of the spinothalamic tract. The case described in question 85 results most likely from an embolic obstruction of the posterior inferior cerebellar artery with infarction of the inferior cerebellum and lateral medulla. The loss of pain and temperature is caused by damage to the trigeminal spinal nucleus and tract, the left limb ataxia is caused by damage of the inferior cerebellar peduncle, the dysarthria and left vocal cord palsy are caused by damage to the left nucleus ambiguus, and the loss of pain and temperature on the right side is caused by damage to the spinothalamic tract on the left side. *(Brazis, Masdeu, and Biller, 371–377)*

86. **(B)** An acute hypothalamic lesion can cause gastrointestinal erosions called neurogenic ulcer that are most often located in the lower esophagus. *(Brazis, Masdeu, and Biller, 390)*

87. **(C)** The medial dorsal nucleus of the thalamus is found to be most consistently associated with memory loss in Wernicke-Korsakoff syndrome. *(Brazis, Masdeu, and Biller, 395–396)*

88. **(D)** Hemiballismus usually occurs with injury to the contralateral subthalamic nucleus or any lesion that disrupts its afferent or efferent fibers. Hemiballismus may also be caused by lesions affecting the caudate, putamen, globus pallidus, precentral gyrus, and thalamic nuclei. *(Brazis, Masdeu, and Biller, 417)*

89. (A) Sensory inattention occurs most commonly with a lesion of the contralateral inferior parietal lobe. Less commonly, it may occur with lesions of the temporo-parieto-occipital junction, dorsolateral frontal lobe, cingulate gyrus, thalamus, and mesencephalic reticular formation. *(Brazis, Masdeu, and Biller, 467–468)*

90. (D)

91. (E)

92. (A)

93. (C)

94. (B)

95. (F)

96. (H)

97. (G)

Explanations 90 through 97

Emotions and their expression depend on the state of arousal of the individual (mediated by the reticular activating system), the vegetative function (mediated in part by the hypothalamus), the previous-experience retrieval system (mediated by the hippocampus and other portions of the limbic system), the ability to perceive, the ability to evaluate stimuli that carry an affective component, and the ability to express emotion. A defect in the ability to perceive stimuli that carry affective components may be seen in right parietotemporal damage. The patient understands the semantic meaning of a verbal threat, but his perception of the emotional overtones that accompany the utterance is impaired. This condition is known as sensory aprosodia. The ability to evaluate properly the importance of stimuli may be impaired in the case of bilateral lesions of the anterior cingulate; the patient may be unconcerned in the presence of painful stimuli. It is also affected with bilateral anterior temporal lesions, where the patient expresses a blunt affect. A lesion of the septal region may cause enhanced irritability and rage reactions.

A lesion of the left dorsofrontal lobe may cause anger and hostility, whereas a lesion of the right orbitofrontal area may cause depression. An epileptogenic right temporal lesion may cause a paranoid behavioral type, whereas an epileptogenic lesion of the left temporal lobe may cause denial, sadness, and elation. *(Brazis, Masdeu, and Biller, 471–474)*

98. (C) Medial frontal lobe syndrome is characterized by the association of mutism, gait disturbance, and urinary incontinence. *(Brazis, Masdeu, and Biller, 474)*

99. (E)

100. (C)

101. (D)

102. (A)

103. (B)

Explanations 99 through 103

Charles Bonnet syndrome may occur in elderly patients with poor vision. It is probably a release phenomenon. It is characterized by hallucinations in the evening of small, brightly colored people or objects with a cartoonlike appearance. The patient is usually aware of the unreality of these hallucinations. Simple visual hallucinations consisting of flashes of light or lines of different colors, but predominantly adopting zigzag or fortification patterns, are suggestive of migraine headache. In occipital epileptic seizures, hallucinations are predominantly multicolored with a circular or spherical pattern. They are also more stereotyped than hallucinations from impaired visual acuity and are associated with other seizure manifestations. A lesion of the upper midbrain bilaterally may cause a complex visual hallucination that has a dreamlike quality. Hallucinations are often hypnagogic, known to be unreal, and may be pleasant to the patient. Focal seizures arising from the neocortex of the temporal lobe may give rise to experiential illusion, "déjà vécu" (already lived) or "jamais vécu" (never experienced before). They may also give rise to visual illusions like "déjà vu" (already seen) or "jamais vu" (never seen before). *(Brazis, Masdeu, and Biller, 477–479)*

104. **(D)** Balint syndrome may result from bilateral parieto-occipital lesions in the convexities of the hemispheres. It is characterized by the following symptoms: (1) simultagnosia: the inability to appreciate the meaning of the whole, though the elemental parts are well recognized; (2) gaze apraxia: failure to shift gaze on command and problems with voluntary redirecting of attention; (3) optic ataxia: disturbance reaching a target under visual control, manifested by clumsiness of object-bound movements of the hand performed under visual guidance; (4) decreased visual attention affecting mainly the peripheral visual field. Altitudinal neglect may also be seen. *(Brazis, Masdeu, and Biller, 485)*

105. **(A)** The presence of left homonymous hemianopia without neglect and preservation of response to threat as well as preservation of drawing and copying ability is highly suggestive of damage to the right occipitoparietal region in area 17 of the occipital cortex. It is usually caused by obstruction of the calcarine branch of the posterior cerebral artery. Right parietal and temporoparietal lesions involving areas 18 and 19 cause lack of awareness of visual loss, contralateral neglect and abnormal optokinetic nystagmus, lack of response to visual threat, and abnormal drawing and copying. Bilateral occipital lesions involving the visual cortex in areas 17, 18, and 19 cause blindness, agitation, and amnesia. A lesion of the inferior calcarine fissure bilaterally causes prosopagnosia, bilateral upper quadranopsia, and achromatopsia. A bilateral lesion of the superior calcarine fissure causes inferior quadranopsia and Balint syndrome. *(Brazis, Masdeu, and Biller, 486)*

106. **(D)** Alien limb signs includes failure to recognize ownership of one's limb when visual cues are removed, feeling that one's body part is foreign, personification of the affected body part, and autonomous activity that is perceived as outside voluntary control. Although the hand is most frequently affected, any limb or combination of limbs may fulfill the alien limb criteria. Alien hand sign should be reserved for cases in which the hand feels foreign, together with observable involuntary motor activity. Etiologies of this syndrome include multiple infarcts and corticobasal degeneration. Two distinct alien hand syndromes have been described: (1) The frontal hand alien limb syndrome occurs in the dominant hand and is associated with reflexive grasping, groping, and compulsive manipulation of tools. It results from damage of the supplementary motor area, anterior cingulate gyrus, medial prefrontal cortex of the dominant hemisphere, and anterior corpus callosum. (2) The callosal form is characterized primarily by intermanual conflict and requires only an anterior callosal lesion. The occurrence of frontal alien hand syndrome in the dominant limb can be explained by an increased tendency for dominant limb exploratory reflexes coupled with release from an asymmetrically distributed, predominant nondominant-hemisphere inhibition. Callosal alien hand syndrome is best explained by hemispheric disconnection manifested during behaviors requiring dominant-hemisphere control. *(Doody and Jankovic, 806–810; Feinberg, Schindler, Flanagan, and Haber, 19–24)*

107. **(A)** Lesions in the peri-rolandic cortex cause impairment of the fine distal movements of the contralateral hand. Picking up small objects by opposing the index finger and the thumb or handling a small coin may become impossible. This type of apraxia has been termed limb-kinetic apraxia. Because separate fine movements of each finger are difficult, these patients pick up a pen or a coin by pressing it against the palm with the proximal portion of the thumb, much as infants do before they develop a pincer grip. *(Brazis, Masdeu, and Biller, 508)*

108. **(E)**

109. **(I)**

110. **(K)**

111. (A)

112. (D)

113. (J)

114. (B)

115. (C)

116. (F)

117. (H)

118. (G)

Explanations 108 through 118

A mesial occipital lesion may cause a visual field defect with visual hallucination, visual agnosia, and alexia without agraphia. A lateral occipital lesion may cause alexia with agraphia, impaired optokinetic nystagmus, and impaired ipsilateral scanning. A bilateral lesion of the anterior tip of the temporal lobe causes Kluver-Bucy syndrome with visual agnosia, oral-exploratory behavior, hypersexuality, hypo-mobility, and a marked tendency to take notice and attend to every visual stimulus. A lesion of the lateroinferior aspect of the dominant temporal lobe causes transcortical sensory aphasia with word selection anomia. The storage of language related information is also impaired. A lesion of the nondominant lobe causes impaired recognition of facial emotional expression and storage of nonverbal patterned materials such as geometric or tonal pattern. A parietal postcentral gyrus lesion causes somatosensory disturbance with contralateral proprioception, pain, and temperature loss with tactile extinction. A lesion of the parietal medial lobe may cause transcortical sensory aphasia when it affects the dominant lobe. A lesion of the lateral parietal lobe results in alexia with agraphia (when the lesion affects the angular gyrus), finger agnosia, acalculia, and right-left disorientation. A lesion of the medial frontal lobe, the cingulate gyrus, causes akinesia, perseveration, and alien hand sign. A lesion of the lateral frontal premotor area

may cause impaired contralateral saccades. An orbitofrontal area lesion may cause blunted affect and impaired appreciation of social nuances. A callosal lesion may cause lack of kinetic transfer with left hand apraxia and agraphia, right hand constructional apraxia, and inability to mimic the position of the contralateral hand. *(Brazis, Masdeu, and Biller, 475, 522–524)*

119. (C)

120. (F)

121. (D)

122. (A)

123. (E)

124. (B)

Explanations 119 through 124

Endarterectomy may cause injury to the cervical plexus. A lesion of the greater auricular nerve causes loss of sensation of the mandible and lower external ear. A lesion of the muscular branches of the cervical nerves causes weakness of the infrahyoid and scalene muscles, resulting in inability to flex the head and rotate it laterally. The C8 and T1 root and the lower trunk of the brachial plexus can be compressed resulting in the rare entity called thoracic outlet syndrome, which may have vascular or neurological signs. Vascular signs are recurrent cyanosis, coldness, and pallor of the hand. Adson's test (turn head to the side of symptoms, extend head, take a deep breath, and pull down on limb) usually reduces or eliminates the radial pulse. Neuropathic signs usually involve the lower trunk of the brachial plexus with pain in the ulnar border of the hand and the medial forearm and arm, and prominent paresis and wasting of thenar muscles.

Erb-Duchenne palsy results from damage to the fifth and sixth cervical roots, which may be caused by sudden forceful depression of the shoulder during contact sports. Muscles supplied by these roots are weak and atrophic.

These include the deltoid, the biceps, the brachioradialis, the brachialis, the supraspinatus, the infraspinatus, and the subscapularis muscles. The limb has a characteristic position: it is internally rotated and adducted because of deltoid, supraspinatus, and infraspinatus (shoulder abduction and arm external rotation) weakness. Therefore the weakness is of forearm flexion and of abduction and external rotation of the arm. The biceps and brachioradialis reflexes may be depressed or absent.

Dejerine-Klumpke palsy results from injury to the eighth cervical and first thoracic roots or the lower trunk of the plexus. Mass compression from a lung tumor may damage the lower brachial plexus (Pancoast syndrome). The patient may present weakness of finger and wrist flexion as well as weakness of the intrinsic hand muscles, causing a claw-hand deformity. A lesion of the lumbar plexus can be caused by a tumor of the pelvis. Its clinical signs include weakness of hip flexion (iliopsoas), leg extension (quadriceps), thigh eversion (sartorius), and thigh adduction. Sensory loss may involve the inguinal region, the lateral, anterior, and medial thigh, and the medial aspect of the lower leg. The patellar and cremasteric reflexes from the femoral nerve and the genitofemoral nerve, respectively, may be decreased or absent.

A lesion of the sacral plexus results in motor disturbances in the field of distribution of the superior gluteal, inferior gluteal, and sciatic nerves. Weakness of dorsiflexion and plantar flexion results in a flail foot. There is weakness of knee flexion, abduction, and internal rotation of the thigh as well as weakness of hip extension. The Achilles reflex is decreased or absent. *(Brazis, Masdeu, and Biller 51–65)*

REFERENCES

Afifi AK, Bergman RA, eds. *Functional Neuroanatomy: Text and Atlas.* New York, NY: McGraw-Hill; 1998.

Brazis PW, Masdeu JC, Biller J. *Localization in Clinical Neurology,* 3rd ed. London, UK: Little, Brown; 1996.

Doody RS, Jankovic J. The alien hand and related signs. *Journal of Neurology, Neurosurgery and Psychiatry* 55(9): 806–810, 1992.

Feinberg TE, Schindler RJ, Flanagan NG, Haber LD. Two alien hand syndromes. *Neurology* 42(1):19–24, 1992.

Goetz CG, Pappert EJ. *Textbook of Clinical Neurology.* Philadelphia, PA: W.B. Saunders; 1999.

Kline and Bajandas. *Neuroophthalmology: Review Manual* (5th ed). Thorofare, New Jersey: Slack; 2001.

Patten J. *Neurological Differential Diagnosis,* 2nd ed. London, New York: Springer; 1996.

Staal A. *Mononeuropathies: Examination, Diagnosis and Treatment.* Philadelphia, PA: W.B. Saunders; 1999.

Thompson HS, Miller NR. Disorders of papillary function, accommodation, and lacrimation. In NR Miller, NJ Newman (eds), *Walsh and Hoyt's Clinical Neuroophthalmology,* 5th ed. Baltimore, MD: Williams and Wilkins; 1998; 1:961–1040.

CHAPTER 3

Pediatrics
Questions

Questions 1 and 2

A 6-year-old fully immunized girl developed a fever of 39°C followed by weakness in her lower extremities and right upper extremity with numbness up to the midthoracic level. Cerebrospinal fluid (CSF) examination showed mild protein and cell elevation with no bacteria on the gram stain.

1. The most likely diagnosis is

   (A) transverse myelitis
   (B) tick-borne paralysis
   (C) poliomyelitis
   (D) botulism
   (E) vascular malformation

2. The most serious complication that may develop in this patient is

   (A) pulmonary emboli
   (B) sphincter compromise
   (C) hypotension
   (D) respiratory failure
   (E) encephalitis

3. Which of the following is true about neonatal seizures?

   (A) They may arise from the hemisphere or brain stem.
   (B) The lack of myelinated pathways facilitates the propagation of seizures from one hemisphere to the contiguous cortex.

   (C) Prolonged epileptiform discharges are often associated with clinical symptoms of seizure.
   (D) Jitteriness is never seen in the newborn.
   (E) Isolated apneic discharge is always a seizure manifestation.

4. Which of the following is the LEAST common among children with cerebral palsy?

   (A) Spasticity
   (B) Seizure
   (C) Mental retardation
   (D) Hearing impairment
   (E) Ataxia

5. Which of the following locations is the LEAST affected in kernicterus, a syndrome associated with cerebral palsy?

   (A) Hippocampus
   (B) Substantia nigra
   (C) Basal ganglia
   (D) Cortex
   (E) Brain stem nuclei

6. A 5-year-old girl was brought to the emergency room because of recurrence of nocturnal right facial twitching and slurred speech over the past 3 weeks. Her parents did not report any change in her mental status during these episodes. Her older brother has absence seizures. Which of the following is true about the patient's condition?

    (A) The patient has absence seizure.
    (B) The patient has complex partial seizure.
    (C) The patient has an autosomal recessive disorder.
    (D) The patient's EEG may show central temporal spikes without overt seizure activity.
    (E) The patient will need lifetime antiepileptic treatment.

7. In a full-term infant, the most frequent cause of neonatal seizure within the first 12 hours is

    (A) hypoxic encephalopathy
    (B) sepsis
    (C) subarachnoid hemorrhage
    (D) trauma
    (E) intraventricular bleed

8. Which of the following is the best predictor of developing cerebral palsy?

    (A) Low birth weight
    (B) Prematurity
    (C) The presence of echodense cystic lesions in the periventricular white matter with a diameter greater than 3 mm
    (D) An Apgar score less than 3 after 10 minutes
    (E) Hyperbilirubinemia

Questions 9 through 14
For each of the following disorders, match the earliest onset of seizures.

    (A) Seizure within the first 24 hours
    (B) Seizure within 24 to 72 hours
    (C) Seizure within 72 hours to the first week
    (D) Seizure within the first week to the first month

9. Neonatal adrenoleukodystrophy

10. Kernicterus

11. Urea cycle disturbances

12. Drug withdrawal

13. Subarachnoid bleed

14. Pyridoxine dependant seizures

Questions 15 through 17
The following conditions may be complicated by a neonatal seizure. Link each condition to its etiology.

    (A) Subdural hemorrhage
    (B) Subarachnoid hemorrhage
    (C) Cerebral venous thrombosis

15. Tear of the tentorium near its junction with the falx

16. Tear of the superficial veins by shearing forces during prolonged delivery

17. May be associated with sepsis or asphyxia

18. A newborn developed generalized seizures in the second week of his life. He was doing well at birth and then progressively became mildly lethargic with feeding difficulties and progressive hypotonia. Serologic studies showed an increased concentration of branched-chain amino acids. The addition of 2,4 dinitrophenylhydrazine reagent colored his urine yellow. The most likely diagnosis is

    (A) carbamyl phosphate synthetase deficiency
    (B) glycine encephalopathy
    (C) bilirubin encephalopathy
    (D) maple syrup urine disease
    (E) isovaleric acidemia

19. All of the following statements are true about DiGeorge syndrome EXCEPT

(A) it results from a microdeletion of chromosome 22q11

(B) there is hypoplasia of the second pharyngeal pouch

(C) hypocalcemia and seizures are among the main features of the syndrome

(D) cardiac defect may be a cause of death

(E) Failure to thrive and recurrent infection may complicate the course of the disease

20. A 12-month-old boy was brought to the emergency room because of multiple episodes of stiffening, upward eye deviation, pupillary dilatation, and alteration of respiratory pattern. Most of these episodes occurred during sleep and were complicated by enuresis. The mother, 1 month ago, reported a brief episode of trembling of the eyelids and mouth with loss of facial tone. An EEG showed a generalized burst of 2.5 spike wave complexes per second. Which of the following is INCORRECT about the patient's condition?

(A) Mental retardation is a usual complication.

(B) Twenty percent of patients with this condition may have a history of infantile spasm.

(C) Seizures in this condition are difficult to control.

(D) An underlying cause is rarely found.

(E) Felbamate may improve seizure control.

21. Which of the following statements is INCORRECT about infantile spasm?

(A) Onset always occurs before the age of 1 year.

(B) Pertussis immunization is a cause of infantile spasms.

(C) It may be associated with agenesis of the corpus callosum.

(D) Hypsarrhythmia is the usual EEG pattern recorded during the early stages of infantile spasm.

(E) Hormone therapy may improve seizures.

22. A 17-year-old male developed daily multiple sleep attacks for the last 2 months. He recently lost his job as a waiter because of multiple falls caused by a sudden loss of tone. Which of the following is true about his condition?

(A) His symptoms are caused by increased latency from sleep onset to rapid eye movement sleep of greater than 90 minutes.

(B) Sleep paralysis rarely complicates this condition.

(C) Vivid and usually pleasant visual and auditory perceptions occur at the transition between sleep and wakefulness.

(D) During the loss of tone, partial paralysis, affecting just the face and hands, is more common than total paralysis.

(E) Clonidine is the treatment of choice.

23. Lafora disease is characterized by

(A) mental retardation complicating myoclonic seizures

(B) ataxia and spasticity occurring early in the course of the disease

(C) age of onset between 3 and 7 years

(D) easily controlled seizures

(E) inclusion bodies present in all stages of the disease

24. A 4-year-old boy with normal language and cognitive abilities developed progressive loss of his cognitive skills. He had difficulty following commands and in language comprehension. This was followed by a reduction in the volume and content of speech. Three months later the patient presented with multiple episodes of staring followed by confusion. Physical examination and brain MRI were normal. The most likely diagnosis is

(A) progressive myoclonic epilepsy

(B) temporal lobe tumor

(C) benign rolandic epilepsy

(D) Landau-Kleffner syndrome

(E) Rasmussen syndrome

25. A 7-year-old boy living in Philadelphia developed the following symptoms over a period of 4 days in January: progressive weakness, clumsiness, and loss of facial expression. Neurological evaluation showed that the patient was ataxic when walking or reaching, with decreased deep tendon reflexes and bilateral facial weakness. Which of the following is true?

  (A) The condition is caused by a block of the neuromuscular junction as a result of a neurotoxin produced by a tick.

  (B) Respiratory failure and autonomic dysfunction may complicate the course of the disease.

  (C) Positive response to edrophonium will be a definitive diagnostic test in this patient.

  (D) Impairment in swallowing, in pupillary reflex response, and in extraocular muscle motility are classic findings in this patient's disease.

  (E) An EMG may show a decremental response after repetitive stimulation in this patient.

26. The most common cause of chorea in a school-aged child is

  (A) Sydenham chorea

  (B) Tourette syndrome

  (C) Huntington disease

  (D) Wilson disease

  (E) lupus erythematosus

27. In which of the following cases would discontinuation of prophylactic antiseizure medications be strongly considered?

  (A) Seizure caused by a surgically treated arteriovenous malformation (AVM) in remission for 6 months

  (B) Absence seizures in remission for 8 months with normal EEG and MRI studies

  (C) Generalized tonic-clonic seizure in remission for 2 years with normal EEG and MRI studies

  (D) Cerebral palsy with seizures in remission for 3 years

  (E) Adolescent onset myoclonic epilepsy in remission for 3 years

28. A newborn developed an asymmetric Moro reflex after a complicated delivery. The poorly responsive arm hung in adduction, rotated internally at the shoulder, extended and pronated at the elbow, and flexed at the wrist. The most likely affected roots are

  (A) C7-C8

  (B) T1-T2

  (C) C3-C4

  (D) T3-T4

  (E) C5-C6

29. A 10-year-old boy was brought for a neurology consultation by his mother because he was disturbing his classmates with sniffing and grunting sounds for the last 2 months. Neurological examination was normal. The most likely diagnosis is

  (A) attention deficit hyperactivity disorder

  (B) anxiety

  (C) tics

  (D) autism

  (E) Sydenham chorea

30. All of the following are signs of ventriculoperitoneal shunt obstruction in a 4-month-old boy EXCEPT

  (A) grade I bruit

  (B) strabismus

  (C) splitting of the sutures

  (D) a setting sun sign

  (E) bulging fontanelle

31. Tourette syndrome is a chronic disease of childhood onset characterized by multiple motor and vocal tic. Criteria for the diagnosis include all of the following EXCEPT

  (A) onset between 2 and 15 years of age

  (B) multiple motor tics

  (C) vocal tics

  (D) inability to temporarily suppress symptoms

  (E) duration of symptoms for more than 1 year

32. You are consulted about a 14-year-old boy complaining of shoulder weakness and change in his facial expression. Physical examination showed a smooth, unlined face, protuberant lips, horizontal smile, and muscle wasting in both shoulders with sparing of the forearms. Lab work-up showed a creatine kinase (CK) level of 600 UI/l. An EMG showed a myopathic pattern. Which of the following is true about the patient's condition?

    (A) This is an autosomal recessive myopathy.
    (B) The abnormal gene is located in Xp 21.2.
    (C) The abnormal gene is responsible for the reduced amount of dystrophin in the muscles.
    (D) Retinal vascular abnormalities may complicate the course of the disease.
    (E) Cardiac arrhythmia is a frequent symptom.

33. A 16-month-old boy with a history of Down syndrome developed his first generalized tonic-clonic seizure lasting 20 minutes. On physical examination, his temperature was 39.5°C and there was no evidence of neurological abnormalities. His older sister had a history of febrile seizure. His risk of developing epilepsy in later life is closest to

    (A) 4%
    (B) 10%
    (C) 30%
    (D) 50%
    (E) 90%

34. A 10-year-old girl developed restless behavior, deterioration in school performance, uncoordinated movements, and angry outbursts. Physical examination showed slow writhing of limbs interrupted by high-amplitude, violent flinging of her upper extremities with an inward compulsion to move. The most likely cause of her condition is

    (A) Wilson disease
    (B) Sydenham chorea
    (C) Tourette syndrome

    (D) attention deficit hyperactivity disorder
    (E) vascular accident

35. A 10-year-old girl was reported by her parents to "space out" at home and in school during the past month. Sometimes these spells had associated lip smacking. Which of the following is the most suggestive of absence seizure rather than complex partial seizure?

    (A) Urinary incontinence during spells
    (B) Centrotemporal spikes on EEG
    (C) Spells lasting 1 to 2 minutes
    (D) Presence of automatism
    (E) Prompt recovery after spells

36. The most frequent cause of athetoid cerebral palsy is

    (A) prematurity
    (B) perinatal asphyxia
    (C) intraventricular bleed
    (D) bilirubin encephalopathy
    (E) low birth weight

37. A preterm newborn male was evaluated in the nursery. He was delivered 8 weeks before the expected date, with an Apgar score of 3 at 5 minutes. Neurological examination demonstrated generalized hypotonia and increased deep tendon reflexes. Which of the following is the correct answer to the mother's concern about her baby developing cerebral palsy?

    (A) His low Apgar score indicates a high risk of cerebral palsy.
    (B) It is very difficult to make the diagnosis of cerebral palsy before the age of 6 months.
    (C) The presence of hypotonia on the initial neurological examination of the newborn is highly suggestive of cerebral palsy.
    (D) The presence of progressive neurological deficit is suggestive of cerebral palsy.
    (E) Seizure is the most frequent complication of cerebral palsy.

38. A newborn with the diagnosis of myelomeningocele should be evaluated for all of the following EXCEPT

    (A) genitourinary dysfunction
    (B) gastrointestinal dysfunction
    (C) orthopedic complications
    (D) Arnold Chiari malformation type II
    (E) noncommunicative hydrocephalus

39. You were asked to see a 10-year-old boy because of facial weakness and increased hand clumsiness progressing over the last 6 months. On physical examination, the patient had an inverted V-shaped upper lip, thin cheeks, and a concave temporalis muscle. The patient was unable to tightly close his eyelids. Hand examination showed mild intrinsic muscle wasting and use of wrist flexor to release grasp. The most likely diagnosis is

    (A) Duchenne muscle dystrophy
    (B) Werdnig-Hoffman disease
    (C) myotonic dystrophy
    (D) myasthenia gravis
    (E) chronic demyelinating polyradiculopathy

40. Which of the following conditions does NOT cause pseudotumor cerebri in a 5-year-old boy?

    (A) Tetracycline
    (B) Hypervitaminosis A
    (C) Hypovitaminosis A
    (D) Nalidixic acid
    (E) Furosemide

41. Which of the following is the latest sign or symptom of an acute rise in intracranial pressure in a 12-year-old boy?

    (A) Decreased consciousness
    (B) Headache
    (C) Vomiting
    (D) Irritability
    (E) Symptomatic papilledema

42. A 15-month-old boy was diagnosed with bacterial meningitis and started on antibiotics. On the third day of his hospitalization, he developed an episode of left side twitching of his arm, face, and leg followed by left side weakness that did not improve over the next 3 days despite the improvement of his general status, appetite, and disappearance of fever. The most likely diagnosis is

    (A) right hemispheric ischemic stroke
    (B) subdural empyema
    (C) focal seizure with Todd's paralysis
    (D) brain abscess
    (E) increased intracranial pressure

43. A premature neonate was diagnosed with gram-negative bacterial meningitis and started on antibiotics. The follow-up exam showed an improvement of his clinical status and CSF examination. On the fourth day the patient presented with episodes of bradycardia and apneic spells. Head CT showed fluid of different contrast densities in the ventricles with an enhancing ependymal rim. A repeat lumbar CSF examination was unchanged. The most likely diagnosis is

    (A) brain abscess
    (B) subdural empyema
    (C) ventriculitis
    (D) idiopathic seizure
    (E) encephalitis

44. A 17-year-old girl experienced 15 pressure-type headaches per month for the last 8 months. Each headache lasted from 2 hours to 2 days. There has been no disturbance of her school performance or attendance. Her neurological examination was normal. The best treatment for her headache is

    (A) low-dose amitriptyline at bedtime
    (B) acetaminophen and codeine
    (C) valproic acid
    (D) propranolol
    (E) clorazepate

45. Familial hemiplegic migraine

(A) is characterized by sudden onset of hemiparesis or hemisensory loss that is usually followed by a controlateral headache

(B) occurs more frequently in adults than in children

(C) improves rapidly, since the neurological impairment lasts no more than a few hours

(D) always affects the same side

(E) is transmitted by an autosomal recessive inheritance

46. Which of the following is NOT a migraine variant?

(A) Recurrent abdominal pain

(B) Benign paroxysmal vertigo

(C) Transient ocular blindness

(D) Paroxysmal torticollis

(E) Choreoathetotic movements

47. A 2-year-old boy developed a 5-minute febrile seizure. Which of the following conditions does NOT increase his risk to develop subsequent epilepsy?

(A) Preexisting cerebral palsy

(B) Family history of epilepsy

(C) History of complex febrile seizure

(D) Two febrile seizures in 1 year

(E) Preexisting development delay

Questions 48 through 52

Link the following causes of encephalitis to their geographic locations.

(A) California La Crosse encephalitis

(B) Eastern equine encephalitis

(C) Japanese B encephalitis

(D) St. Louis encephalitis

(E) Western equine encephalitis

48. It is the major form of encephalitis in Asia.

49. Most cases have been reported in Wisconsin, Minnesota, and Indiana.

50. Human cases follow epidemic in horses from the eastern seaboard.

51. It is an endemic encephalitis in the western United States.

52. Recent cases of encephalitis have been reported in North and South Dakota.

53. A 10-year-old boy developed an episode of fever, headache, nausea and vomiting, and irritability. Three days later, he was brought to the emergency room because of a brief episode of twitching of his right face and arm with decreased consciousness. Neurological examination showed mild right arm and leg weakness. An EEG demonstrated periodic lateralizing epileptiform discharge. The most likely diagnosis is

(A) measles encephalitis

(B) Reye syndrome

(C) Herpes simplex encephalitis

(D) postinfectious encephalitis

(E) St. Louis encephalitis

54. All of the following are appropriate measures to decrease intracranial pressure EXCEPT

(A) head elevation

(B) hypothermia

(C) osmotic diuretics

(D) hyperventilation to lower the arterial carbon dioxide pressure from 40 mm Hg to 20 mm Hg

(E) pentobarbital coma

55. A 15-year-old boy consulted because of exacerbation of headache and difficulties of accommodation. Neurological examination demonstrated loss of pupillary light reflex, palsy of upward gaze with preservation of downward gaze, retraction convergence nystagmus when upward gaze is attempted, and loss of accommodation. Head MRI showed an enlarged, dense, noncalcified pineal gland area with irregular margins. Which of the following is NOT true about this condition?

    (A) Pineal germinoma is the most likely diagnosis.
    (B) Pineal germinoma is more common in males than in females.
    (C) Pineal germinoma is less sensitive to radiotherapy than any other tumor of the pineal area.
    (D) Hydrocephalus may complicate the clinical picture.
    (E) Pineal tumors with abundant amounts of calcium are likely to be benign.

Questions 56 through 58
Link the symptoms to the extensions of a pineal mass.

    (A) Clinical symptoms as described above in question 55
    (B) Loss of vision, diabetes insipidus, and precocious puberty
    (C) Ataxia with cranial nerve deficit

56. Hypothalamus compression

57. Midbrain compression

58. Posterior fossa extension

Questions 59 through 62
The following chromosomal defects may cause mental retardation. Link each chromosomal defect to the appropriate clinical features.

    (A) 5 p monosomy
    (B) trisomy 21
    (C) Fragile X syndrome
    (D) trisomy 18

59. A 5-year-old boy with autistic behavior, long face, enlarged ears, and macro-orchidism

60. A 3-year-old boy with hypotonia and round flat face and flat nape of neck

61. A 6-month-old girl with pointed ears micrognathia, occipital protuberance, narrow pelvis, and rocker bottom feet

62. A 3-year-old boy with "cri du chat" cry

63. A 3-year-old boy was evaluated for mental retardation. He was found to have bilateral hearing loss, interstitial keratitis, and peg-shaped upper incisors. The most likely cause of his mental retardation is

    (A) trisomy 21
    (B) CMV infection
    (C) amino acid–abnormal metabolism
    (D) congenital syphilis
    (E) toxoplasmosis

64. Among the following lysosomal disorders, cherry red spots is least likely to occur in:

    (A) GM1 gangliosidosis
    (B) metachromatic leukodystrophy
    (C) Niemann Pick disease
    (D) sialidosis type III
    (E) Gaucher disorder

Questions 65 through 69
Link the following diseases to the corresponding enzyme deficit.

    (A) GM1 gangliosidosis type II
    (B) Tay-Sachs disease
    (C) Krabbe disease
    (D) Metachromatic leukodystrophy
    (E) Niemann Pick disease

65. Hexosaminidase deficiency

66. Beta galactosidase deficit

67. Sphingomyelinase deficit

68. Arylsulfatase deficit

69. Galactosylceramidase deficit

70. Which of the following is true about Leigh disease?

   (A) It is a disorder caused by multiple sulfatase deficiency.
   (B) Hurler phenotype is prominent in affected patients.
   (C) Hypotonia, ocular motility, and respiratory abnormalities are typical features of the disease.
   (D) Glucose load may improve symptoms.
   (E) The brain stem and basal ganglia are typically spared.

Questions 71 through 75
Link each of the following diseases to its corresponding molecular abnormality.

   (A) Defect in intestinal transport of copper
   (B) Sphingomyelinase deficit
   (C) Glucocerebrosidase deficit
   (D) Mitochondrial abnormalities
   (E) Lack of regulation of fusion of primary lymphocytes

71. Subacute necrotizing encephalomyelopathy

72. Gaucher disease

73. Menkes syndrome

74. Chediak-Higashi syndrome

75. Niemann Pick syndrome

76. A 4-year-old mentally retarded girl was brought by her mother to the neurology clinic because she developed new onset of seizure. Skin examination demonstrated leaf-shaped hypochromic nevi on her left buttock and an angiokeratoma on her face. The most likely diagnosis is

   (A) cerebral palsy
   (B) tuberous sclerosis
   (C) neurofibromatosis type I

   (D) Down syndrome
   (E) Gaucher disease

77. Which of the following is NOT a criterion for the diagnosis of neurofibromatosis type I?

   (A) Six "café au lait" spots greater than 15 mm in the postpubertal individual
   (B) Optic glioma
   (C) Iris hamartoma
   (D) Acoustic neurinomas
   (E) Sphenoid dyplasia

78. Which of the following is a necessary criterion for the diagnosis of Rett syndrome?

   (A) Retinopathy
   (B) Severe progressive dementia
   (C) Microcephaly at birth
   (D) Optic atrophy
   (E) Evidence of acquired neurological disease

79. The most likely diagnosis of a newborn with vomiting, hepatomegaly, cataract, and the presence of reducing substances in the urine is

   (A) mucopolysaccharide enzyme deficit
   (B) Krabbe disease
   (C) Gaucher disease
   (D) Tay Sachs disease
   (E) galactosemia

80. Zellweger syndrome is caused by

   (A) mitochondrial defect
   (B) hypoxic ischemic encephalopathy
   (C) acid maltase deficiency
   (D) neuromuscular transmission defect
   (E) peroxisomal disorder

81. Which of the following is INCORRECT about spinal muscular atrophy type I?

   (A) The age of onset is between birth and 6 months.
   (B) Arthrogryposis is usually present.
   (C) Facial expression is relatively preserved.
   (D) There is a hypertrophy of type I fibers.
   (E) DNA analysis of chorion villi may be used for prenatal diagnosis.

82. A male newborn with normal development started to have poor feeding, constipation, and failure to thrive after the age of 4 weeks. Neurological examination demonstrated generalized hypotonia with areflexia, weak cry, ptosis, and dilated pupils that reacted poorly to light. An EMG showed an incremental response to repetitive stimulation between 20 and 50 Hz. The most likely diagnosis is

   (A) Guillain-Barré syndrome
   (B) myasthenia gravis
   (C) infantile spinal muscle atrophy
   (D) botulism
   (E) Lowe syndrome

83. Congenital myotonic dystrophy in newborns is characterized by all the following EXCEPT

   (A) autosomal dominant disorder
   (B) more than 50 DNA triplets repeat on chromosome 19
   (C) myotonia usually elicited by muscle percussion
   (D) a high incidence of polyhydramnios during pregnancy
   (E) repeat DNA triplets size change greater from mother to child than from father to child

84. Which of the following is NOT true about Duchenne's muscle dystrophy?

   (A) The gene defect is located at chromosome X p21.
   (B) The dystrophin content in Duchenne muscle dystrophy is more reduced than in Becker dystrophy.
   (C) The incidence of Duchenne dystrophy is 1/3500.
   (D) Motor function declines sharply between the age of 3 and 6 years.
   (E) Respiratory failure is a contributing factor for death.

Questions 85 through 92
Link the following gene locations to the appropriate neuromuscular disease.

   (A) 17q23-35
   (B) 1q 31-32
   (C) Xp21.2
   (D) 17q23
   (E) 17p11
   (F) 19q 13.3
   (G) Xq28
   (H) 1p35

85. Myotonic dystrophy

86. Duchenne dystrophy

87. Acid maltase deficiency

88. Familial hyperkalemia periodic paralysis

89. Familial hypokalemia periodic paralysis

90. Dejerine-Sottas disease   V

91. Charcot-Marie-Tooth type II

92. Emery-Dreifuss syndrome

93. A 12-year-old boy consulted because of recurrent numbness and tingling in his lower extremities with unsteady gait over several months. His parents reported that the patient had decreased nocturnal visual acuity that started 3 months ago. Neurological examination showed cerebellar ataxia, nystagmus, and decreased deep tendon reflexes. Cerebral spinal fluid examination showed a protein level of 300 mg/dl. Nerve conduction study showed a marked decrease in conduction velocity throughout. EMG results were consistent with chronic denervation. The most likely diagnosis is

   (A) Refsum disease
   (B) Dejerine-Sottas disease
   (C) Charcot-Marie-Tooth neuropathy
   (D) metachromatic leukodystrophy
   (E) Emery-Dreifuss muscular dystrophy

94. A 12-year-old boy consulted because of muscle stiffness and difficulty when moving. Neurological examination demonstrated a painless myotonia at rest that improved with activity, and generalized muscle hypertrophy. EMG showed myotonic discharges. CK level was normal. The most likely diagnosis is

(A) myotonia congenita

(B) Stiffman syndrome

(C) hypothyroidism

(D) Schwartz-Jampel syndrome

(E) neuromyotonia

95. A 7-year-old boy was evaluated for pain, muscle weakness with exercise, and recurrent rhabdomyolisis. Neurological examination and EMG were normal. CK level was 600 UI/L. An ischemic exercise test showed failure to generate ammonia and normal lactate level. The most likely diagnosis is

(A) Kearns-Sayre syndrome

(B) Menkes syndrome

(C) myoadenylate deaminase deficiency

(D) carnitine palmitoyl transferase deficiency

(E) Brody disease

96. Child ataxia with pellagra-like skin rash after exposure to sunlight may be seen in

(A) Hartnup disease

(B) basilar migraine

(C) maple syrup urine disease

(D) Miller Fisher syndrome

(E) myoclonic encephalopathy

97. Which of the following causes of progressive child ataxia is associated with an increased blood level of very long chain fatty acids?

(A) Ataxia telangiectasia

(B) Sulfatide lipidosis

(C) Hypobetalipoproteinemia

(D) Ramsay Hunt syndrome

(E) Adrenoleukodystrophy

Questions 98 through 103

Link the following diagnosis to the appropriate clinical description.

(A) Tardive dyskinesia

(B) Fahr disease

(C) Hallervorden-Spatz disease

(D) Neuroacanthocytosis

(E) Sydenham chorea

(F) Harp syndrome

98. A 15-year-old boy developed night blindness, mental retardation, and dystonic dysarthria. Head MRI showed eye-of-tiger appearance of the pallidum. Acanthocytes were seen in washed erythrocytes.

99. A 10-year-old girl developed progressive dystonic rigidity and choreoathetotic movements. Head MRI showed, on T2-weighted images, low-intensity signal images from the globus pallidus with a central area of increased intensity.

100. This is the most common cause of acquired chorea in children.

101. There is an association of encephalopathy and progressive calcification of the basal ganglia.

102. A 13-year-old boy with a history of asthma treated by theophylline developed tongue and face abnormal movements. There was a tongue protrusion and lip smacking.

103. A 7-year-old boy developed dystonia of the face and limbs associated with self-mutilation of the lips. Lab work-up showed abnormal erythrocytes with thorny projection from the cell surface. There were no lipoprotein abnormalities.

Answers and Explanations

1. **(A)**

2. **(D)**

Explanations 1 through 2

The acute onset of symptoms in this child is most likely related to acute transverse myelitis. This diagnosis is supported by the occurrence of a rapid asymmetric neurological deficit and a sensory level that suggests a cross-sectional involvement of the spinal cord. MRI of the spinal cord would be the procedure of choice to confirm the diagnosis. It may show evidence of cord swelling at the level of demyelination and rule out any acute cord compression in the epidural space. Transverse myelitis is an acute demyelination of the spinal cord that may progress over hours or days. It may be associated with optic neuritis in Devic disease and uncommonly with multiple sclerosis in childhood. The mean age of onset is 9 years. The level of demyelination is usually thoracic. The motor deficit is commonly asymmetric, and the maximum weakness is reached within 48 hours. Recovery begins after 6 days. Fifty percent of patients make a full recovery, 10% have no recovery, and 40% recover incompletely. Relapsing myelitis may occur. Corticosteroids remain the most common treatment despite the absence of controlled studies. Poliomyelitis may cause asymmetric weakness, but the presence of a sensory level excludes this diagnosis. Tick bite paralysis is unlikely to be the diagnosis because of the presence of fever and the abnormal CSF. The absence of ophthalmoplegia, the presence of fever, and abnormal CSF results are against the diagnosis of botulism. Finally, a spinal cord vascular malformation is unlikely to be the diagnosis because of the presence of fever and the absence of red blood cells in the CSF. In this case, respiratory failure is the major concern because of the involvement of the thoracic spinal cord. Vital capacity should be measured multiple times per day. Pulmonary emboli are a rare complication during acute paralysis. Hypotension and sphincter incontinence, like other autonomic instabilities, are usually not life-threatening. However, cardiac rhythm and blood pressure should be monitored closely. *(Fenichel, 267)*

3. **(A)** Newborns with hydranencephaly or atelencephaly are able to generate seizures, supporting the fact that the brain stem may generate seizure activity. These seizures are confined to the brain stem because of the absence of myelinated fibers. Propagation of seizure activity to a contiguous cortical area is enhanced by the maturity of myelinated pathways. Fifty percent of prolonged epileptiform discharges are not associated with visible clinical seizures. Jitteriness is an excessive response to stimulation by low-frequency, high-amplitude shaking of limbs and jaw. It may occur in a newborn with perinatal asphyxia. It may be confused with myoclonic seizures when it occurs without any apparent stimulation. The absence of eye movement or alteration in respiration pattern and the normal EEG can distinguish the two entities. However, the most practical way to distinguish between seizures and jitteriness is in the following maneuver: grasping the jittering limb will stop normal jitteriness but not seizure activity. Apneic spells

of 10 to 15 seconds may be seen in the premature newborn. They should be considered as a sign of brain stem immaturity rather than a pathologic condition. Apnea is seldom a seizure manifestation unless it is associated with tonic deviation of the eyes or body stiffness. (*Fenichel, 1–4*)

4. **(E)** Cerebral palsy refers to a spectrum of static lesions of the central nervous system that produces chronic problems with motor strength and/or control, and is not the result of a recognized malformation. While the lesion is static by definition, it appears in a central nervous system that is undergoing developmental change during a period of rapid growth. As a result, its manifestations are not stable. Motor disability is the most frequent symptom, and it is the first disability to be identified in affected children. Other central nervous system impairments may be associated with the motor deficit. Mental retardation is the most common associated disability, estimated to occur in 50% to 66% of patients with cerebral palsy. Hearing deficits may be seen in up to 30% of affected children, with higher prevalence in those who have the athetoid form of cerebral palsy. Seizures are seen in 30% to 50% of children with cerebral palsy, especially in hemiplegic patients. Ataxic cerebral palsy is the rarest form of cerebral palsy, most likely denoting dysfunction of the cerebellum or its pathways. Truncal and gait ataxia are more striking than limb ataxia. (*Fenichel, 243–245; Nelson, 73–80; Rosenbloom, 350–354*)

5. **(D)** Kernicterus is a syndrome associated with cerebral palsy. Unbound bilirubin can cross the blood-brain barrier in the neonatal period, enter the nervous system, and produce neuronal damage. Neuronal necrosis and bilirubin staining in specific neuronal regions are the specific pathological features of kernicterus. The most commonly affected regions of the brain are the basal ganglia, hippocampus, substantia nigra, cranial nerve, brain stem nuclei, cerebellar nuclei, and anterior horn cells of the spinal cord. Cortical neurons are the least affected in kernicterus. This reflects the predominance of extrapyramidal, gaze, and auditory abnormalities as clinical symptoms of kernicterus. (*Ahdab-Barmada and Moossy, 45–56*)

6. **(D)** The patient in this case developed a motor seizure with preservation of consciousness, most likely involving the left cortical areas controlling speech and right face movements. Benign rolandic epilepsy is the most likely diagnosis. It is an autosomal dominant condition with incomplete penetrance occurring typically between the age of 3 and 12 years. The area of the brain around the sensory motor fissure is involved in the genesis of seizure. In around 40% of cases, a family history of febrile seizure or epilepsy is found. Seventy percent of children have seizures only while asleep, and 15% only when awake. Interictal EEG may show unilateral or bilateral spike discharges in the central or centrotemporal region. Seizures resolve spontaneously by the age of 14 in most cases. Treatment of benign rolandic seizure is indicated only in the case of frequent seizures or the occurrence of major motor seizures. Carbamazepine is a popular choice because of its effectiveness in treating partial complex seizures and its lack of cognitive side effects. Absence seizure is unlikely to be the diagnosis. It generally occurs during the daytime with brief stares with or without eyes blinking. The preservation of consciousness rules out a complex partial seizure in this patient. Other patients with benign rolandic epilepsy may have complex partial seizures. (*Fenichel, 32–33*)

7. **(A)** Seizures may complicate any brain disorder in full-term infants. The time of onset of the first seizure is helpful in establishing the cause. Hypoxic-ischemic encephalopathy is the most frequent cause of seizure in the first 12 hours, followed by sepsis, meningitis, and subarachnoid hemorrhage. Trauma and intrauterine infection may cause a seizure in the first 24 hours. Pyridoxine dependency, intraventricular bleed in a term infant, and direct drug effects are rare causes of seizure in the first 24 hours. (*Fenichel, 4*)

8. **(C)** Despite taking a comprehensive genetic history, doing a complete physical examination, and performing extensive metabolic,

chromosomal, and neuroimaging studies, 50% of patients with cerebral palsy have no evident cause of their brain damage. Although prematurity is the most common antecedent of cerebral palsy, the majority of infants who develop cerebral palsy are full term. Lower birthweight increases the risk of developing cerebral palsy; however, even for very low birthweights (less than 1500 g), the risk of developing cerebral palsy is only 15% to 20%. Preterm infants who develop intraventricular hemorrhage with extension to the white matter are at the greatest risk for developing cerebral palsy. It seems that in premature infants the best predictor of cerebral palsy is the presence of echodense cystic lesions in the periventricular white matter with a diameter greater than 3 mm, which increases the risk of developing diplegic spastic cerebral palsy to 90%. The Apgar score has been a poor indicator of babies at risk of cerebral palsy. Only 10% to 15% of newborns have an Apgar score of 3 or less at 10 to 15 minutes, and the majority of full-term newborns who develop cerebral palsy have normal Apgar scores. Bilirubin encephalopathy may cause athetoid cerebral palsy. Bilirubin is especially toxic to the basal ganglia and auditory nuclei in the brainstem. It makes the infant with athetoid cerebral palsy at high risk of developing neurosensory hearing loss. It is not the best predictor of cerebral palsy. *(Pidcock et al., 417–422; Taft, 411–418)*

9. **(D)**

10. **(C)**

11. **(D)**

12. **(B)**

13. **(A)**

14. **(A)**

Explanations 9 through 14

The time of onset of seizures is helpful in determining their causes during the neonatal period.

Neonatal adrenoleukodystrophy is an autosomal recessive inheritance characterized by poor adrenal function with accumulation of very long chain fatty acids in the plasma. Initial symptoms are hypotonia and failure to thrive. Seizures generally appear between the first and fourth week. An excessive level of unconjugated free bilirubin in the blood causes kernicterus during the neonatal period. Unconjugated free bilirubin is neurotoxic, especially to the basal ganglia and hippocampus. Seizures may occur from the third day of birth during the second phase of bilirubin encephalopathy. The newborn shows increasing tone with opisthotonos. Urea cycle disturbances are related to a defect in the enzyme systems responsible for urea synthesis. Symptoms are caused by ammonia intoxication. Seizures may complicate the initial hypotonia and lethargy after the first week of birth. The most common drug withdrawal in the newborn is narcotic withdrawal. Tremor, irritability, hyperactivity, and autonomic instability are the earlier symptoms, which may be complicated by seizures in up to 5% of cases. First seizures typically occur from 24 to 72 hours after birth. Subarachnoid hemorrhage may cause unexpected seizures during the first day. Pyridoxine dependency is a rare autosomal recessive disorder that may result from an impairment of glutamic acid decarboxylase activity. Seizures may begin immediately after birth or anytime thereafter. *(Fenichel, 4–14)*

15. **(A)**

16. **(B)**

17. **(C)**

Explanations 15 through 17

Subdural hemorrhage is the consequence of a tear in the tentorium near its junction with the falx. Excessive vertical molding of the head in vertex presentation or anteroposterior elongation of the head in face and brow presentation may be the cause of the tear. The accumulation of blood in the posterior fossa may produce a delayed compression of the brain stem.

Subarachnoid hemorrhage results from tearing of the superficial veins by shearing forces during a prolonged delivery with the head engaged. Seizures occurring in a normal newborn in the first or second day of life may be the only clinical manifestation. Cerebral venous thrombosis may complicate sepsis, asphyxia, and coagulopathy. Superior sagittal thrombosis may occur without known predisposing factors. Head MRI is the best examination to assess the involved vessels. *(Fenichel, 6–7; Rivkin, Anderson, and Kaye, 51–56)*

18. **(D)** The decarboxylation of leucine, isoleucine, and valine is accomplished by a complex enzyme system, branched-chain alpha-ketoacid dehydrogenase. Deficiency of this enzyme causes maple syrup urine disease. Affected newborns are normal at birth but develop poor feeding and vomiting during the first week of life, in addition to hypotonia. Convulsion and hypoglycemia are frequent complications. The correction of hypoglycemia does not improve the clinical condition. The diagnosis is suspected by the odor of maple syrup found in the urine, sweat, and cerumen. It is confirmed by finding increased plasma concentration of the three branched-chain amino acids or enzyme deficiency in peripheral leukocytes. The urine contains a high level of branched-chain amino acids and their keto acids. These keto acids may be detected by adding 2,4 dinitrophenylhydrazine to the urine; if the result is the formation of yellow precipitate, maple syrup urine disease is the most likely diagnosis. Lowering the branched-chain amino acids may be attempted by exchange transfusions, peritoneal dialysis, and special diet.

Isovaleric acidemia is a rare autosomal recessive condition related to a deficiency of isovaleryl CoA dehydrogenase. Clinical manifestations include lethargy, vomiting, convulsion, and severe acidosis in the first few days of life. The characteristic odor of sweaty feet may be present. The diagnosis is established by demonstrating marked elevation of isovaleric acid or its metabolites in urine.

Glycine encephalopathy is an autosomal recessive disorder caused by a defect of the glycine cleaving system. Affected newborns are normal at birth but become irritable with hiccuping usually within 48 hours to several weeks. Myoclonic seizures, hypotonia, and lethargy may follow. The diagnosis is made after seeing hyperglycinemia and a high glycine concentration in the cerebrospinal fluid.

Carbamyl phosphate synthetase deficiency may cause progressive lethargy, vomiting, and hypotonia in the first day of life. The diagnosis is made by demonstrating serum hyperammonemia without organic acidemia.

Bilirubin encephalopathy results from the neurotoxic effect of a high unconjugated free bilirubin level. It may cause hypotonia, lethargy, and seizures. The branched-chain amino acid level in the serum is normal but the bilirubin level is high. *(Behrman, 410–412; Fenichel, 8–12)*

19. **(B)** DiGeorge syndrome is a congenital hypoplasia of organs derived from the third and fourth pharyngeal pouches. It results in hypoplasia or agenesis of the thymus and parathyroid glands, the auricle, and the external auditory canal, congenital cardiac anomalies, cleft palate, and short stature. It is associated with microdeletion of chromosome 22q11. The main features are hypocalcemia, seizures, congenital heart disease, lymphocytopenia, and multiple minor anomalies. Affected newborns may die from cardiac causes during the first month. Frequent infections due to a defect of cell-mediated immunity and failure to thrive may complicate the course of the surviving newborn. *(Behrman, 694; Fenichel, 8–9)*

20. **(D)** The patient described in this case developed symptoms of tonic seizures and atypical absence seizures. The EEG pattern is compatible with absence or atonic seizures. The association of these symptoms to the EEG findings makes Lennox-Gastaut syndrome (which is characterized by the triad of seizure, slow spike wave complexes on EEG, and mental retardation) the most likely diagnosis. Mental retardation will appear later, since more than 90% of patients will be mentally retarded by the age of 5 years. Sixty percent of patients with Lennox-Gastaut syndrome may have an identified underlying cause, and 20% have a history of

infantile spasms. EEG during a tonic seizure may show a one-spike wave per second followed by generalized rapid discharges without postictal depression. Seizures are difficult to control. Valproate and clonazepam are the drugs of choice. Felbamate may reduce seizure frequency in refractory cases. *(Fenichel, 22–23)*

21. **(B)** Infantile spasms are age-dependent myoclonic seizures always seen before the age of 1 year with a peak age of onset between 4 and 7 months. An underlying cause is found in 75% of cases. Perinatal asphyxia, congenital malformations, and tuberous sclerosis are common causes. The association of infantile spasms, agenesis of the corpus callosum or other midline cerebral malformations, and retinal malformation is called Aicardi syndrome. Pertussis immunization is not a cause of infantile spasms. Spasms can be extensor or flexor movements and generally occur in clusters after the infant awakens from sleep. EEG may show hypsarrhythmia and a chaotic and continuously abnormal background of very high voltage and slow waves and spikes. ACTH or corticosteroids may be effective in the control of infantile spasms. *(Fenichel, 19–20)*

22. **(D)** The symptoms of this patient are consistent with the diagnosis of narcolepsy and cataplexy: a sleep disorder characterized by abnormal latency from sleep onset to rapid eye movement (REM) sleep. REM sleep is attained in less than 20 minutes. Hypotonia and dreaming occur normally during REM sleep. In narcolepsy and cataplexy, these phenomena occur during wakefulness. This may induce hypnagogic hallucinations: vivid, frightening visual and auditory perceptions occurring at the transition between wakefulness and sleep. The sudden loss of tone in cataplexy may be induced by excitement; the paralysis most commonly affects the face or hands more than the total body. Sleep paralysis, a generalized hypotonia occurring in the transition between sleep and wakefulness, complicates two-thirds of cases of narcolepsy and cataplexy and is generally experienced once or twice each week. The diagnosis of narcolepsy and cataplexy is made by a multiple sleep latency test showing a REM onset sleep latency of less than 4 to 5 minutes. Pharmacological treatment of narcolepsy has depended on the use of central nervous system stimulants to increase wakefulness, vigilance, and performance. The medications considered effective in the treatment of narcolepsy include dextroamphetamine, pemoline, methylphenidate, and methamphetamine. These stimulants are associated with sympathomimetic side effects, limitations in efficacy, and negative effects on nighttime sleep. Modafinil, a new wakefulness-promoting agent, has been shown to be effective and is well tolerated. *(US Modafinil in Narcolepsy Multicenter Study Group, 43–48)*

23. **(A)** Lafora disease is a progressive myoclonic epilepsy probably transmitted by autosomal recessive inheritance. The age of onset is between 11 and 18 years. Mental retardation appears early in the course of the disease, whereas ataxia, spasticity, and involuntary movements occur late. In later stages of the disease, EEG may show nonspecific generalized polyspike discharges that are not activated by sleep. Seizures are generally refractory to most anticonvulsant drugs as the disease progresses. Inclusion bodies, an aggregate of filaments composed of polyglucosans, are seen on liver biopsy. In rare cases, they may be absent even in late stages of the disease. *(Fenichel, 29–30)*

24. **(D)** This case describes a previously normal child with progressive loss of language skills associated with a seizure disorder. The most likely diagnosis is Landau-Kleffner syndrome. This is a condition of unknown cause, more common in boys, with a mean onset of 5.5 years. At least 70% have an associated seizure disorder. The aphasia may be primarily receptive or expressive, and auditory agnosia may be so severe that the child is unaware of everyday sounds. Hearing is normal, but behavioral problems, including irritability and poor attention span, are particularly common. Formal testing often shows normal performance and visual-spatial skills despite poor language. The seizures are of several types, including focal or generalized tonic-clonic, atypical absence, partial complex, and occasional myoclonic.

High-amplitude spike and wave discharges predominate and tend to be bitemporal but can be multifocal or generalized. In the very early stages of the condition, the EEG findings may be normal. The spike discharges are always more apparent during non-REM sleep; thus, a child suspected of Landau-Kleffner syndrome should have an EEG during sleep, particularly if the awake record is normal. CT and MRI studies typically yield normal results. Microscopic examination of surgical specimens has shown minimal gliosis but no evidence of encephalitis. Progressive myoclonic epilepsy is unlikely to be the diagnosis because of the speech involvement in this patient and the absence of myoclonus, cerebellar ataxia, or involuntary movements. Temporal lobe tumor is a rare diagnostic possibility that may cause seizures with speech disturbance. The normal head MRI rules out that diagnosis. In the Rasmussen syndrome, the affected children have progressive motor seizures that are resistant to anticonvulsive treatment. Progressive hemiplegia may develop in the body side of seizures and may persist after seizures have stopped. *(Behrman, 1998–1999; Fenichel, 31)*

25. (B) The most likely diagnosis in this case is Guillain-Barré syndrome (GBS), which is the most common cause of acquired paralysis in an otherwise well child. A nonspecific viral or bacterial infection may occur prior to the onset of paralysis, but in 25% of cases there is no antecedent of infection or vaccination. Typically the onset of weakness is insidious, following an ascending progression from lower extremities to upper extremities, and may involve the trunk or the cranial nerves. Pain in the extremities is reported in 80% of cases. The patient in this case developed symmetric weakness in all extremities that caused an ataxic gait, decreased deep tendon reflexes, and no sensory level: these are key findings for the diagnosis of GBS. The facial paresis reported in this patient reflects the involvement of the facial nerve, which is the most frequent cranial nerve affected by this disease. Respiratory failure, unstable blood pressure, and arrhythmia are less common but grave complications of GBS. Activation of T cells, cytokine synthesis,

demyelination of the peripheral nervous system by antibodies, and axonal damage by antiglycolipid antibodies are key features of the pathogenesis of Guillain-Barré syndrome.

Tick bite paralysis results from a neuromuscular blockage by a tick-produced neurotoxin. It may cause paralysis that may mimic GBS, but it is unlikely to be considered a first diagnosis in a child living in Philadelphia in January.

Edrophonium, a cholinesterase inhibitor, is used for the diagnosis of myasthenia gravis. The type of weakness described in this patient is unlikely to be seen in myasthenia gravis, in which ptosis, extraocular muscle paresis, dysphagia, and fluctuant weakness are prominent features. In myasthenia, the EMG may show a decremental response on repetitive stimulation. Impairment of pupillary response, paresis of the extraocular muscles, dysphagia, hypotonia, descending paralysis, and constipation are classic findings in botulism. The diagnosis is made by an EMG showing an incremental response to repetitive stimulation and by isolation in the stool of Clostridium botulinum or its toxin. *(Bradshaw and Jones, 500–506; Ropper, 1130–1136)*

26. (A) Sydenham chorea (chorea minor, St. Vitus dance, rheumatic encephalitis), described by Thomas Sydenham in 1686, is considered the most common cause of chorea in a school-age child. Clinically it is characterized by involuntary movements, hypotonia, dysarthria, emotional disorders, and less frequently by other neurological manifestations, such as weakness and headache. The motor disorders may be generalized or unilateral, in which circumstance they constitute a hemichorea. Chorea may present with other rheumatic fever manifestations during an acute episode, or it may present in isolated form in the so-called pure chorea. Its etiology and pathophysiological mechanisms are still unclear, although its relation with a previous group A beta-hemolytic streptococcus infection, is well established. There is also evidence of the participation of immunological mechanisms in its pathogenesis, such as the finding of serum anticaudate and subthalamic nuclear antibodies and an increase in IgG levels in the cerebrospinal fluid of patients with chorea. *(Goldenberg et al., 152–157; Nausieda et al., 331–334)*

27. **(C)** Prophylactic treatment of epilepsy is indicated if there is major motor seizure, if two or more seizures occur in close temporal proximity, or if the seizures are associated with falls. The age and situation of the patient may influence the decision to prescribe antiseizure medications. Most authors agree to discontinue anticonvulsant medication if the patient is free of major motor seizures or absence seizures for 1 or 2 years with normal EEG and brain MRI studies. In Janz syndrome, a variant of myoclonic epilepsy, antiseizure medications should not be stopped even after a remission as long as 3 years, because seizures often recur. Seizure medications should be a lifelong treatment if the seizures are caused by permanent damage of the brain, such as in many cases of cerebral palsy or operated arteriovenous malformations. *(Callaghan, Garrett, and Goggin, 942–946; Shinnar et al., 534–565)*

28. **(E)** The patient described in this case has the classic signs of Erb palsy, a paralysis of the muscles innervated by the C5-C6 roots. It occurs in approximately 0.6% of all vaginal deliveries; shoulder dystocia is typically diagnosed when there is impaction of the anterior fetal shoulder behind the symphysis pubis. The spinal roots have approximately one-tenth the tensile strength of the peripheral nerves because of lesser amounts of collagen and the absence of epineurial and perineurial sheaths in the roots. Therefore, the nerve roots are the weak link in the nerve root-spinal, nerve-plexus complex, and nerve root. Avulsion from the spinal cord may result from the severe traction injury caused by a shoulder dystocia. Brachial plexus injury complicates approximately 8% to 23% of shoulder dystocia cases. Nearly 80% of brachial plexus injuries involve the nerve roots of C5-C6. Clinical findings in Erb palsy may include C5 root avulsion signs, which result in virtually complete paralysis of the rhomboids and spinatus muscles and a varying degree of weakness of the deltoid,

biceps, brachioradialis, and serratus anterior, which receive additional innervation from C6. More than 90% of these injuries will resolve by 1 year of life, with only a 5% to 8% rate of persistent nerve injury. Dejerine-Klumpke palsy occurs less frequently than Erb palsy and involves the lower trunk of the brachial plexus, C8, and T1 roots. It accounts for only 2.5% of brachial plexus injuries. Clinical findings include weakness in the flexor of the wrist and fingers, absent grasp reflex, and possible unilateral Horner syndrome. C3-C4 and T2-T4 nerve root lesions will not affect the muscles of the upper extremity. *(Pollack et al., 236–246)*

29. **(C)** The patient described in this case developed repetitive sniffing and grunting over a period of time, which are most likely related to verbal tics. Tics are defined as sudden, rapid, recurrent, and nonrhythmic stereotyped movements or vocalizations. Motor tics are characterized as simple, such as eye blinking, facial grimacing, and head turning, or complex, such as jumping, thumping, echopraxia, and copropraxia. Simple vocalizations can consist of grunts, coughing, and throat clearing, while examples of complex vocalizations include echolalia, word repetitions, and coprolalia. Tics are unusual examples of movement disorders in that the abnormal movements are often preceded by a feeling of inner tension and a compulsion to move, or in some cases by unpleasant focal sensory symptoms, sometimes termed sensory tics. The subsequent performance of the tic temporarily relieves the sensory symptoms. Some individuals claim that their tics are voluntary, in response to dysphoric sensory symptoms. Tics can usually be suppressed but only at the expense of increasing internal tension, which often causes a rebound exacerbation of the tic. The type, severity, location, and frequency of tics often vary as the years pass. While tics are common in childhood, they are usually a transient phenomenon, and if persistent, they tend to improve during adolescence. Tourette syndrome is the most severe form of the spectrum of tic disorders and is defined by the presence of both motor and vocal tics for a duration of a year or more, with onset before the age of 18 years.

The vast majority of cases are idiopathic. There is a close relationship between tics and obsessive-compulsive disorder. The reported prevalence of obsessive-compulsive disorder in Tourette syndrome patients is approximately 50%, and there is also an increased prevalence of obsessive-compulsive disorder in relatives of tic patients. (*Weeks, Tujanski, and Brooks, 401–408*)

30. **(A)** Grade I cerebral bruit is usually a physiologic murmur heard in cases of hyperdynamic states such as anemia or fever. Cerebral bruit may indicate an arteriovenous malformation of the vein of Galen or increased intracranial pressure by a subdural effusion or other causes. Of the five choices mentioned in this question, cerebral bruit is the least reliable sign of increased intracerebral pressure. Setting sun sign is a downward deviation of the eyes. It is thought to be caused by compression of the upward gaze center in the upper part of the brain stem by the dilated third ventricle. Setting sun sign, strabismus, bulging of fontanelle, and splitting of the sutures are signs of increased intracranial pressure in a 4-month-old patient. (*Fenichel, 222*)

31. **(D)** Tourette syndrome arises during childhood or early adolescence, usually between the age of 2 and 15 years, with a mean age of 7 years. It occurs in boys four times as often as in girls. The most common initial symptoms are motor tics involving the cranial region, especially around the eyes. Subsequently, patients develop a constellation of motor and vocal tics, of either a simple or complex nature. Tics occur many times a day, usually daily for at least one year, and there is never a tic-free period of more than three consecutive months. Tics are increased during time of stress and disappear during sleep. Patients may suppress their tics during a period of time, which leads to increased dysphoric sensation. Two points about the course of Tourette syndrome are notable. One is the changing display of tics, and the other is the tendency toward periodic remissions and exacerbations. A high frequency of various behavioral abnormalities attends Tourette syndrome, and these are often the most disabling aspects of the clinical picture.

Given the usual age of onset, they may translate into poor school performance caused by disruptive activity and attentional difficulty; such patients may be relegated to special education. (*Behrman, 81; Fenichel, 294–296*)

32. **(D)** The patient described in this case has the features of fascioscapulohumeral syndrome. This is an autosomal dominant myopathy that affects mainly the muscles of the face, shoulder girdle, and upper arms. The gene, localized in chromosome 4q35, has a complete penetrance but variable expression. The patient may give a history of inability to whistle or difficulty using straws or inability to fully close his eyes during sleep. As the extraocular muscles are intact, the Bell phenomenon remains and consequently the cornea is protected. The diagnosis is made by the association of insidious muscle weakness involving the shoulder girdle and the face, normal or mildly increased CK level, and myopathic pattern on EMG. Histological examination may show inflammatory signs in addition to the degenerative changes. Retinal telangiectasia, exudation, and detachment are the most severe retinal vascular abnormalities that may be seen by angiography in most patients with fascioscapulohumeral syndrome. (*Fenichel, 336–337; Patterson and Gomez, 73–82*)

33. **(B)** The patient described in the vignette presented a febrile seizure. Typically, it is a generalized type of seizure, occurring between the age of 6 months and 3 years, at a temperature greater than 38°C. The risk factors that may increase the recurrence of febrile seizures or the development later in life of epilepsy include long duration of seizure more than 15 minutes, a known developmental disorder, a positive family history of febrile seizure or epilepsy, focal seizures, repeated febrile seizures within a single illness, and occurrence of febrile seizures outside the usual age range (6 months to 3 years). The patient in the vignette has three risk factors that increase his risk to develop epilepsy in later life, from approximately 4% to 10–15%. (*Annegers et al., 493–498*)

34. **(B)** The patient described in the vignette developed choreoathetotic movements associated

with episodes of ballismus and akathisia. The most common cause of new-onset chorea in that age is Sydenham chorea. It occurs most frequently in females between the age of 5 and 15 years. Cardiac disease may not be evident at the time of chorea. Careful cardiac examination with echocardiogram and electrocardiogram is recommended to assess the extent of cardiac involvement. The differential diagnosis of Sydenham chorea may include attention deficit hyperactivity disorder because restlessness may be confused with mild chorea. The careful history given by the parents, the cardiac findings, and the relatively short-term progression of the disease (few days to weeks compared to the month-to-years chronic progression of attention deficit hyperactivity disorder) suggest Sydenham chorea. Tourette syndrome is a combination of motor and verbal tics. These latter findings are not seen in Sydenham chorea. Wilson disease may present with chorea. The association of Kayser-Fleischer rings, low ceruloplasmin level, and liver function abnormalities suggest the diagnosis of hepatolenticular degeneration. Vascular accident is rare in this age. It could be considered in the differential diagnosis in the case of unilateral chorea. An MRI of the brain is helpful to rule out a stroke. *(Fenichel, 285–286)*

35. **(E)** Prompt recovery after spells is most suggestive of absence seizures rather than partial complex seizure. Urinary incontinence is rare in absence seizure and is occasionally present in complex partial seizure. The spells last 5 to 10 seconds in absence seizure and up to a few minutes in complex partial seizure. Automatism may complicate absence seizure when prolonged and is more frequently present in complex partial seizures. An EEG reveals generalized three-per-second spike wave discharges in absence seizures, whereas in complex partial seizure it shows (in 60% of cases) variably located focal spikes. *(Fenichel, 26–28; Panayiotopoulos, 351–355)*

36. **(B)** Athetosis, a distal slow writhing movement of the extremities, is usually a manifestation of damage to the basal ganglia. Bilirubin encephalopathy selectively involves the globus pallidus and subthalamic nuclei, and characteristically produces athetotic cerebral palsy. Perinatal asphyxia has become the most frequent cause of athetotic cerebral palsy because kernicterus has become less common with better prevention and management of hyperbilirubinemia in the newborn period. *(Fenichel, 13–14)*

37. **(B)** The diagnosis of cerebral palsy is difficult to establish before the age of 6 months because abnormalities in tone, reflexes, or involuntary movements rarely manifest during the newborn period. The primary reason for this is that most of the movements observed in newborns are of reflex origin and not under voluntary control. The maturation of the cortex allows the clinical picture of cerebral palsy to emerge clearly. Also, tone and reflex abnormalities occurring after a perinatal insult to the brain may falsely suggest permanent damage to the central nervous system, since they may improve after 2 to 12 months. The presence of progressive neurological deficit excludes the diagnosis of cerebral palsy because the latter condition is defined as an abnormal control of movement and posture that begins early in life and is not the result of an underlying progressive condition. Clues to a progressive disorder may include mental or motor regression, neurocutaneous signs, and skeletal anomalies. A low Apgar score at 5 minutes does not correlate with high risk of developing cerebral palsy or any other neurological disease. *(Fenichel, 270–271; Taft, 411–418)*

38. **(B)** Myelomeningocele is a congenital defect of the spinal cord closure. The defect is most commonly located in the lumbar region. It may contain spinal cord or nerve roots involved in the innervation of the urinary bladder. To avoid urologic problems and to ensure timely and appropriate intervention, the genitourinary system must be evaluated in all infants who have this malformation. Myelomeningocele may be accompanied by cerebellar tonsillar herniation as part of a Chiari II malformation or aqueductal stenosis, which occurs in approximately 80% of cases and leads to a noncommunicating hydrocephalus that may need a shunt within the first 2 weeks of life. Orthopedic

or physical therapy referral may be appropriate with complications such as talipes equino-varus. *(Behrman, 1984–1985)*

39. **(C)** The patient described in this vignette has a long, thin face because of wasting of the temporal and masseter muscles, and hand intrinsic muscles wasting with muscle relaxation difficulties. These findings are compatible with the diagnosis of myotonic dystrophy. It is an autosomal dominant multisystem disorder with variable penetrance. The disease is caused by amplification of an unstable DNA region in chromosome 19. In addition to the striated muscle, which is primarily involved in this disease, smooth muscle of the digestive tract, cardiac muscle, the endocrine system, the immune system, vision (cataract), and intelligence may be affected. Myotonia can be demonstrated by percussion of the thenar eminence, which remains dimpled at the site of the percussion with thumb abduction for several seconds. In this vignette, the myotonia is demonstrated by the use of wrist flexors to force the flexors of the fingers to open. In Duchenne muscular dystrophy, muscle deficit in dystrophin causes an unsteady gait in males always before the age of 5 years. Myasthenia gravis, Werdnig-Hoffman disease, and chronic demyelinating polyradiculopathy are unlikely to cause myotonia. *(Fenichel, 190–191)*

40. **(E)** Pseudotumor cerebri is a chronic condition characterized by an increase in the intracranial pressure, normal cerebrospinal fluid content, and normal brain with normal or small ventricles on brain-imaging studies. A specific cause can usually be found in children younger than 6 years, while most idiopathic cases occur after the age of 12 years. Administration of tetracycline or nalidixic acid has been postulated as a cause of pseudotumor cerebri. Hypervitaminosis A as well as hypovitaminosis A has been documented as a cause of pseudotumor cerebri, but not furosemide administration. *(Fenichel, 114–115)*

41. **(E)** The most sensitive and one of the earliest signs of critically increased intracranial pressure is decreased level of consciousness. Headache, vomiting, irritability, and abducen

nerve palsy may, sequentially, develop. Headache is caused by traction on the intracranial arteries. Pain fibers from supratentorial intracranial vessels are innervated by the trigeminal nerve and pain is referred to the eyes, forehead, and temple. Infratentorial vessels are innervated by cervical nerves and pain is referred to the occiput and neck. Papilledema is a passive swelling of the optic disk, probably caused by the obstruction of venous return from the retina and nerve head. It does not develop in all patients with acute increased intracranial pressure. Early papilledema is asymptomatic, and only when it is advanced or chronic does the patient experience a transitory decrease in his vision. This preservation of visual acuity may differentiate papilledema from a primary optic nerve disturbance such as optic neuritis. *(Fenichel, 92–95)*

42. **(A)** The patient described in the vignette showed the emergence of a left side focal seizure during the course of his meningitis, followed by the persistence of left side weakness despite the improvement of his meningitis. Cerebral ischemic event is the most likely cause. It complicates the course of bacterial meningitis in 2% to 19% of cases. It may be caused by focal brain ischemia due to venous thrombosis or arterial vasculitis. Brain abscess is an uncommon complication of bacterial meningitis in children and unlikely to be the right diagnosis in this case, where all signs of infection improved. Transient paresis may complicate a focal seizure. However, such neurological deficit classically improves within a few hours. Persistent motor deficit suggests an underlying structural lesion rather than Todd paralysis. Subdural empyema and hydrocephalus with increased intracranial pressure may complicate meningitis. These entities are expected to cause generalized rather than focal seizures. *(Fenichel, 108–109)*

43. **(C)** The patient in the vignette has a clinical worsening of his symptoms, with ependymal rim enhancing and fluid of different contrast in the ventricles. The most likely diagnosis in this case is ventriculitis. It is a common complication in gram-negative meningitis in newborns.

Necrotic bits of choroid plexus can block the cerebral aqueduct, making the lateral cerebral ventricles a closed space. The diagnosis is confirmed by a neurosurgical ventricular puncture, which might yield the infecting organism. Subdural empyema usually occurs in an infant with a gram-negative severe meningitis. Head CT with contrast will reveal the subdural collection of fluid surrounded by an enhancing rim. Brain abscess is an uncommon complication of bacterial meningitis in the newborn. It may occur as a complication of severe Haemophilus influenzae infant meningitis. Surgical drainage is indicated if the abscess is large and accessible. *(Smith, 11–18)*

44. **(A)** The frequency and the duration of headaches described in this vignette suggest the diagnosis of chronic tension-type headaches. A pressure or tightening quality that is dull and nonpulsatile is typical of these headaches. Depression is a common comorbidity of this condition and should be assessed appropriately. The frequency of the headaches in this case warrants the administration of a prophylactic treatment. Amitriptyline has been the most successful medication with patients who have tension-type headaches. Sedation that may interfere with daytime activity and anticholinergic side effects can be avoided by administrating the drug at bedtime and using low dosages. *(Fenichel, 85)*

45. **(A)** Familial hemiplegic migraine is characterized by a sudden onset of hemiplegia or hemisensory loss that is usually followed by a contralateral headache. The trait is transmitted by an autosomal dominant inheritance. The gene is located on chromosome 19p. Attacks are stereotyped, occur primarily in childhood or adolescence, and may be precipitated by minor head trauma. The hemiplegia, although more severe in the face and arm, affects the leg and may be present on alternate sides during different episodes. Aphasia may occur when the dominant hemisphere is affected. Stupor, confusion, and psychosis may complicate attacks. The episode may last two or three days and may suggest a strokelike syndrome. The neurological deficit usually resolves completely,

but permanent sequelae, such as gaze-evoked nystagmus, may persist between attacks. *(Fenichel, 254–255)*

46. **(E)** Abdominal migraine refers to children who have recurrent abdominal pain, nausea, and vomiting, as well as recurrent headaches. This problem ceases by the teenage years and often is replaced by more conventional headaches. Benign paroxysmal vertigo is seen predominantly in children between 2 and 6 years of age. Episodes, which last only minutes, are characterized by the sudden onset of vertigo, pallor, and nystagmus. There is a positive family history of migraine. Most patients will develop a typical migraine by adolescence. Recurrent episodes of head tilt associated with headache, nausea, and vomiting, are characteristic of paroxysmal torticollis, an uncommon benign disorder. Ocular migraine consists of episodes of transient monocular blindness in a patient who previously has had migraine attacks or a history of migraine in the family. Most attacks last for only minutes, but permanent ocular changes have been reported. There is no choreoathetotic movement disorder attributed to migraine variant. *(Singer, 94–101)*

47. **(D)** In a child with febrile seizure, the risk of developing subsequent epilepsy increases if there is a family history of epilepsy or a history of febrile seizures in parents or siblings. A history of complex febrile seizure, which is defined as a seizure that lasts longer than 15 minutes or occurs in a prolonged series for more than 30 minutes, may increase the risk of having subsequent epilepsy. A preexisting neurological disease such as cerebral palsy or developmental delay may also increase the risk of epilepsy. Children who have one of the above risk factors have a 2% chance of developing epilepsy by the age of 7 years. Those who have two or more risk factors have a 10% chance. Having two febrile seizures in one year does not increase the risk of developing epilepsy but increases the risk of having a third febrile seizure, as 50% of children who experience a second seizure will experience a third one within the next 6 to 12 months. *(Berg et al., 1122–1127; Fenichel, 18–19; Verity and Golding, 1373–1376)*

48. (C)

49. (A)

50. (B)

51. (D)

52. (E)

Explanations 48 through 52

LaCrosse virus is the most common cause of encephalitis by California subgroup viruses in the United States. Most cases were reported in Wisconsin and Minnesota before 1984. Later epidemics occurred in Indiana. Small woodland mammals serve as a reservoir and mosquitoes as the vector. Eastern equine encephalitis is a perennial infection of horses from New York to Florida. Human cases follow epidemics in horses. Wild birds serve as a reservoir and mosquitoes as a vector. Japanese B encephalitis is a major form of encephalitis in Asia and is an important health hazard to nonimmunized travelers during summer months. St. Louis encephalitis is endemic in the western United States. The vector is a mosquito and birds are the major reservoir. Western equine encephalitis is a rare disorder. All recent cases have been reported in North Dakota, South Dakota, and Canada. *(Fenichel, 57–58)*

53. (C) The patient described in the vignette developed complex febrile seizure complicated by right side hemiparesis and periodic lateralizing epileptiform discharge. These findings are consistent with the diagnosis of herpes encephalitis. Herpes simplex is the single most common cause of nonepidemic encephalitis and accounts for 10% to 20% of cases. The annual incidence is estimated at 2.3 cases per million people. Thirty-one percent of cases occur in children. Primary infection is the most common cause of encephalitis in children, and only 22% of patients give a history of recurrent labial herpes infection. The diagnosis is made by the examination of cerebrospinal fluid, which may show a pleocytosis in 97% of cases. Up to 500 red blood cells/mm³ may be present with a median protein concentration of 80 mg/dL. The demonstration of lateralizing epileptiform discharges on EEG is considered presumptive evidence of herpes encephalitis. However, MRI has proved to be an early indicator of herpes encephalitis; the T2-weighted images show increased signal intensity in one or both temporal lobes. The identification of the organism in the cerebrospinal fluid has been made possible by a polymerase chain reaction, which obviates the need for brain biopsy to confirm the diagnosis.

Measles encephalitis is a rare complication of measles, since compulsory immunization has almost eliminated natural measles infection in the United States. Symptoms of encephalitis are usually abrupt, following the rash by 1 day to 3 weeks, and are characterized by lethargy that may rapidly progress to coma; generalized seizure occurs in 50% of patients. Hemiplegia, ataxia, involuntary movement disorders, and acute transverse myelitis may occur.

Postinfectious encephalomyelitis is unlikely to be the diagnosis in this case. The clinical picture would be lethargy and weakness followed by declining consciousness, seizures, optic neuritis, and/or transverse myelitis. Postinfectious encephalomyelitis is a demyelinating disorder that occurs during or after a systemic viral illness and is presumed to be an immune-mediated disease. The diagnosis is based on a T2-weighted MRI scan that shows a marked increase in signal intensity throughout the white matter. Reye syndrome is a systemic disorder of mitochondrial function that occurs during or following a viral infection and/or after the use of salicylate. The clinical picture may progress from vomiting and lethargy to flaccid coma. Typical blood abnormalities include hypoglycemia, hyperammonemia, and increase in hepatic enzymes. Cerebrospinal fluid is normal except for increased pressure. EEG shows diffuse encephalopathy. The diagnosis is confirmed by liver biopsy, which may show on electron microscopy characteristic mitochondrial abnormalities. St. Louis encephalitis may present with headache, fever, and a spectrum of neurological illness that varies from aseptic meningitis to severe encephalitis.

Decreased consciousness is common, but seizures or focal neurological disturbances are rare. *(Fenichel, 58–59)*

54. **(D)** Hyperventilation immediately reduces the intracranial pressure through vasoconstriction, induced by lowering the arterial pressure of carbon dioxide. However, excessive lowering of carbon dioxide below 25 mm Hg is contraindicated because it may cause brain ischemia. Elevation of the head of the bed 30 to 45 degrees above horizontal decreases intracranial pressure by improving jugular venous drainage. Mannitol and glycerol are the most widely used osmotic diuretics in the United States. These agents remain in the plasma and create an osmotic gradient that draws water from the brain into the capillaries. Hypothermia between 27°C and 31°C reduces cerebral blood flow. It is frequently used with pentobarbital, which also decreases cerebral flow and edema formation at a dosage causing burst suppression on EEG. *(Fenichel, 96–97)*

55. **(C)** The patient described in this question has Parinaud syndrome, which results from dysfunction of the midbrain by periaqueductal compression by a pineal region tumor. Tumors of the pineal region are most frequently derived from germ cells. They are more frequent in boys than girls and generally become symptomatic during the second decade. Symptoms of pineal tumors are caused either by tumor mass effect on local tissues, or by hydrocephalus (from the tumor blocking the normal CSF drain pathway). Head MRI is a valuable tool in assessing the location and extension of pineal tumors, and in some cases it may suggest the tumor's histological type. Germinomas are isodense and have irregular margins. Teratomas may appear lobulated and have both hyperdense and multicystic areas. Tumors that spread into the ventricles and that show intense contrast enhancement are likely to be malignant. Tumors with abundant amounts of calcium are likely to be benign. Pineal germinomas are more radiosensitive than other pineal tumors, with a 5-year survival rate up to 80%. *(Fenichel, 101)*

56. **(B)**

57. **(A)**

58. **(C)**

Explanations 56 through 58

Pineal tumors compressing the anterior hypothalamus may cause diabetes insipidus, precocious puberty (exclusively in males), loss of vision, and emaciation. Midbrain compression in the periaqueductal gray matter causes Parinaud syndrome, as described in question 55. Extension of the tumor to the posterior fossa causes ataxia and cranial nerve dysfunction, whereas lateral extension may cause hemiparesis. *(Fenichel, 101)*

59. **(C)**

60. **(B)**

61. **(D)**

62. **(A)**

Explanations 59 through 62

The patient described in question 59 has the features of fragile X syndrome. It is the most common chromosomal cause of mental retardation in boys. The unstable chromosomal fragment contains a trinucleotide repeat that becomes larger in successive generations, causing more severe phenotype expression. Because folic acid antagonists must be added to the culture medium (to create a folate-free culture) to detect the abnormality, high doses of folate have been used to treat children with fragile X syndrome, with some behavioral improvement. Hypotonia, mongoloid facies, flat nape of neck, and brushfield spots are features of trisomy 21. The patient described in question 61 has the features of trisomy 18. 5p monosomy is characterized by moonlike face, hypertelorism, microcephaly, and "cri du chat" cry. *(Fenichel, 120)*

63. **(D)** Hutchinson triad, defined as the combination of deafness, interstitial keratitis, and peg-shaped upper incisors, is characteristic of congenital syphilis. The more common features

in symptomatic infants with congenital syphilis are condylomata lata, periostitis or osteochondritis, persistent rhinorrhea, and maculopapular rash. *(Fenichel, 121)*

64. **(E)** A cherry red spot of the macula develops as retinal ganglial cells in the parafoveal region accumulate stored material, swell, and burst. The red color of the normal fundus can then be seen. GM1 ganglioside storage disorder results from a deficit of lysosomal enzyme beta galactosidase. The beta galactosidase gene is on chromosome 3, and the deficiency state is transmitted by autosomal recessive inheritance. A cherry red spot of the macula is present in 50% of patients with GM1 gangliosidosis type 1. Metachromatic leukodystrophy is an inherited disorder of myelin metabolism caused by deficient activity of the enzyme arylsulfatase A. A cherry red spot may be found in patients with this disease, as well as in patients with sialidosis type III, a disease characterized by a deficit in sialidase. A cherry red spot is also found in Niemann-Pick disease, as well as in Farber lipogranulomatosis. Gaucher disease, an autosomal recessive disorder, is caused by a deficit in glucocerebrosidase. Type I does not affect the central nervous system. Type II is the acute and devastating infantile form, affecting the brain and viscera. Type III is like type II, with childhood onset and slow progression. A cherry red spot is not present in any form of Gaucher disease. *(Fenichel, 128–130)*

65. **(B)**

66. **(A)**

67. **(E)**

68. **(D)**

69. **(C)**

Explanations 65 through 69

Tay-Sachs disease results from a deficit of hexosaminidase A or the GM2 activator of hexosaminidase A. It is transmitted by an autosomal recessive inheritance in Ashkenazi Jews. Beta

galactosidase deficiency is seen in GM1 gangliosidosis. The defective gene is located on chromosome 3. It is transmitted by an autosomal recessive inheritance. Niemann-Pick disease is transmitted by autosomal recessive inheritance and is caused by a deficit in sphingomyelinase Arylsulfatase deficiency causes metachromatic leukodystrophy, and a galactosylceramidase deficit causes Krabbe disease. *(Fenichel, 128–130)*

70. **(C)** Leigh disease is a syndrome of progressive dystrophy primarily affecting neurons of the brain stem, thalamus, basal ganglia, and cerebellum. The disease is transmitted by an autosomal recessive inheritance or X-linked inheritance. The disease may be caused by an enzyme deficit, either in pyruvate metabolism or in respiratory chain complexes. Onset of the disease occurs in 60% of cases in the first year. The initial symptoms are developmental delay, failure to thrive, hypotonia, and seizures. Intercurrent infection or a heavy carbohydrate meal may worsen symptoms. During infancy the patient may show three typical features: respiratory disturbance, hypotonia, and ocular motility abnormalities. Hypotonia results from a combination of peripheral neuropathy and disturbed cerebellar function. Ocular motility disturbance varies from nystagmus to ophthalmoplegia. Respiratory disturbance can be characterized by Cheyne-Stokes breathing, ataxic breathing, or central hyperventilation. *(Fenichel, 133–134)*

71. **(D)**

72. **(C)**

73. **(A)**

74. **(E)**

75. **(B)**

Explanations 71 through 75

Subacute necrotizing encephalomyelopathy is a mitochondrial disease characterized by a degeneration of the brain stem, thalamus, basal ganglia, and cerebellum. The blood level of pyruvate and lactate is high and may become higher with clinical exacerbation or oral glucose load. MRI may show lesions in the brain stem and around the third ventricle. Gaucher disease results from a deficit of glucocerebrosidase. The diagnosis is made by the presence of Gaucher cells in the reticuloendothelial system. Menkes syndrome is believed to result from a primary defect in the intestinal transport of copper. Symptoms are attributed to a secondary deficit of copper-dependent enzymes, especially cytochrome c oxidase. Chediak-Higashi syndrome is an autosomal recessive disorder resulting from lack of regulation of the fusion of primary lymphocytes. Recurrent infection during infancy, skin and hair pigmentation defects, peripheral neuropathy, seizures, and developmental retardation may be seen in affected patients. Niemann-Pick disease is caused by a sphingomyelinase deficiency. *(Fenichel, 131–134)*

76. **(B)** The association of skin lesions and neurological symptoms suggests a neurocutaneous disorder. The association of developmental delay, seizures, and hypopigmented area is highly suggestive of tuberous sclerosis. The disease is transmitted by an autosomal dominant inheritance with a genetic linkage to chromosome 9 and 16. The seizures and mental retardation are caused by disturbed histogenesis in the brain. Leaf-shaped hypochromic nevi are only present in around 18% of patients. Besides the skin, other organs may be affected, such as the retina, kidney, bone, and lungs. Neurofibromatosis type I is unlikely. It is characterized by the presence of at least two of the following: 6 or more "café au lait" spots greater than 5 mm (in prepubertal age), 2 or more neurofibromas, freckling in the axillary or inguinal region, optic glioma, 2 or more iris hamartoma, bone dyplasia, and a first-degree relative with neurofibromatosis type I. The patient in the vignette does not correspond to these criteria. *(Fenichel, 135–136)*

77. **(D)** Bilateral acoustic neurinomas are a characteristic of type II neurofibromatosis. The other conditions listed in the question are characteristic of type I neurofibromatosis. Other features of type I neurofibromatosis include a first-degree relative with this diagnosis, neurofibroma, and freckling in the inguinal or axillary region. *(Fenichel, 134–135)*

78. **(B)** Rett syndrome is an X-linked dominant disorder affecting girls almost exclusively (it is lethal to the male fetus). It has a prevalence of 1–2/20,000. Development proceeds normally until approximately 1 year of age, at which time language and motor development regress and acquired microcephaly becomes apparent. These girls present with midline hand-wringing and unusual sighing. Autistic behaviors are typical. Postmortem examinations have revealed greatly reduced brain size and weight as well as a reduced number of synapses. The Rett syndrome Diagnosis Criteria Work Group divided the diagnostic criteria into necessary criteria, supportive criteria, and exclusion criteria. Severe progressive dementia is a part of the necessary criteria. Exclusion criteria include intrauterine growth retardation, microcephaly at birth, organomegaly or sign of storage disease, retinopathy, optic atrophy, and evidence of acquired identifiable neurological disease. *(Behrman, 2034; Fenichel, 137–138)*

79. **(E)** The association of vomiting, hepatomegaly, cataract, and the presence of reducing substances in the urine, especially after feeding, is highly suggestive of galactosemia. It is a serious disease with early onset of symptoms. Its incidence is around 1/60,000. It results from galactose-1-phosphate uridyl transferase deficiency. The newborn infant normally receives up to 20% of caloric intake as lactose, which consists of glucose and galactose. Without the transferase enzyme, the infant is unable to metabolize galactose-1-phosphate, the accumulation of which results in injury to parenchymal cells of the kidney, liver, and brain. High concentrations of intracellular galactose-1-phosphate can function as a competitive inhibitor of phosphoglucomutase. This inhibition transiently impairs the conversion of glycogen to glucose and produces hypoglycemia. Injury to parenchymal cells may begin prenatally in the affected fetus by transplacental galactose derived from the

diet of the heterozygous mother or by endogenous production of galactose in the fetus.

The diagnosis of galactose-1-phosphate uridyl transferase deficiency should be considered in newborns with any of the following features: jaundice, hepatomegaly, vomiting, hypoglycemia, convulsions, lethargy, irritability, feeding difficulties, aminoaciduria, cataracts, or vitreous hemorrhage. The preliminary diagnosis of galactosemia is made by demonstrating a reducing substance in several urine specimens collected while the patient is receiving human milk, cow's milk, or another formula containing lactose. The deficient activity of galactose-1-phosphate uridyl transferase is demonstrable in hemolysates of erythrocytes, which also exhibit increased concentrations of galactose-1-phosphate.

Krabbe disease is a rapidly progressive demyelinating disorder caused by a deficit of the activity of galactosylceramidase. Diffuse demyelination suggests the diagnosis on MRI; prolonged motor nerve conduction velocity and increased cerebrospinal fluid protein content are supportive. The diagnosis is confirmed by showing decreased galactosylceramidase activity in leukocytes.

Gaucher disease is a multisystemic lipidosis characterized by hematologic problems, organomegaly, and skeletal involvement. It is the most common lysosomal storage disease and the most prevalent genetic defect among Ashkenazi Jews. There are three clinical subtypes, delineated by the absence or presence and progression of neurological manifestations: type 1 or the adult, non-neuronopathic form; type 2, the infantile or acute neuronopathic form; and type 3, the juvenile form. All subtypes are autosomal recessive traits. Gaucher disease type 2 is much less common and does not have a striking ethnic predilection. It is characterized by a rapid neurodegenerative course with extensive visceral involvement and death, often within the first 2 years of life. It presents in infancy with increased tone, strabismus, and organomegaly. Failure to thrive and stridor due to laryngospasm are typical. After a several-year period of psychomotor regression, death occurs secondary to respiratory complications.

Tay-Sachs disease results from the deficiency of hexosaminidase activity and the lysosomal accumulation of GM2 gangliosides, particularly in the central nervous system. Patients with clinical manifestations of the infantile form of Tay-Sachs disease present with loss of motor skills, increased startle reaction, and the presence of macular pallor and a cherry red spot on retinoscopy. Macrocephaly, not associated with hydrocephalus, may develop. In the second year of life, seizures requiring anticonvulsant therapy develop. Mucopolysaccharidoses result from a deficit of enzymes involved in the catabolism of dermatin sulfate, heparan sulfate, or keratin sulfate. The clinical picture of these diseases is different from the clinical picture presented in the vignette. (*Behrman, 475–476; Fenichel, 138–139*)

80. **(E)** Zellweger syndrome, or cerebrohepatorenal syndrome, is a rare and lethal disorder. It is inherited as an autosomal recessive trait. It represents the prototype of a group of peroxisomal disorders that have overlapping symptoms, signs, and biochemical abnormalities. Infants with this syndrome have dysmorphic facies consisting with frontal bossing and a large anterior fontanel. The occiput is flattened, and the external ears are abnormal. A high-arched palate, excessive skinfolds of the neck, severe hypotonia, and areflexia are usually evident. Examination of the eyes reveals searching nystagmoid movements, bilateral cataracts, and optic atrophy. Generalized seizures become evident early in life, associated with severe global developmental delay and significant bilateral hearing loss. The cause of the severe neurologic abnormalities is related to an arrest of migrating neuroblasts during early development, resulting in cerebral pachygyria with neuronal heterotopia. Patients with Zellweger syndrome rarely survive beyond 1 year of age. (*Behrman, 439–440*)

81. **(B)** Spinal muscular atrophy is a genetic disorder in which anterior horn cells in the spinal cord and motor nuclei of the brain stem are progressively lost. Two clinical syndromes of infantile spinal muscular atrophy can be distinguished: spinal muscular atrophy type I,

which is the acute fulminant form appearing in the first 6 months, and spinal muscular atrophy type II, which is the more chronic form. Affected newborns in spinal muscular atrophy type I have generalized weakness more proximal than distal, hypotonia, and areflexia. Facial expression is relatively well preserved, as are extraocular movements. Despite intrauterine hypotonia, arthrogryposis is not present. Creatinine kinase is normal or mildly elevated. The diagnosis is established by a histological examination that shows hypertrophy of type I fibers by the myosin ATPase reaction. Prenatal diagnosis can be accomplished by DNA analysis of chorion villus biopsy. *(Fenichel, 173–175)*

82. **(D)** The association of constipation, poor feeding, and incremental response to repetitive stimulation between 20 and 50 Hz is highly suggestive of infantile botulism. It is an age-limited disorder in which *Clostridium botulinum* is ingested, colonizes the intestinal tract, and produces toxin in situ. The exotoxin prevents the release of acetylcholine, causing a cholinergic blockade of skeletal muscles and the end organs innervated by autonomic nerves. Infected infants at the age of 4 weeks are usually living in a dusty environment adjacent to construction or agricultural soil disruption. The prodromal signs are poor feeding and constipation. Typically the newborn may present with diffuse hypotonia, ptosis, dysphagia, weak cry, and dilated pupils that react sluggishly to light. Electrophysiology studies show an incremental response to repetitive stimulation at a frequency between 20 and 50 Hz. The diagnosis is confirmed by isolation of organisms or toxin from the stool. Infantile botulism may suggest Guillain-Barré syndrome. The clinical differential diagnosis may be difficult, but electrophysiology testing establishes the diagnosis. Infantile botulism differs from infantile spinal muscular atrophy by the early appearance of facial and pharyngeal weakness, the presence of ptosis and dilated pupils, and the occurrence of severe constipation. Infants with generalized myasthenia do not have dilated pupils, absent reflexes, or severe constipation. Lowe syndrome, or oculocerebrorenal syndrome, is an X-linked disease characterized by hypotonia and hyporeflexia and sometimes cataracts. Later in infancy mental retardation and defects in urine acidification appear. *(Behrman, 947–995)*

83. **(C)** Myotonic dystrophy is a multisystem disorder transmitted by autosomal dominant inheritance. It is caused by an unstable DNA triplet on chromosome 19 that repeats 50 to several thousand times in successive generations. The number of triplets correlates with the severity of the disease. Repeat size changes from mother to child are greater than from father to child. For this reason, the mother is the most often affected parent when a child has a myotonic dystrophy. The main feature during pregnancy is reduced fetal movements and polyhydramnios. Prominent clinical features in the newborn include facial diplegia, generalized muscular hypotonia with more proximal than distal weakness, and arthrogryposis. Myotonia is not elicited by percussion and may not be demonstrable by EMG. *(Fenichel, 194–195)*

84. **(D)** Duchenne and Becker muscular dystrophies are variable phenotypic expressions of a gene defect at the Xp21 site. The abnormal gene produces a reduced muscle content of dystrophin, a structural muscle protein. In Duchenne muscular dystrophy, the dystrophin content is less than 3% of normal, whereas in Becker muscular dystrophy, the dystrophin content is between 3% and 20% of normal. The incidence of Duchenne dystrophy is 1/3500 male births. The initial feature of the disease is gait disturbance. Toe-walking and frequent falling before the age of 5 years are typical. The decline in motor function is linear throughout childhood. Motor function appears static between the age of 3 and 6 years because of cerebral maturation. The immediate cause of death may be caused by arrhythmia, aspiration, and intercurrent infection. Respiratory insufficiency is a contributing factor in most cases. *(Fenichel, 176–178)*

85. **(F)**

86. **(C)**

87. **(D)**

88. (A)

89. (B)

90. (E)

91. (H)

92. (G)

Explanations 85 through 92

Myotonic dystrophy is an autosomal dominant multisystem degenerative disease characterized by myotonia, progressive muscular weakness, gonadal atrophy, cataracts, and cardiac dysrhythmias. The molecular basis of myotonic dystrophy is an unstable trinucleotide repeat sequence, cytosine, thymine, and guanidine (CTG) in the protein kinase-encoding gene (DMK), located at 19q13.3. The repeat is present 50 to several thousands of times in patients with myotonic dystrophy rather than the 5 to 30 times in the normal population. The size of the repeat correlates with the severity of symptoms.

Duchenne muscular dystrophy is the most common hereditary neuromuscular disease affecting all races and ethnic groups. This disease is inherited as an X-linked recessive trait. The abnormal gene is on the X chromosome at the Xp21 locus and is one of the largest genes identified. The gene defect in deficiency of the glycolytic lysosomal enzyme acid maltase is located at locus 17q23. Periodic paralyses have been traditionally divided into those associated with a high or normal serum potassium concentration, hyperkalemic periodic paralysis, and those associated with a low serum potassium concentration, hypokalemic periodic paralysis. Hypokalemic periodic paralysis is transmitted by an autosomal dominant inheritance and is caused by a gene defect in chromosome 1q31-32 encoding for L type calcium channel. Hyperkalemic periodic paralysis is transmitted by an autosomal dominant inheritance and is caused by a defect in chromosome 17q23-35, causing abnormal inactivation of sarcolemmal sodium channels. Emery-Dreifuss muscular dystrophy is characterized by early contractures and cardiomyopathy. Generally it is transmitted by X-linked inheritance. The gene is located in Xq28. Hereditary motor and sensory neuropathy type II, or Charcot-Marie-Tooth type II, is transmitted by an autosomal dominant inheritance. The defective gene is located on chromosome 1 at 1p35 1p36. Hereditary motor and sensory neuropathy type III, or Dejerine-Sottas disease, is transmitted by an autosomal recessive inheritance. The defective gene is located on 17p11. (*Goetz, 776–778, 787–789; Fenichel, 176–192*)

93. (A) The patient described in the vignette has signs of chronic polyneuropathy, cerebellar ataxia, decreased deep tendon reflexes, and night blindness. These signs are highly suggestive of Refsum disease. It is hereditary motor and sensory polyneuropathy type IV, which is an autosomal recessive disorder caused by inborn error in the metabolism of phytanic acid. The clinical picture may include, beside the symptoms described in the vignette, progressive hearing loss, cardiomyopathy, ichthyosis, and pes cavus. The diagnosis is confirmed by showing reduced oxidation of phytanic acid in cultured fibroblasts. (*Fenichel, 186–187*)

94. (A) The patient described in this case has a generalized myotonic syndrome. The association of generalized muscle hypertrophy and myotonic discharges on EMG examination is suggestive of myotonia congenita. Transmission of the disorder is either autosomal dominant or recessive. The abnormal gene is located on chromosome 17q23-35. Clinical features are stereotyped. At rest, muscles are stiff with difficulty in moving, which improves with activity. The myotonia causes generalized muscle hypertrophy, which gives the infant a Herculean appearance. The diagnosis is established by EMG, which shows repetitive discharges at rates of 20–80 Hz when the needle is inserted into the muscle or on voluntary contraction (myotonic discharges). Muscle biopsy shows the absence of type II fibers. The absence of involuntary muscle twitching, excessive sweating, and the improvement of stiffness by exercise make the diagnosis of neuromyotonia unlikely. The absence of skeletal deformities rules out Schwartz-Jampel syndrome. Stiff-person syndrome is an autoimmune mediated condition that is extremely rare in children. It is characterized by involuntary truncal muscle tightness without spinal deformity. Abdominal wall rigidity and contraction of the thoracolumbar paraspinal muscles cause a hyperlordosis that is characteristic of the disease. The patient described in the vignette does not have the features of stiff-person syndrome. *(Fenichel, 202)*

95. **(C)** The patient described in this case has pain and muscle weakness associated with mild rhabdomyolysis and failure to generate ammonia on an ischemic exercise test. These features are suggestive of myoadenylate deaminase deficiency. It is an autosomal recessive disease. The defective gene is located on chromosome 1p. Myoadenylate deaminase deficiency most commonly presents with isolated muscle weakness, fatigue, and myalgias following moderate-to-vigorous exercise. Myalgias may be associated with an increased serum creatine kinase level and detectable electromyelographic abnormalities. Muscle wasting or histologic changes on biopsy are absent. The age of onset may be as early as 8 months of life. The enzyme defect has been identified in asymptomatic family members. The disorder may be screened for by performing an exercise test. The normal elevation of venous plasma ammonia following exercise that is seen in normal subjects is absent in myoadenylate deaminase deficiency. The final diagnosis is made by histochemical or biochemical assays of a muscle biopsy. The absence of external ophthalmoplegia, pigmentary degeneration of the retina, and heart block make the diagnosis of Kearns-Sayre syndrome unlikely. Brody disease is caused by a deficiency of calcium-activated ATPase in the sarcoplasmic reticulum. Stiffness becomes worse with exercise. Ischemic exercise results are normal. Muscle biopsy results reveal type II atrophy. Biochemical studies confirm the diagnosis. The age of onset and the absence of myoclonic seizures rule out Menkes syndrome, a disorder of intestinal copper transport that starts at the age of 3 months. Most patients die before the

age of 18 months. Carnitine palmityl transferase deficiency causes exercise intolerance and reduced production of ketone bodies in the blood or urine when fasting. *(Behrman, 492; Fenichel, 208)*

96. **(A)** The association of limb ataxia with photosensitivity indicates the diagnosis of Hartnup disease. It is a disorder transmitted by an autosomal recessive inheritance. It is caused by a defect of neutral amino acid transport in cells in the proximal cell tubules and small intestine. The result is massive aminoaciduria and retention of amino acids in the small intestine, where they may be converted into absorbed toxic products. Clinical features include limb ataxia, nystagmus, decreased tone, and pellagra-like skin lesions after exposure to sunlight because of nicotinamide deficiency. Mental change may occur, ranging from emotional instability to delirium. Administration of nicotinamide may prevent the rash. *(Fenichel, 226)*

97. **(E)** Progressive ataxia with increased blood level of very long chain fatty acids occurs in adrenoleukodystrophy. It is an X-linked disorder associated with the accumulation of saturated very long chain fatty acids and a progressive dysfunction of the adrenal cortex and nervous system white matter. Excess hexacosanoic acid is the most striking and characteristic feature. This accumulation of fatty acids is due to genetically determined deficient degradation of fatty acids, which is a normal peroxisomal function. Sulfatide lipidosis is a disorder of central and peripheral myelin metabolism caused by deficient activity of the enzyme Arylsulfatase A. Abetalipoproteinemia is a disorder of lipid metabolism transmitted by autosomal recessive inheritance. Apolipoprotein B is essential for the synthesis and integrity of low density and very low density lipoproteins. Its absence results in fat malabsorption and a progressive deficiency of vitamins A, E, and K. Clinical features include progressive cerebellar ataxia, delayed psychomotor development, and retinitis pigmentosa. Laboratory features include severe anemia, the presence of acanthocytes, low cholesterol, and low triglyceride levels. Ataxia telangiectasia is a multisystem disorder

affecting the nervous and immune system. It is transmitted by autosomal recessive inheritance. The abnormal gene is located on chromosome 11. Clinical features include chronic sinopulmonary infections, truncal ataxia, oculomotor apraxia, and telangiectasis. Ramsay Hunt syndrome is a progressive degeneration of the dentate nucleus and superior cerebellar peduncle characterized by myoclonus and cerebellar ataxia without elevation of very long chain fatty acids. *(Behrman, 2032–2033; Fenichel, 145–146)*

98. (F)

99. (C)

100. (E)

101. (B)

102. (A)

103. (D)

Explanations 98 through 103

The clinical picture described in question 98 is suggestive of Harp syndrome. It is a genetic disorder transmitted by autosomal recessive inheritance. Clinical features of the disease include retinitis pigmentosa, mild mental abnormalities, dystonic dysarthria, and decreased facial expression. Head MRI shows eye-of-the-tiger appearance of the pallidum. Acanthocytes and echinocytes are seen in preparations of washed erythrocytes.

The patient described in vignette 99 is highly suggestive of Hallervorden-Spatz disease. It is a rare degenerative disorder inherited as an autosomal recessive trait. Linkage analysis indicates that the gene is located on chromosome 20p13. The condition usually begins during childhood and is characterized by progressive dystonia, rigidity, and choreoathetosis. Spasticity, extensor plantar responses, dysarthria, and intellectual deterioration become evident during adolescence, and death usually occurs by early adulthood. Head MRI shows lesions of the globus pallidus, including low signal intensity in T2-weighted images

(corresponds to iron pigments) and an anteromedial area of high signal intensity or "eye-of-the-tiger" (sign corresponding to areas of vacuolation). Neuropathologic examination indicates excessive accumulation of iron-containing pigments in the globus pallidus and substantia nigra.

Sydenham chorea (question 100) is the most common acquired chorea of childhood and is the sole neurologic manifestation of rheumatic fever. The pathogenesis of Sydenham chorea is probably an autoimmune response of the central nervous system to group A streptococcal organisms. The majority of children with Sydenham chorea have antineuronal antibodies, which develop in response to group A beta-hemolytic streptococcal infections. Antineuronal antibodies cross-react with the cytoplasm of subthalamic and caudate nuclei neurons.

The combination of encephalopathy and progressive calcification of the basal ganglia is seen in Fahr disease (question 101). Affected children may have dwarfism, senile appearance, retinitis pigmentosa, mental retardation, choreoathetotic movements, ataxia, dysarthria, and seizures. Head CT may show calcification that appears first in the dentate nuclei and pons, then in the basal ganglia, and finally in the corpus callosum.

Tardive dyskinesia (question 102) is characterized by stereotypical facial movements, particularly by lip smacking and protrusion and retraction of the tongue. These are drug-induced choreiform movements. The condition is most often associated with drugs used to modify behavior or antiemetics. It can occur in children with asthma treated with theophylline.

Neuroacanthocytosis (question 103) is a rare disorder with autosomal dominant, recessive, or even X-linked inheritance and is manifested by chorea, tics, dystonia, parkinsonism, self-mutilatory behavior, amyotrophy, areflexia, and elevated creatine phosphokinase. One of the most distinguishing features of Neuroacanthocytosis is an eating dysfunction that is due to orolingual dystonia and is manifested by expulsion of food from the mouth by a protruding tongue. Involuntary vocalizations and parkinsonism also occur. *(Behrman, 2020–2023; Fenichel, 283–292; Goetz, 725)*

REFERENCES

Ahdab-Barmada M. Moossy J. The neuropathology of kernicterus in the premature neonate: diagnostic problems. *J Neuropathol Exp Neurol.* 1984;43:45–56.

Annegers JF, Hauser WA, Shirts SB, Kurland LT. Factors prognostic of unprovoked seizures after febrile convulsions. *N Engl J Med.* 1987;316:493–498.

Behrman, RE: *Nelson Textbook of Pediatrics.* 16th ed. Philadelphia, Pa: W.B. Saunders; 2000.

Berg AT, Shinnar S, Hauser WA, Alemany M, Shapiro ED, Salomon ME, Crain EF. A prospective study of recurrent febrile seizures. *N Engl J Med.* 1992;327:1122–1127.

Bradshaw DY, Jones HR Jr. Guillain Barre syndrome in children: clinical course, electrodiagnosis, and prognosis. *Muscle Nerve.* 1992;15:500–506.

Callaghan N, Garrett A, Goggin T. Withdrawal of anticonvulsant drugs in patients free of seizures for two years. A prospective study. *N Engl J Med.* 1988; 318:942–946.

Fenichel Gerald M: *Clinical Pediatric Neurology. A signs and Symptoms Approach.* 4th ed. Philadelphia, Pa: WB Saunders; 2001.

Goetz CG, Pappert EJ. *Textbook of Clinical Neurology,* Philadelphia, Pa: W.B. Saunders; 1999.

Goldenberg J, Ferraz MB, Fonseca AS, Hilario MO, Bastos W, Sachetti S. Sydenham chorea: clinical and laboratory findings. Analysis of 187 cases. *Rev Paul Med.* 1992; 110(4):152–157.

Nausieda PA, Grossman BJ, Koller WC, Weiner WJ, Klawans HL. Sydenham chorea: an update. *Neurology.* 1980;30:331–334.

Nelson KB. Epidemiology and etiology of cerebral palsy. In: Capture AJ, Accardo PJ, eds. *Developmental Disabilities in Infancy and Childhood.* 2nd ed. Baltimore, Md: Paul H Brookes; 1996:73–80.

Panayiotopoulos CP. Typical absence seizures and their treatment. *Arch Dis Child.* 1999;81:351–355.

Patterson MC, Gomez MR. Muscle disease in children: a practical approach. *Ped Rev.* 1990;12:73–82.

Pidcock FS, Graziani LJ, Stanley C, Mitchell DG, Merton D. Neurosonographic features of periventricular echodensities associated with cerebral palsy in preterm infants. *J Pediatr.* 1990;116:417–422.

Pollack RN, Buchman AS, Yaffe H, Divon MY. Obstetrical brachial palsy: pathogenesis, risk factors, and prevention. *Clin Obstet Gynecol.* 2000;43:236–246.

Rivkin MJ, Anderson ML, Kaye EM. Neonatal idiopathic cerebral venous thrombosis: an unrecognized cause of transient seizures or lethargy. *Ann Neurol.* 1992; 32:51–56.

Ropper AH. The Guillan-Barre syndrome. *N Engl J Med.* 1992;326:1130–1136.

Rosenbloom L. Diagnosis and management of cerebral palsy. *Arch Dis Child.* 1995;72:350–354.

Shinnar S, Berg AT, Moshe SL, Kang H, O'Dell C, Alemany M, Goldensohn ES, Hauser WA. Discontinuing antiepileptic drugs in children with epilepsy: a prospective study. *Ann Neurol.* 1994;35:534–545.

Singer HS. Migraine headaches in children. *Ped Rev.* 1994;15:94–101.

Smith AL. Bacterial meningitis. *Ped Rev.* 1993;14:11–18.

Taft LT. Cerebral palsy. *Ped Rev.* 1995;16:411–408.

US Modafinil in Narcolepsy Multicenter Study Group. Randomized trial of modafinil as a treatment for the excessive daytime somnolence of narcolepsy: Treatment modalities for narcolepsy. *Neurology.* 1998; 50(2 Suppl 1): S43–48.

Verity CM, Golding J. Risk of epilepsy after febrile convulsions: a national cohort study. *BMJ.* 1991;303:1373–1376.

Weeks RA. Turjanski N. Brooks DJ. Tourette's syndrome: a disorder of cingulate and orbitofrontal function? *QJM.* 1996;89:401–408.

CHAPTER 4

Neurophysiology, Epilepsy, Evoked Potentials, and Sleep Disorders
Questions

1. What is the frequency of the posterior dominant rhythm at the age of 3 months?

    (A) 9 Hz
    (B) 7 Hz
    (C) 6 Hz
    (D) 8 Hz
    (E) 4 Hz

2. Which of the following statements is true about Mu rhythm?

    (A) Mu activity is increased with movements of the contralateral arm.
    (B) Mu amplitude is usually higher than the amplitude of alpha rhythm.
    (C) It is always unilateral.
    (D) Mu activity should be considered normal, even if it is persistent in a region of focal slowing.
    (E) Mu activity may slow gradually with aging.

3. Which of the following drugs have the LEAST effect on beta rhythm?

    (A) Phenobarbital
    (B) Valproic acid
    (C) Clonazepam
    (D) Chloral hydrate
    (E) Amitriptyline

4. Which of the following cardinal features of stage II sleep is NOT seen in stage I sleep?

    (A) Alpha attenuation
    (B) Positive occipital sharp transient
    (C) Sleep spindles
    (D) Vertex sharp transient
    (E) Increased frontocentral beta rhythm

5. All of the following statements are true about the photomyoclonic response EXCEPT

    (A) It occurs in the frontal area when the flashing light evokes facial musculature contraction.
    (B) It is reduced in case of barbiturate withdrawal.
    (C) It is enhanced in case of ethanol withdrawal.
    (D) Stimulation rate of 12 to 18 Hz is most effective in producing a photomyoclonic response.
    (E) The amplitude of muscle contraction increases as the photic stimulation continues.

6. Well-formed synchronous sleep spindles appear at the age of

    (A) 1 month
    (B) 3 months
    (C) 4 months
    (D) 6 months
    (E) 2 years

Questions 7 through 10
Link the following EEG patterns to the gestational age at which when they first appear

    (A) 30 weeks
    (B) 36 weeks asleep
    (C) 40 weeks awake
    (D) 46 weeks asleep

7. Trace alternant

8. Trace discontinue

9. Activité moyenne

10. Continuous slow wave sleep

11. Asynchronous burst of hemispheric activity is defined as activity in one hemisphere leading the other by more then

    (A) 5 seconds
    (B) 0.5 second
    (C) 1 second
    (D) 1.5 seconds
    (E) 3 seconds

12. Delta brushes are characterized by all of the following EXCEPT

    (A) They represent the fusion of underlying delta transient with a superimposed rhythmic fast activity.
    (B) They occur only during active sleep.
    (C) They disappear by the age of one month.
    (D) Frontal delta brushes are rare at any age.
    (E) They are more common in the rolandic area at the conceptual age of 29 weeks.

13. Sleep spindles appear for the first time at a conceptual age of

    (A) 32 weeks
    (B) 36 weeks
    (C) 40 weeks
    (D) 46 weeks
    (E) 50 weeks

14. Which of the following is true about active sleep in a full-term neonate?

    (A) Eyes are always closed
    (B) Increased muscle tone
    (C) No body or facial movement
    (D) Irregular respiration
    (E) Active sleep comprises 30% of the time spent in sleep in a full-term neonate

15. Photomyogenic response is

    (A) an epileptiform discharge triggered by photic stimulation
    (B) a spike-like driving response
    (C) of noncerebral origin
    (D) less frequent than the flashing stimulus
    (E) felt to be an abnormal response to high intensity of light

Questions 16 through 20
Link the following.

    (A) Alpha activity
    (B) Alpha rhythm
    (C) Temporal transient
    (D) Bancaud phenomenon
    (E) Posterior slowing of youth

16. Posterior predominant activity during wakefulness blocked by eye opening

17. Failure of alpha rhythm to block on eye opening

18. Sail wave

19. EEG activity between 8 and 13 Hz

20. Sylvian theta activity that seems to be related to normal aging

21. Triphasic waves are not seen in

    (A) renal failure
    (B) hepatic failure
    (C) hyponatremia
    (D) hypoglycemia
    (E) hypoparathyroidism

22. Which of the following EEG waves is the LEAST likely to be seen in anoxic encephalopathy?

    (A) Burst suppression pattern
    (B) Periodic spike or sharp waves
    (C) Alpha coma pattern
    (D) Delta brushes
    (E) Bihemispheric epileptiform discharges

23. The EEG pattern most commonly seen in dialysis dementia is:

    (A) bilateral spike and wave complex
    (B) triphasic waves
    (C) alpha pattern
    (D) bihemispheric lateral epileptiform discharges
    (E) burst suppression pattern

24. Benzodiazepine overdose typically shows an EEG pattern of

    (A) triphasic wave
    (B) widespread high amplitude beta activity
    (C) burst suppression pattern
    (D) alpha coma
    (E) spontaneous epileptiform spike and wave

25. In which stage of Rett syndrome does the EEG show background slowing with focal spike or sharp waves, most commonly over the centroparietal region?

    (A) Stage 1
    (B) Stage 2
    (C) Stage 3
    (D) Stage 4
    (E) None of the above

26. EEG guidelines in the determination of brain death in adults include all of the following EXCEPT

    (A) minimum of 8 scalp and 2 ear electrodes
    (B) electrode impedances between 10,000 and 100 ohms
    (C) instrument sensitivity set at 2 microvolts per millimeter
    (D) interelectrode distance of 8 cm or less
    (E) monitoring for artifact, EMG and EKG

27. Which of the following EEG patterns has the best prognosis in case of anoxic encephalopathy?

    (A) Nearly isoelectric record
    (B) Dominant alpha rhythm with scattered theta activity

    (C) Dominant theta activity with rare alpha activity
    (D) Invariant low amplitude delta activity unresponsive to stimulus
    (E) Continuous polymorphic slow delta waves with little activity and fast frequency

28. In which of the following conditions does alpha coma cause the abnormal alpha rhythm to have some reactivity and to be more prominent over the posterior head region?

    (A) Ventral pons ischemic stroke
    (B) Cardiorespiratory arrest
    (C) Barbiturates overdose
    (D) Benzodiazepine overdose
    (E) Methaqualone overdose

Questions 29 through 33
Link each EEG to its appropriate description.

    (A) Mu rhythm
    (B) Positive occipital sharp transients
    (C) Lambda waves
    (D) Wicket spikes
    (E) Benign epileptiform transients of sleep

29. Monophasic triangular waves in the occipital region

30. Small sharp spikes seen in adult during drowsiness without distortion of the background activity

31. Arc-like waves typically occurring in trains. They are often mistaken for a temporal spike.

32. They may represent an evoked cerebral response to visual stimulus produced from shifts of images across the retina in the course of saccadic eye movements.

33. Rolandic alpha activity

Questions 34 through 42
Link the following evoked potential waves to their anatomical generation location.

(A) P 100
(B) N9
(C) Wave III
(D) N20
(E) P38
(F) Wave I
(G) N22
(H) N14
(I) Wave V

34. Distal part of the auditory nerve

35. Cortical response to visual evoked potential

36. Trapezoid body

37. Midbrain

38. Erb's point

39. Caudal medial lemniscus

40. Primary sensory cortex from median nerve stimulation

41. Lumbar cord

42. Cortical response from posterior tibial nerve stimulation

Questions 43 through 47
Link each of the following conditions to the appropriate EEG variety.

(A) Bancaud's phenomenon
(B) Breach rhythm
(C) Stage I sleep
(D) Stage III sleep
(E) Stage IV sleep

43. Sleep spindle

44. Skull defect causes enhanced beta activity

45. Presence of occipital sharp transient

46. Delta slowing is present in 20% to 50% of its record

47. Unilateral failure of alpha wave blocking on eye opening

48. All of the following are side effects of valproic acid EXCEPT

(A) hair loss
(B) weight gain
(C) essential tremor
(D) acute pancreatitis
(E) aplastic anemia

49. Which of the following is true about carbamazepine?

(A) It is highly soluble in water.
(B) In the naïve patient, the half-life of the drug is about 30 hours and decreases to 10 hours within a few weeks.
(C) Skin rash is seen less with carbamazepine than phenytoin.
(D) Hypernatremia may complicate the chronic use of carbamazepine.
(E) It may cause elevation of hepatic enzymes that predispose to hepatitis.

50. Which of the following antiseizure medications is NOT metabolized by the liver?

(A) Zonisamide
(B) Levetiracetam
(C) Topiramite
(D) Lamotrigine
(E) Tiagabine

51. A 45-year-old man with a history of seizure disorder and ethanol abuse was admitted to the neurology floor because of phenytoin intoxication. His admission phenytoin level was 45 μg/mL. In the second and third day of admission, his level drops to 35 and 25 μg/mL, respectively. What would be his level in the fourth day of his admission?

(A) 15 μg/mL
(B) 10 μg/mL

(C) Unpredictable because phenytoin follows zero-order kinetics

(D) Unpredictable because phenytoin follows first-order kinetics

(E) Unpredictable because the patient is an ethanol abuser

52. A 25-year-old man was diagnosed with a complex partial seizure and started on carbamazepine 200 mg po qid. In the first week of treatment, he developed blurred vision, nystagmus, dizziness, fatigue, and headache that progressively improved. He consulted about these symptoms 2 weeks later. His carbamazepine level was 8 µg/mL. The cause of the initial symptoms is

(A) physiologic effect of carbamazepine

(B) carbamazepine intoxication

(C) idiosyncratic reaction to carbamazepine

(D) psychogenic symptoms not related to carbamazepine administration

(E) none of the above

53. Which of the following is true about lamotrigine?

(A) The half-life of the drug is not affected by other antiepileptic drugs.

(B) It acts through prolonging inactivation of voltage-sensitive calcium channels.

(C) Cutaneous rash may occur in 10% of cases.

(D) Its antiseizure activity correlates with its ability to inhibit dihydrofolate reductase activity.

(E) It is about 95% protein bounded.

54. In case of renal failure, which of the following drugs needs the LEAST adjustment?

(A) Ethosuximide

(B) Carbamazepine

(C) Phenytoin

(D) Phenobarbital

(E) Topiramate

55. Which of the following antiepileptic drugs is NOT removed by dialysis?

(A) Ethosuximide

(B) Phenobarbital

(C) Gabapentin

(D) Phenytoin

(E) Lamotrigine

56. Which of the following drugs is the treatment of choice for infantile spasm?

(A) Carbamazepine

(B) ACTH

(C) Phenobarbital

(D) Topiramate

(E) Phenytoin

Questions 57 through 64
Link each of the following antiepileptic drugs to its side effect.

(A) Phenytoin

(B) Phenobarbital

(C) Carbamazepine

(D) Valproic acid

(E) Gabapentin

(F) Lamotrigine

(G) Felbamate

(I) Zonisamide

57. Somnolence, headaches, and ataxia

58. Poor memory, cognitive impairment and Dupuytren's contracture with chronic use

59. Cutaneous rash occurs in up to 10% of cases, especially with concomitant administration of valproic acid.

60. Weight gain is seen in 50% of cases

61. Cerebellar atrophy and gum hypertrophy is seen with long-term use

62. Hyponatremia

63. Aplastic anemia

64. Renal stones

65. Which of the following drugs is removed by dialysis?

(A) Carbamazepine
(B) Topiramate
(C) Valproic acid
(D) Phenytoin
(E) None of the above

66. All of the following antiepileptic drugs inhibit voltage dependent sodium channels EXCEPT

(A) Tiagabine
(B) Phenytoin
(C) Carbamazepine
(D) Valproic acid
(E) Zonisamide

67. The overall risk of having a baby with a major malformation from a mother taking a single antiepileptic drug is

(A) 2%
(B) 5%
(C) 10%
(D) 15%
(E) 20%

68. Which of the following drugs increases the level of phenytoin?

(A) Reserpine
(B) Sucralfate
(C) Amiodarone
(D) Verapamil
(E) Erythromycin

69. Which of the following drugs decreases the level of carbamazepine?

(A) Cimetidine
(B) Fluoxetine
(C) Isoniazid
(D) Theophylline
(E) Propoxyphene

70. Which of the following drugs may increase EEG beta activity?

(A) Olanzapine
(B) Phenytoin
(C) Carbamazepine
(D) Topiramate
(E) Lorazepam

71. What is the most likely EEG pattern seen in a 56-year-old man with acute left parietal ischemic stroke?

(A) Left triphasic wave
(B) Beta asymmetry
(C) Generalized temporal theta
(D) Hypsarhythmia
(E) PLEDs (periodic lateralizing epileptiform discharges)

72. Which of the following is an inhibitor neurotransmitter?

(A) Aspartic acid
(B) Cysteic acid
(C) Glutamic acid
(D) GABA
(E) Homocysteic acid

73. Hyperventilation is most helpful in which of the following conditions?

(A) 65-year-old man with recurrence of stroke
(B) 8-year-old girl with staring spells
(C) 40-year-old woman with history of depression
(D) 53-year-old woman with history of cerebral aneurysm
(E) 10-year-old boy with history of ADDH

74. Which of the following is true about REM parasomnia?

(A) It shows marked female predominance.
(B) It usually occurs in preschool children.
(C) It often occurs in the first portion of sleep.
(D) It results from lack of normal atonia of REM sleep.
(E) It responds well to treatment with tricyclic antidepressant.

75. Which of the following is more characteristic of complex partial seizure rather than absence seizure?

(A) 3 Hz spike and wave on EEG

(B) Photic stimulation induces seizure activity in 10% to 30% of cases.

(C) Brief period of confusion, emotional disturbance, and headache is seen in the postictal phase.

(D) Hyperventilation most likely increases the seizure activity in the EEG.

(E) The most likely age of onset is childhood or early adulthood.

76. Which of the following is more suggestive of lateral temporal seizure rather than medial temporal seizure?

(A) A history of febrile seizure

(B) Autonomic signs or symptoms

(C) Motionless stare

(D) Structured hallucination of visual type during the aura period

(E) Postictal confusion

77. Which of the following is NOT characteristic of frontal seizure?

(A) Frequent attacks with clustering

(B) Presence of psychiatric aura

(C) Absence of postictal confusion

(D) Frequent secondary generalization

(E) EEG may show no focal abnormalities ictally or interictally

78. The incidence of epilepsy is greater in which of the following degenerative diseases?

(A) Alzheimer's disease

(B) Pick's disease

(C) Huntington's disease

(D) Wilson's disease

79. The most frequent inducing factor for reflex epilepsy is

(A) Menstruation

(B) Visual stimuli

(C) Music

(D) Eating

(E) Bathing in hot water

80. Which of the following is true about West syndrome?

(A) Phenobarbital is the treatment of choice.

(B) EEG typically shows burst suppression pattern.

(C) Seizures remit only on antiepileptic medications.

(D) Patients typically show spasms that take the form of sudden brief contractions of the head, neck or trunk, usually in flexion but sometimes in extension.

(E) Long-term prognosis is good, with improvement of mental retardation after the spasms cease.

81. In a benign rolandic epilepsy

(A) seizures have a strong tendency to occur during wakefulness

(B) typical seizures are primarily generalized

(C) typical EEG shows focal high-amplitude mid-temporal spikes

(D) cognitive function is usually mildly affected

(E) seizures may persist for 5 years after their onset in 90% of cases

82. Lennox-Gastaut syndrome is characterized by all of the following EXCEPT

(A) the age of onset is between 1 and 7 years

(B) multiple seizures type

(C) occurrence of progressive mental retardation

(D) seizures are precipitated by hyperventilation

(E) there is a poor response to antiepileptic drugs

83. Which of the following is true about childhood absence epilepsy?

    (A) Monozygotic twins develop absence as frequently as dizygotic twins.
    (B) Hyperventilation may precipitate absence more than photic stimulation.
    (C) Ten precent of patients with childhood absence epilepsy develop generalized tonic-clonic seizures within 5 to 10 years after the onset of absence seizures.
    (D) Typical EEG in childhood absence epilepsy shows generalized bilateral synchronous, symmetric 3 Hz spikes, and slow wave discharges with abnormal background.
    (E) By adulthood, remission occurs in only 20% of cases.

84. Which of the following is NOT a progressive myoclonic epilepsy?

    (A) Juvenile myoclonic epilepsy
    (B) Lafora disease
    (C) Unverricht-Lundborg disease
    (D) Juvenile neuronal ceroid lipofuscinosis
    (E) Myoclonic epilepsy with ragged-red fibers

Questions 85 through 90
Link each of the following epilepsy syndromes with the appropriate EEG pattern.

    (A) Idiopathic generalized epilepsy
    (B) Temporal lobe epilepsy
    (C) Infantile spasm
    (D) Benign rolandic epilepsy
    (E) Benign occipital epilepsy
    (F) Lennox-Gastaut syndrome

85. Generalized epileptiform discharges of 3 Hz maximum in the parasagittal region. Normal background. Photic stimulation often induces occipital spikes.

86. Bitemporal spikes are usually maximal over the temporal frontal region. Ictal EEG shows rhythmic theta at onset.

87. Posterior 1.5 to 3 spikes and slow waves per second discharges that usually attenuate with eye opening

88. Hypsarrhythmia

89. Triphasic large amplitude spikes maximum in the centrotemporal area

90. Slow disorganized background. EEG with superadded 1 to 2.5 Hz generalized interiorly predominant and slow wave discharges

Questions 91 through 100
Link each of the following causes of seizures with impairment of cognitive function to its corresponding defect.

    (A) GM2 gangliosidosis
    (B) GM1 gangliosidosis
    (C) Niemann-Pick disease
    (D) Gaucher disease
    (E) Sialidosis
    (F) Lafora bodies
    (G) Adrenoleukodystrophy
    (H) Metachromatic leukodystrophy
    (I) Globoid leukodystrophy
    (J) Canavan's disease

91. Reduced N-acetylneuraminidase activity in leukocytes

92. Spongiform leukodystrophy with deficiency in aspartoacylase

93. Polyglucosans are found in the peripheral muscle and liver

94. Sphingomyelinase activity is decreased in leukocytes

95. Reduced arylsulfatase activity

96. Reduced beta glucocerebrosidase activity in leukocytes

97. Reduced beta galactosidase activity in leukocytes

98. Reduced galactocerebroside beta-galactosidase in leukocytes

99. Reduced hexosaminidase activity in leukocytes

100. Defective lignoceroyl CoA

Questions 101 through 105
Link each of the following neurometabolic causes of seizures to its feature.

(A) MELAS syndrome (myopathy, encephalopathy, lactic acidosis, stroke)
(B) Non-ketotic hyperglycinemia
(C) Wilson's disease
(D) Porphyria
(E) Menkes' disease

101. X-linked disorder characterized by abnormal copper metabolism

102. Kayser-Fleischer ring

103. Reduced activity of glycine cleavage enzyme

104. Respiratory chain enzymes defect

105. Carbamazepine may exacerbate seizures in this condition

106. Failure of oral contraception may be caused by which of the following antiepileptic drugs?

(A) Vigabatrin
(B) Carbamazepine
(C) Valproate
(D) Gabapentin
(E) Benzodiazepine

107. Which of the following causes of seizures carries the best prognosis after surgical resection?

(A) Hippocampal sclerosis
(B) Large arteriovenous malformation
(C) Gross cortical dysplasia
(D) Small low-grade glioma
(E) Trauma

Questions 108 through 112
Link each of the following polysomnographic patterns to its cause.

(A) Short sleep latency, excessive disruption of sleep with frequent arousals, reduced total sleep time, excessive body movement, and reduced slow-wave sleep
(B) Reduction of slow-wave, reduced REM and total sleep time, increased sleep latency, and increased number of awakenings during sleep
(C) Reduced total sleep time, decreased REM and slow-wave sleep, reduction of sleep spindle and K complexes, and increased sleep fragmentation
(D) Absence of muscle atonia during REM sleep, with increased muscle tone activity in upper and lower limbs
(E) Periodic limb movements

108. REM sleep behavior disorder

109. Multiple system atrophy

110. Restless leg syndrome

111. Narcolepsy

112. Alzheimer's disease

Questions 113 through 119
Link each EEG pattern to the appropriate description.

(A) Hepatic failure
(B) Hypsarrhythmia
(C) K complexes
(D) Stage I of sleep
(E) Absence seizures
(F) Porencephaly
(G) Normal EEG pattern at the conceptional age of 29 weeks

113. EEG1

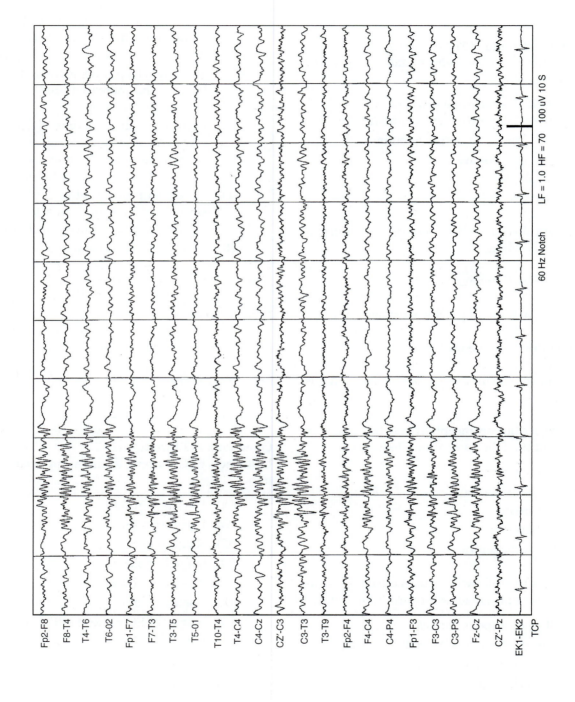

Fp2-F8
F8-T4
T4-T6
T6-02
Fp1-F7
F7-T3
T3-T5
T5-01
T10-T4
T4-C4
C4-Cz
CZ'-C3
C3-T3
T3-T9
Fp2-F4
F4-C4
C4-P4
Fp1-F3
F3-C3
C3-P3
Fz-Cz
CZ'-Pz
EK1-EK2
TCP

60 Hz Notch   LF = 1.0 HF = 70   100 uV 10 S

96

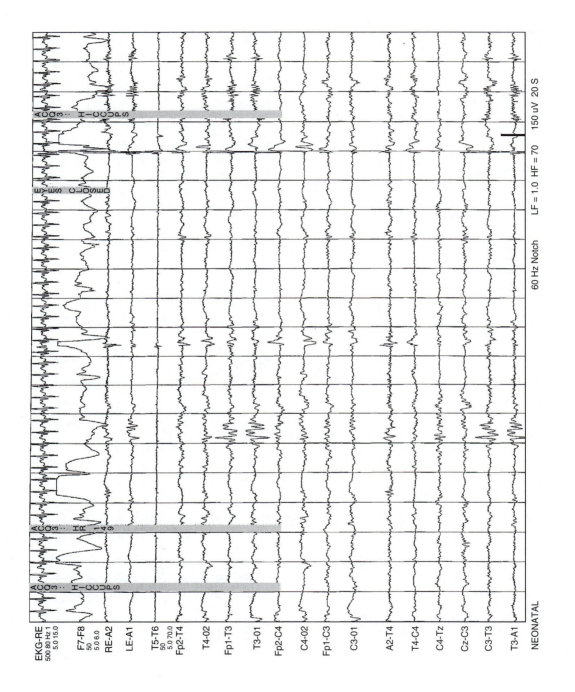

114. EEG2

NEONATAL

60 Hz Notch   LF = 1.0 HF = 70   150 uV 20 S

115. EEG3

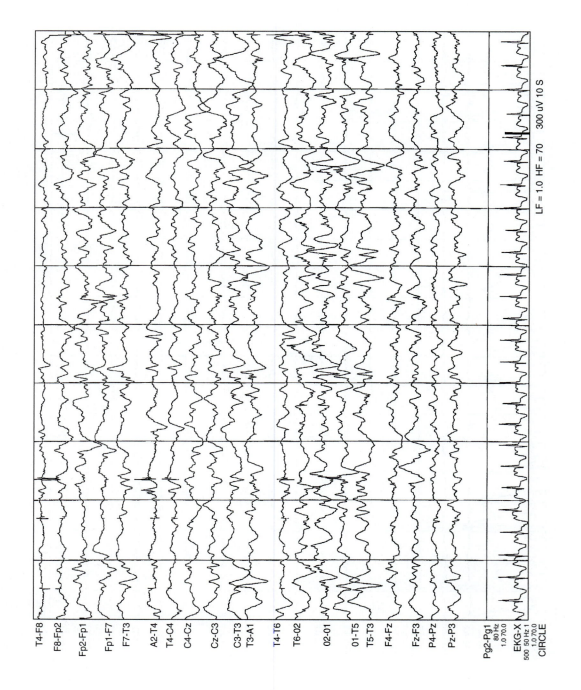

T4-F8
F8-Fp2
Fp2-Fp1
Fp1-F7
F7-T3
A2-T4
T4-C4
C4-Cz
Cz-C3
C3-T3
T3-A1
T4-T6
T6-02
02-01
01-T5
T5-T3
F4-Fz
Fz-F3
P4-Pz
Pz-P3
Pg2-Pg1
EKG-X

80 Hz
1.0 70.0
500 50 Hz 1
1.0 70.0
CIRCLE

LF = 1.0 HF = 70   300 uV 10 S

116. EEG4

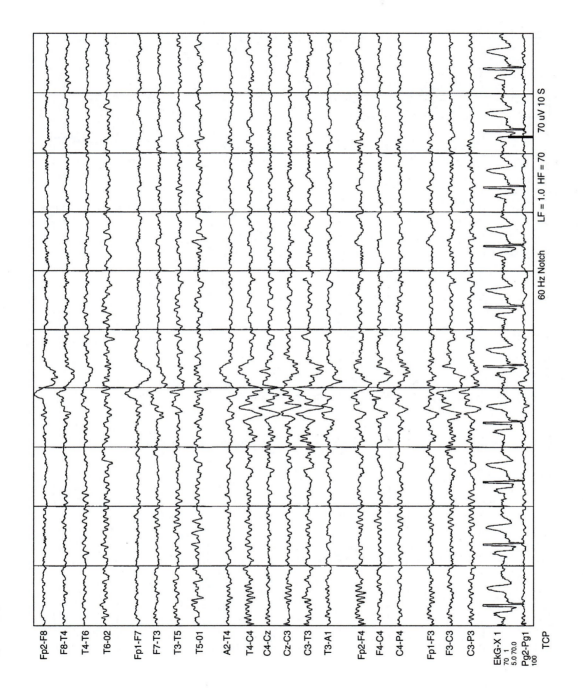

Fp2-F8
F8-T4
T4-T6
T6-02
Fp1-F7
F7-T3
T3-T5
T5-01
A2-T4
T4-C4
C4-Cz
Cz-C3
C3-T3
T3-A1
Fp2-F4
F4-C4
C4-P4
Fp1-F3
F3-C3
C3-P3
EkG-X 1
70 1
5.0 70.0
Pg2-Pg1
100
TCP

60 Hz Notch   LF = 1.0 HF = 70   70 uV 10 S

117. EEG5

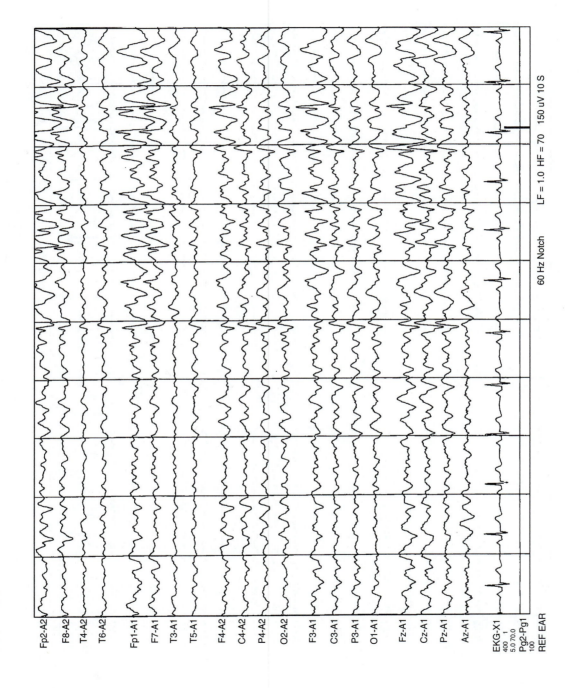

Fp2-A2
F8-A2
T4-A2
T6-A2

Fp1-A1
F7-A1
T3-A1
T5-A1

F4-A2
C4-A2
P4-A2
O2-A2

F3-A1
C3-A1
P3-A1
O1-A1

Fz-A1
Cz-A1
Pz-A1
Az-A1

EKG-X1
400   1
5.0 70.0
Pg2-Pg1
100

REF EAR   60 Hz Notch   LF = 1.0 HF = 70   150 uV 10 S

118. EEG6

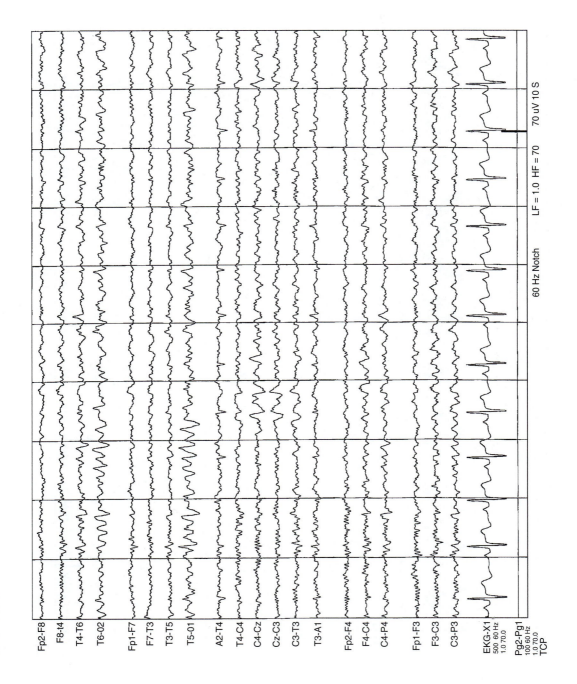

Fp2-F8
F8-t4
T4-T6
T6-02

Fp1-F7
F7-T3
T3-T5
T5-01

A2-T4
T4-C4
C4-Cz
Cz-C3
C3-T3
T3-A1

Fp2-F4
F4-C4
C4-P4

Fp1-F3
F3-C3
C3-P3

EKG-X1
500 60 Hz
1.0 70.0

Pg2-Pg1
100 60 Hz
1.0 70.0
TCP

60 Hz Notch   LF = 1.0 HF = 70   70 uV 10 S

101

119. EEG7

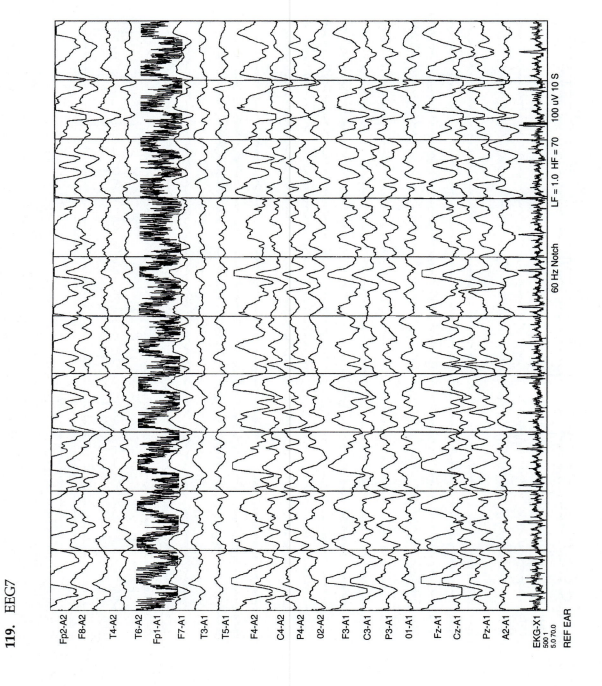

Fp2-A2
F8-A2
T4-A2
T6-A2
Fp1-A1
F7-A1
T3-A1
T5-A1
F4-A2
C4-A2
P4-A2
O2-A2
F3-A1
C3-A1
P3-A1
O1-A1
Fz-A1
Cz-A1
Pz-A1
A2-A1

EKG-X1
500 1
5.0 70.0

REF EAR

60 Hz Notch   LF = 1.0 HF = 70   100 uV 10 S

Answers and Explanations

1. **(E)** The posterior dominant rhythm is located over the occipital, parietal, and posterior temporal regions of both hemispheres. The typical alpha frequency is 8–13 Hz, usually 9–11 Hz in adults. Age affects alpha frequency. A reactive posterior dominant rhythm first appears at the age of 3–4 months. The typical frequency at that age is 3.5–4.5 Hz.

Age	Frequency in Hz
3–4 months	3.5–4.5
1 year	5–7
2 years	6–8
3 years	7–9
7–9 years	9
Mid teens	10

Frequency of posterior dominant rhythm by age.

(Spehlman, 170–173)

2. **(E)** Mu rhythm is a centrally located alpha frequency activity that diminishes with movement of the contralateral arm or body. Tactile stimuli and the thought of movement can also attenuate Mu activity. Its morphology is often arch-shaped and the rhythm can be unilateral or bilateral. Mu activity may slow with aging. It should be considered abnormal if it is persistent or nonreactive in a region of focal slowing. *(Spehlman, 191–192)*

3. **(B)** Beta rhythm is defined by a frequency greater than 13 Hz. It is best seen when the subject is relaxed or drowsy. Beta activity can increase with cognition or stage I sleep, especially in children. Beta activity is enhanced by the use of barbiturates, benzodiazepines, and chloral hydrate. Occasionally, antidepressants, antihistamines, and neuroleptics may enhance beta activity in routine EEG. Valproic acid does not modify beta activity. *(Aminoff, 43)*

4. **(C)** Stage II sleep has all the features of stage I sleep with the addition of sleep spindles and K complexes. Sleep spindles can be located centrally at a frequency of 14–15 Hz. They can be frontally located, especially in younger individuals, often at a frequency of 12 Hz. Spindles first appear at the age of 2 months at a frequency of 8–12 Hz. They are asynchronous before the age of 18 months. They later become symmetric in amplitude and frequency. They become less frequent with aging. They are seen in stages II and III of sleep.

K complexes are diphasic waves, which consist of an initial sharply contoured transient followed by high amplitude, slow waves, usually of delta frequency, maximal in the frontocentral region. They are seen in sleep stages II to IV. They appear at the age of 5 months. Vertex sharp transients can be seen in the deeper portion of stage I of sleep and in stages II and III of sleep. They are diphasic sharp transients maximal centrally at C3 and C4 with prominent negative phase reversal at the midline in the coronal bipolar montages. They are first seen at the age of 2 months with synchronous and symmetric appearance. A consistent lateralization of vertex waves is abnormal. Positive occipital sharp transients are surface positive, bisynchronous sharp transients, occasionally followed by low amplitude surface negativity. They occur in stages I or II, predominantly in the occipital region singly or in runs. Alpha attenuation and increased frontocentral beta are features of stages I and II. *(Spehlman, 203–204)*

5. **(B)** Intermittent photic stimulation is used as an activating procedure in the diagnostic evaluation of epilepsy. A photomyoclonic response occurs frontally when the flashing light evokes muscle contraction of the facial musculature about 50–60 msec after each flash. The amplitude of this muscle artifact increases as photic stimulation continues. The response can be enhanced in case of barbiturate or ethanol withdrawal. Photic stimulation rates from about 12 to 18 Hz are most effective in producing a photomyoclonic response. *(Spehlman, 448–449)*

6. **(E)** Sleep spindles consist of sinusoidal waves, from 12 to 15 Hz, which develop in the central regions during the first few weeks of life and are well established by the age of 6 to 8 weeks. Spindle bursts are commonly asynchronous in the 2 hemispheres until the age of 2 years. *(Aminoff, 108)*

7. **(B)**

8. **(A)**

9. **(C)**

10. **(D)**

Explanations 7 through 10

The neonatal EEG is characterized by an age-specific bioelectric rhythm. Between the ages of 24 and 28 weeks conceptional age, the entire EEG is essentially discontinuous. Whether the child is clinically awake, or asleep, active or quiet, the EEG itself is composed of discontinuous background. Stimulation of the newborn or spontaneous state changes provokes minor qualitative changes in the discontinuity of the background. After 32 weeks of age, EEG discontinuity is mostly confined to quiet sleep. The voltage of the interburst activity remains less than 25 μV. With advancing maturity, the voltage of the interburst period exceeds 25 μV. The label assigned to this more mature discontinuous quiet sleep activity is trace alternant.

It is seen by the age of 36 weeks. The distinction between trace discontinue and trace alternant is arbitrary, except for the higher interburst voltage. By the age of 44 to 46 weeks of conceptional age, the trace discontinue and trace alternate gradually yield to more mature and continuous slow-wave sleep during which nonstop high voltage and activity dominate the tracing. Activité moyenne appears during wakefulness, by the age of 36 to 40 weeks gestational age. It is formed by a continuous low to medium voltage mixed frequency signal. *(Spehlman, 159–170)*

11. **(D)** Lambroso has proposed an operational definition of interhemispheric synchrony that has been widely adopted. In a synchronous burst, the signal begins in both hemispheres within 1.5 seconds. Excessive interhemispheric asynchrony of burst activity may be seen in prematurity, diffuse encephalopathy, and cerebral dysgenesis. *(Lombroso, 460–474)*

12. **(B)** Delta brushes are the quintessential waveforms of prematurity. The brush represents a pattern of the simultaneous fusion of two subunits, the underlying delta transient and the superimposed rhythmic fast activity. Brushes occur during wakefulness, active sleep, and quiet sleep. At a very premature age, brushes are more common in the rolandic region. When they achieve their highest expression, between the age of 32 and 34 weeks conceptional age, brushes are seen in the occipital, temporal, and rolandic regions. Frontal brushes are rare at any age. By the age of 1 month after term, brushes largely disappear as greater maturity emerges. *(Aminoff 86)*

13. **(D)** By 44 to 46 weeks of conceptual age, quiet sleep sheds its immature trace alternate pattern and establishes its mature foundation as continuous slow wave sleep. Sleep spindles appear from the midline or the central region. They are asynchronous between the 2 hemispheres and remain so until the age of 2 years. *(Spehlman, 175)*

14. **(D)** A full-term neonate expresses the following behavioral sleep states:

1. Waking state: the full-term neonate spends one-third of the time in this state. It is characterized by eye opening, body and facial movements, muscle activity, and irregular breathing.
2. Active sleep: the full-term neonate spends 50% to 60% of the time in this state. It is characterized by closed eyes, most of the time with occasional opening, slower facial and body movements, decreased muscle tone, and irregular respiration.
3. Quiet sleep represents 30% to 40% of sleep time with regular respiration, few body and face movements, and muscle tone similar to the waking state.
4. Transitional sleep. *(Spehlman, 165–170)*

15. **(C)** The photomyogenic response is a noncerebral response characterized by brief repetitive muscle spikes in the frontal leads with the same frequency as the flash stimulus. This may be associated with fluttering and twitching movements of the forehead and eyelid muscles. The photomyogenic response shows recruitment and ceases when the photic stimulus stops. It is most prominent when the eyes are closed, but can occur when the eyes are open. It is believed by some to represent a physiologic response to high-intensity light. *(Aminoff, 53–54)*

16. **(B)**

17. **(D)**

18. **(E)**

19. **(A)**

20. **(C)**

Explanations 16 through 20

Alpha activity refers to an activity in the range of 8–13 Hz, whereas alpha rhythm is 8–13 Hz activity occurring during wakefulness over the posterior head region, which is present when the eyes are closed and the patient relaxed, and is blocked by eye opening or alerting the patient. Bancaud phenomenon results from failure of alpha rhythm to block on one side of the brain. It indicates an abnormality on the side that fails to attenuate. Posterior slowing of youth consists of single 2–4 Hz triangular contoured slow waves (also called sail waves) interspersed with alpha activity over the posterior head regions and occurring maximally over the occipital head regions. Temporal transients consist of episodic slow-wave components ranging from 2 to 5 Hz, occurring singly or in brief trains over the temporal region. This is usually maximal over the mid-Sylvian area. Temporal transients are seen in normal subjects after the age of 40 with left side preponderance. They occur in about 35% of individuals between the fifth and sixth decades. They appear to be related to a normal aging process, although some studies suggest cerebrovascular ischemia as the origin of this activity. *(Spehlman, 215; Aminoff 42–43, 109)*

21. **(E)** Triphasic waves are 100 to 300 μV positive sharp waves, preceded and followed by lower amplitude negative waves. They are bilaterally synchronous, generalized in distribution, and usually predominant in the frontal region. Triphasic waves occur more commonly from hepatic encephalopathy than from other causes. They may occur in hypoglycemia, renal failure, hyponatremia, hypercalcemia, hyperthyroidism, drug intoxication, and anoxia. There is no specific EEG finding in hypoparathyroidism. EEG may show irregular high-voltage delta activity that is increased on hyperventilation. Paroxysmal abnormalities may also occur during wakefulness and sleep. *(Spehlman, 327)*

22. **(D)** Patients with anoxic encephalopathy exhibiting the following EEG patterns are gravely ill and may have a poor prognosis.

- The burst suppression pattern consists of generalized high voltage-mixed frequency waveforms of variable duration, usually with admixed spike and sharp waves.
- The periodic spikes or sharp waves are usually seen at a rate of 0.5 to 2 Hz. They are often associated with multifocal or bilateral myoclonus.

- The alpha coma pattern in cerebral anoxia describes monotonous unreactive alpha activity with diffuse and frontal predominance. This pattern carries a poor prognosis in anoxic encephalopathy.
- Bihemispheric periodic lateralized epileptiform discharges pattern carries also a poor prognosis. About 60% of patients showing this pattern do not recover.
- Delta brushes are seen in prematurity.

(Spehlman, 389–392; Prior 770)

23. **(A)** Dialysis dementia is a progressive condition that develops in patients on chronic hemodialysis. It is characterized by confusion, progressive dementia, dysarthria, myoclonus, and seizure. It is caused by toxic accumulation of aluminium in the brain. Hughes et al. found bilateral spike and wave complexes in 77% of patients with dialysis dementia. Based on the presence or absence of that pattern, 91% of the patients, along with 91% of their EEGs, were correctly placed by Hughes et al. into either clinical category of dialysis dementia or dialysis without chronic encephalopathy. *(Hughes and Schreeder, 1148–1154)*

24. **(B)** Benzodiazepines acutely induce widespread fast activity with a maximum in the central and frontal region. This persists during wakefulness until stages I and II of sleep and become more conspicuous when the alpha rhythm disappears. *(Spehlman, 428)*

25. **(B)** Rett syndrome is caused by mutations in the MECP2 gene, which is found on the X chromosome, occurs exclusively in girls, and has a prevalence of approximately 1/15,000 to 1/22,000. The hallmark of Rett syndrome is repetitive hand-wringing movements, loss of purposeful and spontaneous use of the hands; these may not appear until 2 to 3 years of age. Autistic behavior is a typical finding in all patients. Generalized tonic-clonic convulsions occur in the majority and are usually well controlled by anticonvulsants. The EEG in Rett syndrome has been extensively studied. In stage 1 of the disease the corresponding EEG is normal or may show minimal slowing of the background. In stage 2 corresponding to a rapid destructive stage, background slowing of the EEG is evident. Focal spikes or sharp waves, most commonly over the centroparietal regions, but sometimes bilateral, multifocal, or diffuse appear. By stage 3, or plateau stage, diffuse intermittent 2–4 Hz slow waves superimposed on background slowing. In stage 4, the motor deterioration stage, the EEG is dominated by monorhythmic 4–5 Hz activity, frequent multifocal, and generalized slow spike wave discharges in both waking and sleep stages. *(Behrman, 2034; Verma et al., 395–401)*

26. **(D)** Electrocerebral inactivity or electrocerebral silence is defined as no EEG activity of more than 2 μV when recording from scalp electrode pairs 10 cm or more apart with interelectrode impedances less than 10,000 ohm, but more than 100 ohm. 10 guidelines for EEG recordings are recommended:

    1. A minimum of 8 scalp electrodes should be utilized.
    2. Interelectrode impedances should be less than 10,000 ohm but more than 100 ohm.
    3. The integrity of the entire recording system should be tested.
    4. Interelectrode distances should be at least 10 cm.
    5. Sensitivity must be increased from 7 μV/mm to at least 2 μV/mm for at least 30 minutes of the recording, with inclusion of appropriate calibrations.
    6. Filter settings should be appropriate for the assessment of electrocerebral silence.
    7. Additional monitoring techniques should be employed when necessary.
    8. There should be no EEG reactivity to intense somatosensory, auditory, or visual stimuli.
    9. Recordings should be made only by a qualified technologist.
    10. A repeat EEG should be performed if there is doubt about electrocerebral silence.

    (Aminoff, 688)

27. **(B)** Hockaday et al. studied the EEG of patients with anoxic encephalopathy, and classified the abnormalities into 5 grades according to the final

outcome. The prognosis for patients belonging to grade 1 was favorable. Severity increases and prognosis worsens from grade 1 to grade 5. In Grade 1, the EEG shows reactive alpha rhythm with scattered theta activity. In stage 2, the EEG shows dominant theta activity with rare alpha activity. In stage 3, there is continuous polymorphic slow delta waves with little activity and faster frequency. In stage 4, there is invariant low amplitude delta activity unresponsive to stimulus or any activity with suppression interval of 1 second or more. Stage 5 shows nearly or completely isoelectric record. *(Hockaday et al., 575)*

28. **(A)** Alpha coma in patients with brain stem lesions is most commonly seen in vascular disease, with lesions noted in the ventral pons, sparing the brain stem tegmentum. This abnormal alpha rhythm tends to be more reactive than that seen after hypoxia or drug overdose and is most prominently seen over the posterior head region. *(Spehlman, 438)*

29. **(B)**

30. **(E)**

31. **(D)**

32. **(C)**

33. **(A)**

Explanations 29 through 33

Positive occipital sharp transients of sleep are monophasic triangular waves in the occipital regions. They may appear at the end of stage 1 of sleep in many subjects. Benign epileptiform transients of sleep are small sharp spikes seen mainly in adults during drowsiness. Unlike true epileptiform discharges, they do not distort the background activity. They go away in deeper levels of sleep. Wicket spikes are arc-like waves that typically occur in train. When they occur as a single waveform, they are often mistaken for a temporal spike. They are not associated with a subsequent slow wave and do not disrupt the background. Lambda waves occur over the occipital head regions when subjects are

engaged actively at something that arouses their interest. They appear to represent an evoked cerebral response to visual stimulus produced from shifts of images across the retina in the course of saccadic eye movements. Mu rhythm has been called rolandic alpha activity and consists of 7–11 Hz arc-shaped waveforms, usually unilateral, present over the central region. It seems to be related to functions of the sensorimotor cortex. It is not attenuated by eye opening but by active movement or the thought movement of the contralateral extremity. *(Spehlman, 191–197)*

34. **(F)**

35. **(A)**

36. **(C)**

37. **(I)**

38. **(B)**

39. **(H)**

40. **(D)**

41. **(G)**

42. **(E)**

Explanations 34 through 42

The clinical interpretation of the pattern reversal visual evoked potential is based on measurement of the latency of the cortical response from the P100 component, the major positive wave having a nominal latency of 100 ms in normal subjects.

The brain stem evoked potentials are signals generated in the auditory nerve and brain stem, following an acoustic stimulus. A normal brain stem evoked response has 5 waves. Waves I and II correspond to the activation of the distal and proximal part of the auditory nerve, respectively. Wave III corresponds to the activation of the superior olive and trapezoid body. The generators of wave IV and V are located in the upper pons and midbrain.

Median nerve somatosensory evoked potentials shows in normal cases, N9 generated at Erb's point, N14 generated in the cervicomedullary region, probably in the caudal medial lemniscus, and N20 in the cortical area processing the stimulus. Somatosensory evoked potential obtained from stimulation of the posterior tibial nerve shows N22 potential generated in the gray matter of the lumbar cord and P38 generated in the cortical area close to the leg representation. *(Aminoff, 421–536)*

43. **(D)**

44. **(B)**

45. **(C)**

46. **(E)**

47. **(A)**

Explanations 43 through 47

Sleep spindles and K complexes are seen in stage II or III of sleep. K complexes are simply a sharp vertex wave associated with a sleep spindle. Positive occipital transients of sleep are seen in deep stage I of sleep. In stage III of sleep, delta slowing is seen in 20% to 50% of sleep. The enhancement of the amplitude of beta activity in the presence of a skull defect is called a breach rhythm. Bancaud phenomenon results from failure of the alpha rhythm to attenuate by eye opening. *(Aminoff, 45–46, 54)*

48. **(E)** Nausea, vomiting, and gastrointestinal distress are among the most frequent adverse effects with valproic acid use. Other common side effects include weight gain in 50% of cases, hair loss, and a tremor in 10% of cases. Hyperammonemia may occur, usually asymptomatic but can cause encephalopathy in the absence of hepatic dysfunction. Mild to moderate hepatic dysfunction may occur in 40% of cases. It is dose related and reversible. Fatal hepatitis may occur as an idiosyncratic reaction, especially in children under the age of 2 years on multiple antiseizure medications.

Acute pancreatitis can be induced by valproic acid in children more than adults. Aplastic anemia is seen after treatment with felbamate. *(Bazil and Pedley 1998, 135–162; Dichter and Brodie, 1531–1590)*

49. **(B)** Carbamazepine has poor solubility in water, a factor that inhibited the development of a parenteral form for clinical use. Carbamazepine is metabolized by the liver. Its pharmacokinetics are characterized by the phenomenon of autoinduction of hepatic microsomal enzymes. In naïve patients, introduction of the drug is associated with a half-life of 30 hours, decreasing within days to weeks to 10–20 hours. Low dose of the drug should be introduced first, then slowly increased to avoid toxicity when starting the treatment. Skin rash occurs in 15% of patients with carbamazepine, whereas it occurs in only 10% of patients with phenytoin. Carbamazepine has a slight antidiuretic effect, which may result in mild to moderate hyponatremia. Mild elevation of hepatic enzymes may occur with carbamazepine use in 5% to 10% of cases. This elevation neither predicts nor predisposes to hepatitis, which is presumed to be an immune hypersensitivity reaction. *(Bazil and Pedley 1998, 135–162)*

50. **(B)** Levetiracetam is not extensively metabolized in humans. The major metabolic pathway is the enzymatic hydrolysis of the acetamide group, which produces the carboxylic acid metabolite (24%) and is not dependent on any of the liver cytochrome P450 isoenzymes. The major metabolite is inactive in animal seizure models. Its plasma half-life in adults is 7 ± 1 hour and is unaffected by either dose or repeated administration. It is eliminated from systemic circulation by renal excretion as unchanged drug, which represents 66% of administered dose. The mechanism of excretion is glomerular filtration with subsequent partial tubular reabsorption. Levetiracetam elimination is correlated to creatinine clearance. Levetiracetam clearance is reduced in patients with impaired renal function.

Zonisamide is 70% metabolized by the liver. Topiramite is 30% metabolized by the liver, whereas lamotrigine and tiagabine are more than 90% metabolized by the liver. *(Patsalos, 123–129)*

51. **(C)** Phenytoin has zero-order kinetics. This means that its process of utilization is not linear. The plasma drug concentration and clearance are independent of drug dose. Furthermore, in this case, one cannot reliably predict the time that will be required for phenytoin concentration to fall into the therapeutic range. *(Bazil and Pedley 1998, 135–162)*

52. **(B)** The patient described in the therapeutic vignette has early symptoms of carbamazepine intoxication. The therapeutic level of carbamazepine is explained by the phenomenon of autoinduction of the drug from its own metabolism by hepatic microsomal enzymes. The patient was started initially on a full dose of the drug, which caused signs of carbamazepine intoxication. Autoinduction of the drug decreases its serum level to a therapeutic range and improves the clinical symptoms. It is recommended that carbamazepine be started at a low dose (100 mg po bid) and increased progressively. *(Bazil and Pedley, 2003, 38–52)*

53. **(C)** Lamotrigine was originally developed because of an observation that some anticonvulsants have antifolate properties. Although lamotrigine weakly inhibits dihydrofolate reductase, there is no correlation between this activity and its anticonvulsant action. Lamotrigine is about 55% bound to protein. It undergoes extensive liver metabolism. Its rate of elimination is influenced by concomitant administration of hepatic inhibitors or inducers. When given in monotherapy, the elimination half-life is about 25 hours. When it is given with enzyme inducers (carbamazepine, phenytoin, phenobarbital) its half-life is reduced to 15 hours. When given with an enzyme inhibitor (valproic acid), the half-life increases to 60 hours. Rash may complicate lamotrigine administration in 10% of cases. It acts through prolonging inactivation of voltage-sensitive sodium channels. *(Bazil and Pedley, 2003, 38–52*

54. **(C)** Phenytoin has minimal renal excretion and does not require adjustment in case of renal failure. Ethosuximide has renal excretion of 10% to 20%. A decrease of 25% of the regular dose is needed if the glomerular filtration is less than 10 ml/min. Phenobarbital has a renal excretion of 25% to 30%. Dose interval needs to be increased by 50% to 100% in case of renal failure. Carbamazepine has minimal renal excretion but its dose needs to be decreased by 25% in case of renal failure with glomerular filtration less than 10 ml/min. Topiramate has renal excretion of 70%. A decrease in the regular dose by 50% is needed in case of renal failure or dialysis. *(Bazil and Pedley 2003, 38–52)*

55. **(D)** All these drugs are removed by dialysis except phenytoin. In case of phenytoin overdose, forced fluid diuresis, peritoneal dialysis, exchange transfusion, hemodialysis, and plasmapheresis are ineffective. They produce little renal elimination and a danger of fluid overload. *(Bazil and Pedley 2003, 38–52)*

56. **(B)** West syndrome is an age-dependent epilepsy with a characteristic EEG pattern known as hypsarrhythmia, infantile spasms, and psychomotor retardation. Infantile spasms occur in 24 to 42 of 100,000 births. Spasms and psychomotor retardation appear in the first year of life in 85% of cases, the majority between 3 and 7 months. Associated abnormalities include generalized hypotonicity, microcephaly, paralysis, ataxia, blindness, and deafness. The typical EEG reveals hypsarrhythmia, a chaotic pattern of high-amplitude, slow waves with multifocal epileptiform discharges, and poor interhemispheric synchrony. ACTH is the treatment of choice for infantile spasm. The dose and duration of steroid therapy has not been standardized. The most common treatment is ACTH 40IU per day administered intramuscularly. Approximately 75% of patients achieve initial seizure control using this regimen. The response rate tends to increase with duration of therapy. Within 2 months of remission, however, approximately 30% to 50% of patients suffer relapse after the first course of steroids. *(Goetz, 1070–1072)*

57. **(E)**

58. **(B)**

59. **(F)**

60. **(D)**

61. **(A)**

62. **(C)**

63. **(G)**

64. **(I)**

Explanations 57 through 64

Gabapentin is typically well tolerated. The most common side effects are headache, fatigue, ataxia, and somnolence. The main limitation of phenobarbital use is its propensity to alter cognition, mood, and behavior. The drug can cause fatigue in adults, and insomnia, hyperactivity, and aggression in children (and sometimes in the elderly). Memory, mood, and learning capacity may be subtly impaired. Depression, arthritic changes, and Dupuytren's contracture can be associated problems.

The most common side effects of lamotrigine are headache, nausea and vomiting, dizziness, diplopia, and ataxia. Tremor can be troublesome at high dosages. In up to 10% of patients in add-on trials, a rash may develop, which subsequently disappears in some patients, despite continued therapy. In a few patients, however, the rash is more serious, and fever, arthralgias, and eosinophilia occur. In rare cases (less than 1%) Stevens-Johnson syndrome develops. The concomitant administration of valproic acid with lamotrigine may increase the likelihood of a serious rash; the gradual introduction of lamotrigine may lower the likelihood of skin reactions. The common side effects of valproic acid are dose-related tremor, weight gain due to appetite stimulation, thinning or loss of hair (usually temporary), and menstrual irregularities, including amenorrhea. Sedation is unusual, although stupor and encephalopathy occur in rare cases. The incidence of hepatotoxic effects, histologically evident as a microvesicular steatosis, is less than 1 in 20,000 patients, but such effects are of concern in children under 3 years of age who are receiving multiple antiepileptic drugs. Approximately 20% of all patients receiving the drug have hyperammonemia without hepatic damage. This effect is usually asymptomatic but occasionally can cause confusion, nausea, and vomiting.

Phenytoin can cause a range of dose-related and idiosyncratic adverse effects. Reversible cosmetic changes (gum hypertrophy, acne, hirsutism, and facial coarsening), although often mild, can be troublesome. Neurotoxic symptoms (drowsiness, dysarthria, tremor, ataxia, and cognitive difficulties) may occur when the plasma drug concentration exceeds 20 µg/mL. Cerebellar atrophy may occur with chronic use.

Carbamazepine can cause a range of idiosyncratic reactions; the most common is a morbilliform rash, which develops in about 10% of patients. Less common skin eruptions include erythema multiforme and Stevens-Johnson syndrome. Reversible mild leukopenia is common but does not generally require discontinuation of therapy. Blood dyscrasias and toxic hepatitis are rare. At high plasma concentrations, carbamazepine has an antidiuretic hormone-like action; the resulting hyponatremia is usually mild and asymptomatic, but if the plasma sodium concentration falls below 125 mmol/L, there may be confusion, peripheral edema, and decreasing control of seizures. Orofacial dyskinesias and cardiac arrhythmias are additional rare side effects.

Felbamate may cause aplastic anemia and hepatic toxicity. Zonisamide is a weak carbonic anhydrase inhibitor, which is probably responsible for increased incidences of symptomatic renal stones, although in clinical trials, the rate was similar to placebo. (*Brodie and Dichter,168–175; Dichter and Brodie, 1583–1590*)

65. **(B)** Carbamazepine, valproic acid, and phenytoin are not removed by dialysis. (*Bazil and Pedley, 2003, 38–52*)

66. **(A)** Tiagabine acts as an inhibitor of GABA reuptake into presynaptic nerve terminals. Because GABA is a major inhibitory neurotransmitter in the central nervous system, the increase of available GABA through this mechanism may be responsible for tiagabine anticonvulsant action. *(Bazil and Pedley 2003, 38–52)*

67. **(B)** The overall risk of having a baby with a major malformation is about 2% to 3% in healthy populations. This is increased to 5% to 6% in women with epilepsy taking a single antiepileptic drug, perhaps to 6% to 7% if the drug is carbamazepine or valproic acid. This rate may be doubled by the use of 2 or more drugs or by a very high plasma level of antiepileptic drugs. *(Bazil and Pedley 2003, 38–52)*

68. **(C)** Many drugs may increase phenytoin levels. Serum level determinations for phenytoin are especially helpful when possible drug interactions are suspected. Drugs that may increase phenytoin serum levels include: acute alcohol intake, amiodarone, chloramphenicol, chlordiazepoxide, diazepam, dicumarol, disulfiram, estrogens, H2-antagonists, halothane, isoniazid, methylphenidate, phenothiazines, phenylbutazone, salicylates, succinimides, sulfonamides, tolbutamide, and trazodone. *(Bazil and Pedley, 2003, 38–52)*

69. **(D)** Theophylline, a CYP3A4 inducer, can increase carbamazepine metabolism, resulting in the potential for decreased plasma carbamazepine levels. *(Bazil and Pedley 2003, 38–52)*

70. **(E)** Barbiturates and benzodiazepines are potent beta activators Chloral hydrate is also another activator of beta activity. Occasionally neuroleptics, antidepressants, and antihistamines can also increase beta activity in routine EEG. Drug-induced beta activity is usually slower than physiologic beta. *(Spehlman, 428–429)*

71. **(E)** Periodic lateralizing epileptiform discharges (PLEDs) are EEG patterns showing complexes consisting of di- or polyphasic spike or sharp waves. They commonly appear in a wide distribution on one side of the head. They are uni- or bilateral but with clear maximum on one side. Clinical conditions causing PLEDs are mainly acute cerebral infarcts, but also encephalitis, cerebral tumors, meningitis, cerebral abscess and other conditions causing acute destruction of an area of the brain. PLEDs usually disappear after days or weeks from the acute phase of the damage. *(Spehlman, 321)*

72. **(D)** Amino acids have been separated into two general classes: excitatory amino acids and inhibitory amino acids. The former group depolarizes neurons in mammalian cells and is formed by aspartic acid, cysteic acid, glutamic acid, and homocysteic acid. The latter group hyperpolarizes neurons in mammals and is formed by GABA, glycine, taurine, and beta-alanine. *(Cooper, 126)*

73. **(B)** Hyperventilation is an activation procedure used to bring out focal slowing or epileptiform abnormalities. The incidence and intensity of hyperventilation response depend on age, blood sugar level, and cerebral oxygen supply. Hyperventilation responses are most common and most extensive in children and teenagers. In children, spike and wave discharges of 3 Hz are particularly seen in absence seizures and are particularly sensitive to hyperventilation, and in many cases appear only during this procedure. The 8-year-old boy with episodes of staring most likely has absence seizures. Hyperventilation may be the only procedure to induce spike and waves, considering his age and the type of seizure that this patient is most likely to have. *(Spehlman, 219–222)*

74. **(D)** REM parasomnias usually occur in middle-aged or elderly patients, and show a marked male predominance. They are due to a lack of normal atonia of REM sleep. Consequently, they occur more often in the later portion of sleep. During REM sleep, patients may have an increase in the severity or the frequency of fragmentary myoclonus. Although REM sleep behavior disorders may occur in healthy elderly subjects, they are also seen with tricyclics, alcohol abuse, or central nervous system diseases affecting the pathways controlling REM atonia, such as multisystem atrophy. REM parasomnias, like other REM

sleep disorders, respond well to clonazepam. *(Duncan, 21)*

75. **(C)** Absence seizures usually occur in childhood or early adulthood, whereas complex partial seizures occur at any age. Absence seizures are idiopathic and generalized, while complex partial seizures can be cryptogenic or caused by focal pathology. The duration of attacks is short in absence seizures, less than 30 seconds, while it is longer in cases of complex partial seizures. There is no postictal state in absence seizures, whereas in complex partial seizures confusion, emotional disturbance or headaches usually occur in the postictal state. The EEG may show spikes and slow waves induced by hyperventilation or, less frequently, by photic stimulation in absence seizures. Photosensitivity induces spikes and waves in only 10% to 30% of cases in absence seizures. In complex partial seizures, photic stimulation does not induce seizure activity on EEG, while hyperventilation has a modest effect. *(Duncan, 35)*

76. **(D)** There is a considerable overlap between the clinical and EEG features of mesio-basal and lateral temporal lobe epilepsy. In lateral temporal seizures there is usually a detectable underlying structural pathology like glioma, angioma, hamartoma, neural migration defect, and posttraumatic changes. There is no association with a history of febrile seizure. Consciousness may be preserved longer than in mesial temporal epilepsy. Typical aura includes structured hallucination of visual, auditory, gustatory, or olfactory forms. Illusion of size, shape, weight, distance, or sound may occur. Automatisms may occur unilaterally and have more motor manifestations than mesial temporal epilepsy. Motor arrest or absence is most often seen in mesial temporal epilepsy. Postictal phenomena and autonomic changes may occur in both mesial and lateral temporal epilepsy. *(Duncan, 44–46)*

77. **(B)** The clinical and EEG features of frontal lobe seizures overlap with complex partial seizures of temporal lobe origin. Nevertheless, there are a number of core features that are strongly suggestive of frontal lobe origin.

Typically, the seizures are frequent with marked tendency to cluster. A brief nonspecific cephalic aura may occur, which is a vague sensation of dizziness, strangeness, and headache. Automatisms are present. They are typical gestural, highly excited, violent, or bizarre, leading to misdiagnosis of nonepileptic attacks. Postictal recovery is rapid, with a shorter period of postictal confusion than in temporal epilepsy. Frontal lobe seizures are more likely to secondarily generalize than partial seizures of temporal lobe origin. The EEG in frontal lobe epilepsy may be normal ictally or interictally, partially because of the large area of frontal cortex covered by the relatively few scalp electrodes and the inaccessibility of scalp electrodes to the medial and inferior frontal lobe surfaces. *(Duncan, 47)*

78. **(A)** Epilepsy, although a relatively common symptom of cerebral degenerative diseases, is seldom the predominant clinical problem. Seizures develop in up to 33% of cases of Alzheimer's disease, late in the course of the illness. Pick disease rarely causes seizures. Epilepsy occurs in 5% of cases of Huntington disease, especially in late stages and juvenile rigid form. Epilepsy occurs in 6% of cases of Wilson disease and may be the presenting feature. *(Duncan, 55–56)*

79. **(B)** Reflex seizures are attacks precipitated by a specific stimulus, such as touch, musical tune, a particular movement, reading, stroboscopic light patterns, or complex visual images. The most common reflex epilepsies are those induced by visual stimuli such as flashing lights and moving patterns. The other answers mentioned cause seizures less frequently. *(Duncan, 66–67)*

80. **(D)** West syndrome is defined by the clinical triad of infantile spasms, arrest of psychomotor development, and hypsarrhythmia on EEG. Its incidence is estimated to be 1 per 4,000–6,000 live births. The identified causes of infantile spasms are divided into prenatal (cerebral dysgenesis, genetic disorders, intrauterine infection), perinatal (anoxic injury, head trauma, infection), and postnatal (metabolic disorders, trauma, infection). No etiology (cryptogenic)

can be identified in as many as 40% of cases. The onset of almost all cases occurs before age 1 year, with peak onset between 3 and 7 months of age. The spasms occur in clusters and are characterized by sudden flexor or extensor movements of the trunk. They have a myoclonic quality but are somewhat longer in duration. Developmental arrest and regression begins with or before the spasms. EEG shows hypsarrhythmia on interictal EEG recordings. In the waking record, hypsarrhythmia consists of disorganized high-voltage slow waves, spikes, and sharp waves that occur diffusely with a somewhat posterior predominance.

The prognosis for children with infantile spasms is extremely poor. Although the spasms cease, 70% to 90% of infants develop mental retardation and 35% to 60% have chronic epilepsy. However, the major determinant of outcome is the underlying cause of the spasms. Only 5% of children develop normally, and these are mainly from the cryptogenic group. Corticosteroids, in the form of adrenocorticotropic hormone (ACTH), prednisone, or prednisolone, are the treatment of choice for infantile spasms. Benzodiazepines, in the form of clonazepam, provide some benefit but are not as effective as corticosteroids. Valproic acid is also effective, but the risk of hepatotoxicity in this age group must be considered. Vigabatrin has been used to treat infantile spasms effectively. *(Bradley, 1757–1758; Duncan, 73–74)*

81. **(C)** Rolandic epilepsy is a well-defined childhood syndrome accounting for up to 15% of all childhood epilepsies. The age of onset is between 3 and 13 years with a peak incidence between 5 and 10 years. The seizures are typically focal, involving the face and oropharynx, often with secondary generalization, and have a strong tendency to occur during sleep. The motor phenomena are usually associated with sensory disturbances and with clonic unilateral jerking of the upper limb. In about two-thirds of patients, secondarily generalized tonic-clonic seizures occur, almost always during sleep. There is generally no associated neurological abnormality, and intellect is usually normal. The diagnosis of rolandic epilepsy

can be made by the typical clinical features and confirmed by characteristic EEG findings. These consist of remarkably focal high-amplitude mid-temporal spikes or spike wave discharges. There is a striking contrast between the active EEG and the benign clinical picture. The prognosis of rolandic epilepsy is good. Only 10% of patients will continue to have seizures 5 years after onset of the disease. *(Duncan, 78–79)*

82. **(D)** Lennox-Gastaut syndrome is responsible for 2% to 3% of childhood epilepsies. The syndrome is characterized by multiple seizure types, slow spike-wave complexes, and diffuse cognitive dysfunction. Seizure onset ranges from 1 to 8 years of age, with a peak incidence between 3 and 5 years of age. Fifty percent of cases have severe mental retardation, preceding the onset of seizures 20% to 60% of the time. In addition, disturbances of behavior and personality are common. The EEG reveals 2.0–2.5 Hz slow spike-wave complexes and multifocal spikes superimposed on abnormal background activity. The complexes are rarely induced by hyperventilation or photic stimulation. Seizures may be precipitated by drowsiness or stimulation. In general, seizures respond poorly to anticonvulsant treatment, and polytherapy is usually required. Benzodiazepines and valproic acid are the most effective agents, although the former may precipitate tonic status. Sedation should be minimized because of the tendency for seizures to increase in sleep. Phenytoin and rectal diazepam are effective for serial tonic seizures and status epilepticus. Refractory cases may benefit from the ketogenic diet or corpus callosotomy, which reduces tonic and atonic seizures in some cases. *(Goetz, 1072–1073)*

83. **(B)** Absence seizures begin between the ages of 3 and 12 years. Patients are more commonly female than male and there is a strong genetic predisposition. Monozygotic twins develop absences in 75% of pairs, as do 5% of dizygotic twins. Typical absence seizure is characterized by sudden behavioral arrest and unresponsiveness that may be accompanied by eyelid or facial clonus; automatisms; and autonomic,

tonic, or atonic features. The interictal EEG in patients with typical absence seizures reveals generalized 3.0 Hz spike-wave complexes superimposed on normal background activity. Bursts of generalized 3.0 to 4.0 Hz spike-wave complexes slowing to 2.5 to 3.0 Hz are observed during seizures. Typical absence seizures are commonly precipitated by hyperventilation and infrequently by photic stimulation. The prognosis of absence seizure is good. Absences become less frequent through adolescence and about 80% remit by adulthood. *(Duncan, 84–85; Goetz, 1063–1064)*

84. **(A)** Progressive myoclonic epilepsies represent a group of disorders of various etiology that collectively account for 1% of all epilepsy syndromes. The natural history varies with the specific disorder from mild neurological impairment to severe disability progressing to death in early childhood.

The disorders comprising the progressive myoclonic epilepsies may be classified into the following categories: (1) those with well-defined biochemical defects such as sialidosis; (2) those with a known pathological or biochemical marker yet poorly defined mechanism, such as Lafora disease and myoclonic epilepsy with ragged-red fibers; (3) the degenerative diseases such as Unverricht-Lundborg disease (Baltic myoclonus) and dentatorubro-pallidoluysian atrophy.

Juvenile myoclonic epilepsy is distinct from progressive myoclonic epilepsy. It usually appears around puberty and is characterized by seizures with bilateral, single or repetitive arrhythmic, irregular, myoclonic jerks, predominantly in the arms. Jerks may cause some patients to fall suddenly. No disturbance of consciousness is noticeable. The disorder may be inherited and sex distribution is equal. Often there are generalized tonic-clonic and, less often, infrequent absences. The seizures usually occur after awakening and are often precipitated by sleep deprivation. Interictal and ictal EEG have rapid, generalized, often irregular spike waves and polyspike waves; there is no close phase correlation between EEG spikes and jerks. Frequently, the patients are photosensitive. Response to

appropriate drugs is good. *(Duncan, 90–92; Goetz, 1073–1074)*

85. **(A)**

86. **(B)**

87. **(E)**

88. **(C)**

89. **(D)**

90. **(F)**

Explanations 85 through 90

The key EEG features of idiopathic generalized epilepsy are: generalized epileptiform discharges that often have a 3 Hz frequency; usually maximum in the anterior parasagittal regions, normal background, and often photosensitive. Photic stimulation may induce occipital spikes, occipital spikes and slow waves with frontal or parieto-occipital regions, and generalized spike and slow-wave discharges. Temporal lobe epilepsy is characterized in the EEG interictally by spikes that are usually maximum over the temporal or frontotemporal regions. The ictal scalp EEG often shows rhythmic theta at the onset that may be bilateral or localized in the affected temporal lobe. In benign occipital epilepsy, the EEG shows posterior 1.5–3 Hz spike and slow-wave discharges, singly or in long runs, may be lateralized, and usually attenuate with eye opening. In infantile spasms, the resting EEG shows a characteristic disorganized high voltage pattern, with generalized attenuation during spasms. This pattern may be seen unilaterally or bilaterally. Benign rolandic epilepsy is characterized by unilateral or bilateral triphasic, large amplitude spikes that are maximum in the central or centrotemporal, without background abnormalities. In Lennox-Gastaut syndrome, the background EEG is usually slow and disorganized, with superimposed 1–2.5 Hz generalized, anteriorly predominant, spike and slow-wave discharges. *(Duncan, 115–119)*

91. (E)

92. (J)

93. (F)

94. (C)

95. (H)

96. (D)

97. (B)

98. (I)

99. (A)

100. (G)

Explanations 91 through 100

GM2 gangliosidosis is an autosomal recessive condition caused by a deficit in the activity of hexosaminidase A. Its clinical picture includes seizures, dementia, blindness, and cherry-red spot in the retina. GM1 gangliosidosis usually presents with failure to thrive in infants, hepatosplenomegaly, mental regression, and seizures. Later onset forms result in seizures, cognitive decline, spasticity, extrapyramidal rigidity, and ataxia. The key diagnostic test is reduced leukocyte beta-galactosidase activity. Niemann-Pick disease is characterized in type A by infant hepatosplenomegaly, slow development, loss of skills, spasticity, and seizures. In type C, Niemann-Pick disease is characterized by tonic-clonic seizures, ataxia, and dementia. Sphyngomyelinase activity in both types is deficient. Although in type C, an impairment of cholestorol esterification is believed to be the primary problem. In Gaucher's disease, the beta-galactocerebrosidase activity is reduced in leukocytes.

Sialidosis is a complex of two types of autosomal recessive disorders associated with deficiencies of N-acetylneuraminidase. Clinical picture includes myoclonic and generalized tonic-clonic seizures, dementia, and visual failure.

Lafora disease usually presents with the phenotype of progressive myoclonic epilepsy with cerebellar ataxia, dementia, and personality changes. Death occurs within 10 to 15 years from the onset. Lafora's bodies consist of polyglucosans and are found in peripheral nerve, liver, and muscle.

Adrenoleukodystrophy is a disorder with several clinically and genetically distinct forms. It is a progressive disease with symptoms referable to myelin loss from the central nervous system and peripheral nerves as well as adrenal insufficiency. In general, forms with earlier onset have a more rapid course. The X-linked form usually presents in the early school years with neurologic symptoms and adrenal insufficiency. The disease is rapidly progressive and fatal. In individuals with later onset, the course is more protracted, and when it develops in adults, it is usually a slowly progressive disorder with predominantly peripheral nerve involvement developing for a period of decades. The adrenoleukodystrophy gene encodes a member of the ATP-binding transporter family of proteins. The disease is characterized by the inability to properly catabolize very long chain fatty acids within peroxisomes because of deficit of lignoceroyl CoA, with elevation of levels of very long chain fatty acids in serum.

Metachromatic leukodystrophy is transmitted in an autosomal recessive pattern and results from a deficiency of arylsulfatase A. Enzyme deficiency leads to an accumulation of the sulfatides, especially cerebroside sulfate. The gene for arylsulfatase A has been localized to chromosome 22q, and a wide range of mutations has been described.

Krabbe disease or globoid cell leukodystrophy is a rare autosomal recessive neurodegenerative disorder characterized by severe myelin loss and the presence of globoid bodies in the white matter. The gene for Krabbe disease is located on chromosome 14q24.3-q32.1. The disease results from a marked deficiency of the lysosomal enzyme galactocerebroside beta-galactosidase.

Canavan's disease, an autosomal recessive disorder characterized by spongy degeneration of the white matter of the brain, leads to a severe form of leukodystrophy. The cause of the disease is a deficit of the enzyme aspartoacylase which leads to the accumulation of N-acetylaspartic acid in the brain. *(Behrman, 2030–2932; Duncan, 160–164; Goetz, 1074)*

101. (E)

102. (C)

103. (B)

104. (A)

105. (D)

Explanations 101 through 105

Menkes' disease is an X-linked disorder of copper metabolism. Clinically, it is characterized by failure to thrive, hypotonia, seizure, ataxia, and extrapyramidal signs. Plasma copper and ceruloplasmin are low. In Wilson's disease, seizures occur in about 6% of cases, and may be associated with disorder of movement, psychiatric and behavioral derangements, and impaired cognition. A slit lamp examination of the cornea shows Kayser-Fleischer ring, which is a peripheral corneal deposition of copper involving Descemet's membrane. In non-ketotic hyperglycinemia, severe epilepsy and mental retardation with abnormal EEG are the key features. Glycine concentration is very high in plasma and urine without ketosis or acidosis. Reduced glycine cleavage enzyme activity is demonstrated in liver biopsy. MELAS syndrome is a mitochondrial disease caused by a defect in respiratory chain enzyme deficiencies. Carbamazepine inhibits uroporphyrinogen-1 synthase, which increases the frequency of seizures in case of porphyria, a condition caused by a defect in uroporphyrinogen-1 synthase, coproporphyrinogen oxidase and protoporphyrine oxydase in erythrocytes. *(Duncan, 165–166)*

106. (B) Carbamazepine increases the rate of metabolism of steroid hormones by inducing the activity of hepatic microsomal enzymes. This will reduce the plasma estrogen level in women taking carbamazepine and birth control pills. As a consequence, there is a reduction of contraceptive efficacy. Vigabatrin, valproate, benzodiazepines, and gabapentin do not induce hepatic enzymes. *(Duncan, 268)*

107. (D) The nature of the underlying pathology is a key determinant of outcome of epilepsy surgery. Small low-grade glioma, dysembryolastic neuroepithelial tumors and small cryptic vascular malformations carry the best prognosis for epilepsy surgery, with about 70% to 80% of cases being rendered seizure-free following adequate resection. In MRI based study, 62% of patients with hippocampal sclerosis become seizure-free after surgery. Large or complex vascular malformations, particularly if they have bled and resulted in deposition of haemosiderin, or traumatic injuries, have a poorer prognosis after epilepsy surgery with less than 50% of patients rendered seizure-free. Cortical dyplasia carries a poor prognosis for surgery, presumably because such abnormalities represent a more diffuse process than is usually apparent. Only a small percent of patients with gross cortical dysplasia become seizure-free following epilepsy surgery. *(Duncan, 359–360)*

108. (D)

109. (B)

110. (E)

111. (A)

112. (C)

Explanations 108 through 112

The characteristic polysomnographic findings in REM behavior disorder (RBD) consists of the absence of muscle atonia and the presence of increased EMG activity in the upper and lower limbs. In multiple system atrophy, polysomnography shows a reduction of slow-wave, REM, and total sleep time, increased sleep latency, and increased number of awakenings during sleep.

In restless leg syndrome, polysomnography documents sleep disturbance and periodic limb movements in sleep, which is found in at least 80% of patients. Diagnosis of periodic limb movements in sleep is based on the periodic limb movements in sleep index (number of periodic limb movements in sleep per hour of sleep), periodic limb movements in sleep of up to 5 is considered normal. High periodic limb movements in sleep index with arousal is more significant than the index without arousal. Narcolepsia is a disorder that rarely begins before adolescence and is characterized by paroxysmal attacks of irrepressible daytime sleep, which is sometimes associated with transient loss of muscle tone. Overnight polysomnography findings include short sleep latency, excessive disruption of sleep with frequent arousals, reduced total sleep time, excessive body movements, and reduced slow-wave sleep.

In Alzheimer's disease (AD), the essential features of sleep architectural alterations are reduced total sleep time, decreased REM and slow-wave sleep, reduction of sleep spindles and K complexes, increased nighttime awakenings, and sleep fragmentation. There is a high frequency of sleep apnea in those with AD compared with age-matched controls. (*Bradley, 1807–1814*)

113. (F)

114. (G)

115. (B)

116. (C)

117. (E)

118. (D)

119. (A)

Explanations 113 through 119

EEG1 shows generalized paroxysmal fast activity that may be seen in porencephaly. Reduced EEG amplitude, focal slow waves, and focal epileptiform activity over areas of atrophic brain may be also seen. EEG2 shows a pattern of discontinuous background activity with a series of bursts separated by lower voltage interburst periods. This is characteristic of trace discontinu, a normal EEG pattern for a 29-week-old premature baby.

Hypsarrhythmia corresponds to the EEG pattern seen in EEG3. It is a disorganized EEG background seen in west syndrome. EEG4 shows K complexes, which are diphasic waves consisting of an initial sharply contoured transient followed by a high amplitude slow wave, usually of delta frequency. EEG5 shows 3 Hz burst of spikes and waves that may be seen in typical absence seizure. EEG6 shows a pattern of positive occipital transient, which are surface positive bisynchronous sharp transient. They occur in stage I of sleep. EEG7 shows triphasic waves, a pattern seen in hepatic failure, renal failure, and drug intoxication. (*Spehlman, 327; 31; 175; 201–205; 254–255*)

REFERENCES

Aminoff MJ. *Electrodiagnosis in Clinical Neurology.* 4th ed. New York, NY: Churchill Livingstone; 1999.

Bazil CW, Pedley TA. Advances in the medical treatment of epilepsy. *Annu Rev Med.* 1998;49:135–162.

Bazil CW, Pedley TA. Clinical pharmacology of Antiepileptic Drugs. *Clin Neuropharmacol.* 2003;26:38–52.

Cooper JR, Bloom FE, Roth RH. *The Biochemical Basis of Neuropharmacology.* 7th ed. New York, NY: Oxford University Press; 1996.

Dichter MA. Brodie MJ. New antiepileptic drugs. *N Engl J Med.* 1996;334:1583–1590.

Duncan JS, Shorvon SD, Fish DR. *Clinical Epilepsy.* New York, NY: Churchill Livingstone; 1995.

Goetz CG, Pappert EJ. *Textbook of Clinical Neurology,* 1st ed. Philadelphia, Pa: WB Saunders; 1999.

Hockaday JM, Potts F, Epstein E, et. al. Electroencephalographic changes in acute cerebral anoxia from cardiac or respiratory arrest. *Electroencephalogr Clin Neurophysiol.* 1965;575:1965.

Hughes JR, Schreeder MT. EEG in dialysis encephalopathy. *Neurology.* 1980;30:1148–1154.

Lombroso CT. Quantified electrographic scales on 10 preterm healthy newborns followed up to 40–43 weeks of conceptional age by serial polygraphic recordings. *Electroencephalogr Clin Neurophysiol.* 1979;46:460–74.

Patsalos PN. The pharmacokinetic characteristics of levetiracetam. *Methods Find Exp Clin Pharmacol.* 2003;25:123–129.

Prior PF. Scott DF. Outcome after severe brain damage. *Lancet.* 1073;1:770.

Spehlman R. *EEG primer.* Elsevier/North-Holland Biomedical. Amsterdam; 1981.

Verma, NP, Chheda, RL, Nigro MA, Hart ZH. Electroencephalographic findings in Rett syndrome. *Electroencephalogr Clin Neurophysiol.* 1986;64:394–401.

CHAPTER 5

Neuromuscular Diseases
Questions

Questions 1 through 5
Link each of the following spontaneous muscle activities to the appropriate definition.

(A) End-plate noise
(B) End-plate spike
(C) Fibrillation
(D) Positive sharp wave
(E) Myotonia

1. Regularly occurring spikes firing at 0.5–10 Hz with a sound similar to rain on a tin roof and an initial positive deflection. They are not specific for muscle fiber damage.

2. The spike is formed by an initial brief positive wave, followed by a slow negative phase. It may be seen in cases of denervation.

3. Low-amplitude, monophasic potentials fire at 20–40 Hz and have a characteristic hissing sound on EMG.

4. Spikes are waxing and waning in both amplitude and frequency.

5. Brief, irregular spikes have a negative initial deflection and a crackling sound on EMG.

Questions 6 through 9
Link the following.

(A) Complex repetitive discharge
(B) Fasciculation
(C) Myokymia
(D) Neuromyotonia

6. There is a spontaneous involuntary discharge of an individual motor unit.

7. They are 150 Hz decrementing discharges of a single motor unit that have a characteristic pinging sound on EMG.

8. It occurs from depolarization of a single muscle fiber, followed by ephaptic spread to adjacent denervated fibers.

9. They are rhythmically grouped repetitive discharges of the same motor unit, often noted in radiation plexitis.

10. Which of the following needle EMG parameters is seen in acute neuropathic axonal damage?

(A) Increased duration of the motor unit action potential
(B) Increased amplitude of the motor unit action potential
(C) Increased phases of the motor unit action potential
(D) Decreased activation of the motor unit action potential
(E) Decreased interference pattern on maximum voluntary effort

11. On needle EMG, early recruitment of the motor unit action potential is seen in the case of

(A) stroke
(B) chronic inflammatory demyelinating polyneuropathy
(C) acute inflammatory demyelinating polyneuropathy
(D) acute myopathy
(E) early reinnervation following severe denervation

12. Which of the following conditions is commonly associated with type I muscle fiber atrophy?

   (A) Corticosteroid-induced myopathy
   (B) Myotonic muscular dystrophy
   (C) Hyperthyroidism myopathy
   (D) Disuse atrophy
   (E) Upper motor neuron disease

13. Which of the following is NOT characteristic of myotonic muscular dystrophy?

   (A) The mutation in the myotonic dystrophy gene is an extension of the trinucleotide CTG.
   (B) The abnormal gene is located on chromosome 19.
   (C) Cardiac conduction abnormalities are rarely seen.
   (D) Testicular atrophy is seen in 60% of cases with myotonic dystrophy.
   (E) Excessive daytime sleepiness is the most common nonmuscular symptom.

14. The third cranial (oculomotor) nerve is most frequently affected in cases of

   (A) diphtheria
   (B) sarcoidosis
   (C) diabetes mellitus
   (D) Lyme disease
   (E) porphyria

15. The most frequent cranial nerve affected in diabetes mellitus is the

   (A) abducens nerve
   (B) trochlear nerve
   (C) oculomotor nerve
   (D) facial nerve
   (E) spinal accessory nerve

16. Primary axonopathy, with secondary demyelination and abnormal marker of the connexin-32 gene, is a characteristic of

   (A) hereditary sensory and motor neuropathy type I
   (B) hereditary sensory and motor neuropathy type II

   (C) hereditary sensory and motor neuropathy type III
   (D) hereditary sensory and motor neuropathy type IV
   (E) X-linked Charcot-Marie-Tooth disease

17. Which of the following myopathies is the most likely associated with arrhythmia?

   (A) Centronuclear myopathy
   (B) Nemaline myopathy
   (C) Acid maltase deficiency
   (D) Carnitine deficiency
   (E) Kearns-Sayre syndrome

18. The asymmetric and bilateral slowly progressive weakness of wrists, ulnar finger flexors, and knee extensors with normal facial muscles in a 55-year-old male is highly suggestive of

   (A) inclusion body myositis
   (B) acid maltase deficiency
   (C) myotonic dystrophy
   (D) polymyositis
   (E) nemaline myopathy

Questions 19 through 22
Link each of the following to the most frequent corresponding disease.

   (A) Chloride channelopathy
   (B) Sodium channelopathy
   (C) Calcium channelopathy

19. Hyperkalemic periodic paralysis

20. Myotonia congenita

21. Hypokalemic periodic paralysis

22. Paramyotonia congenita

Questions 23 through 31
Link the following.

   (A) Charcot-Marie-Tooth neuropathy type I A
   (B) Charcot-Marie-Tooth neuropathy type I B
   (C) Both
   (D) Neither

23. Autosomal dominant disorder.

24. Autosomal recessive disorder.

25. Hammertoes and pes cavus are seen in up to 75% of patients.

26. In nerve conduction studies, definite conduction block is characteristically present.

27. Tandem DNA duplication on the short arm of chromosome 17 is seen in up to 90% of patients.

28. Peripheral myelin protein 22 is defective.

29. Presence of onion bulbs on histologic examination of the nerve.

30. It is linked to chromosome 1.

31. Myelin protein 0 is defective, causing an abnormal compaction of peripheral nerve myelin.

32. Which of the following is true of the dominant form of X-linked Charcot-Marie-Tooth disease?

   (A) It is primarily a demyelinating disorder with secondary axonal degeneration.
   (B) Mental retardation is commonly seen.
   (C) The autosomal recessive form is more frequent than the autosomal dominant form.
   (D) Cranial nerves are frequently involved.
   (E) The connexin-32 gene is defective.

33. Multifocal motor neuropathy is characterized by all the following EXCEPT

   (A) Anti GM1 antibodies are elevated in about 50% of patients.
   (B) Bulbar function, as well as cranial nerves, are affected early.
   (C) Upper motor neuron function is normal.
   (D) Nerve conduction studies show conduction block and temporal dispersion.
   (E) Cyclophosphamide and intravenous immunoglobulin are the most effective therapies, while corticosteroids are ineffective.

34. Which of the following excludes a diagnosis of chronic inflammatory demyelinating polyradiculoneuropathy?

   (A) Hyporeflexia or areflexia in four limbs
   (B) Sensory level
   (C) Evidence of demyelination and remyelination on histological examination of the nerve
   (D) Prolonged distal latencies in two or more nerves on nerve conduction studies
   (E) Negative VDRL in the cerebrospinal fluid

Questions 35 through 41
Link the following.

   (A) Multifocal motor neuropathy (MMN)
   (B) Chronic inflammatory demyelinating polyradiculoneuropathy (CIDP)
   (C) Both
   (D) Neither

35. Symmetric distribution of weakness

36. Prolonged F wave on nerve conduction study

37. Possibility of relapse

38. Usually elevated CSF protein

39. Normal sensory nerve conduction studies

40. High anti-GM1 antibody titers

41. Prednisone is an effective treatment

42. Which of the following may cause a predominantly sensory neuropathy?

   (A) Arsenic exposure
   (B) N-hexane exposure
   (C) Dapsone
   (D) Pyridoxine intoxication
   (E) Nitrofurantoin

43. Which of the following is true about polymyalgia rheumatica?

    (A) It is the most common cause of pain in young adults.
    (B) It is more common in males than females by a ratio of 3 to 1.
    (C) High CK is commonly found.
    (D) The sedimentation rate is high.
    (E) The response to steroids is poor.

44. Which of the following muscles is spared in facioscapulohumeral dystrophy?

    (A) Latissimus dorsi
    (B) Trapezius
    (C) Rhomboid
    (D) Serratus anterior
    (E) Deltoid

45. Which of the following myopathies is caused by a defective synthesis of dysferlin AND is linked to an abnormal gene located on chromosome 2p13?

    (A) Miyoshi myopathy
    (B) Nonaka myopathy (distal myopathy with rimmed vacuoles)
    (C) Bethlem myopathy
    (D) Emery-Dreifuss muscular dystrophy
    (E) Oculopharyngeal muscle dystrophy

46. In Duchenne muscular dystrophy, the biochemical defect is based on a deficit of which of the following proteins?

    (A) Dystrophin
    (B) Myotonia protein kinase
    (C) Laminin alpha 2
    (D) Myelin basic protein
    (E) Ryanodine receptor channels

47. Which of the following myopathies is related to a chloride channel defect?

    (A) Becker myotonia
    (B) Myotonic dystrophy
    (C) Paramyotonia congenita
    (D) Hyperkalemic periodic paralysis
    (E) Potassium-aggravated myopathy

48. Which of the following is NOT true about congenital myotonic dystrophy?

    (A) Myotonia is the cardinal clinical sign in the neonatal age.
    (B) It is caused by an abnormal unstable trinucleotide repeat on chromosome 19.
    (C) There is a frequent history of hydramnios.
    (D) Hypotonia is one of its clinical signs.
    (E) The defective gene expresses a serine/threonine kinase.

49. Which of the following statements is true about hyperkalemic periodic paralysis?

    (A) It is an autosomal recessive disease.
    (B) It is caused by a mutation on 1q32.
    (C) The first occurrence of symptoms is usually at birth.
    (D) Muscle exercise with subsequent rest may trigger symptoms.
    (E) Spironolactone is an effective treatment for the disease.

Questions 50 through 56
Link the following.

    (A) Leber hereditary optic neuropathy
    (B) Mitochondrial neurogastrointestinal encephalopathy
    (C) Leigh syndrome
    (D) Alpers disease
    (E) Myoclonic epilepsy with ragged-red fibers
    (F) Kearns-Sayre syndrome
    (G) Mitochondrial encephalomyelopathy with lactic acidosis and stroke-like episode

50. A 7-month-old male infant died following a progressive neurological illness over 6 weeks, with somnolence, blindness, deafness, and generalized limb spasticity. Autopsy showed bilateral symmetric necrotic lesions of the thalamus, pons, inferior olive, and spinal cord.

51. A 25-year-old male developed recurrent episodes of nausea, vomiting, and diarrhea, concomitant with decreased ocular motility, weakness, and numbness in his lower extremities. Neurological examination demonstrated symmetric extraocular ophthalmoplegia. EMG/NCS showed a generalized sensorimotor neuropathy.

52. A 25-year-old male developed a painful decrease of his visual acuity with decreased ocular motility over 6 weeks. Neurological examination demonstrated bilateral external ophthalmoplegia, bilateral centrocecal scotoma, abnormal color vision, bilateral optic atrophy, and a visual acuity of 20/400 bilaterally.

53. A 2-year-old female infant was brought to the emergency room by her mother because of intractable seizures, developmental delay, failure to thrive, and episodes of vomiting. Neurological examination showed developmental delay and generalized hypotonia. CT scan of the head showed bilateral occipital and temporal hypodensities with cortical atrophy. EEG showed generalized slow wave activity. Lab work-up showed increased liver enzymes. Liver biopsy showed fatty degeneration.

54. A 15-year-old male consulted because of recurrence of headache, vomiting, and transient right hemiparesis. He also reported two episodes of generalized tonic-clonic seizures. Neurological examination was not focal. MRI of the head revealed multiple subacute small vessel ischemic lesions in the parietal lobes. Lab work-up showed elevated lactic acid level in the serum and the cerebrospinal fluid.

55. A 17-year-old male came to the emergency room because of an episode of syncope. He reported a decrease in his visual acuity and ocular motility over the past few weeks. Neurological examination demonstrated bilateral retinal degeneration, mild bilateral extraocular ophthalmoplegia, and mild cerebellar ataxia. The rest of the physical examination was unremarkable. EKG showed a Mobitz type II atrioventricular block.

56. A 30-year-old male developed progressive ataxia, myoclonic seizures, and severe myopathy.

57. All of the following descriptions are true about Kearns-Sayre syndrome EXCEPT

   (A) progressive external ophthalmoplegia
   (B) retinal degeneration
   (C) age of onset after 20 years
   (D) cardiac conduction defect
   (E) diabetes mellitus

58. Hypertrophic cardiomyopathy is NOT associated with which of the following mitochondrial diseases?

   (A) Kearns-Sayre syndrome
   (B) Leigh syndrome
   (C) Myoclonic epilepsy with ragged-red fibers
   (D) Mitochondrial encephalomyelopathy with lactic acidosis and strokelike episodes
   (E) The dominant form of progressive external ophthalmoplegia

59. A 30-year-old male consulted because of exercise intolerance, especially when lifting heavy weights and walking uphill. He also complained of myalgia, premature fatigue, and muscle swelling (relieved by rest). The patient reported increased shortness of breath and palpitation on exercise. Neurological examination was normal. Laboratory evaluation showed normal pyruvate and lactate levels in the serum, myoglobinuria with exercise, CK 1200 UI/Ml, normal CBC, liver function tests, and electrolytes. The administration of epinephrine induced a normal rise of the blood sugar. Which of the following is true about this condition?

   (A) There is a decrease of the ADP level in the muscle cells during exercise.
   (B) Glucose infusion may cause a substantial drop in patient exercise capacity.
   (C) It is caused by a myophosphorylase deficiency.
   (D) It is caused by a phosphofructokinase deficiency.
   (E) Phosphorous magnetic spectroscopy may detect a high phosphomonoester peak.

60. Which of the following is true about acquired myasthenia?

(A) The loss of acetylcholine receptors results in increased postsynaptic sensitivity to acetylcholine.

(B) Within 1 year of its onset, the disease remains purely ocular in 80% of cases.

(C) Bulbar symptoms are present in about 16% of patients at the onset of the disease.

(D) Magnesium-containing drugs may improve the symptoms of myasthenia gravis.

(E) Repetitive stimulation study at 50 Hz shows a decremental response.

61. Which of the following is NOT characteristic of Lambert-Eaton myasthenic syndrome?

(A) Antibodies to the N type of voltage-gated calcium channel is detected in 70% of Lambert-Eaton myasthenic syndrome cases associated with malignancy.

(B) The first symptom is usually lower extremity weakness.

(C) Autonomic symptoms are usually prominent.

(D) An incremental response at a rate of 3 Hz is highly suggestive.

(E) Postactivation stimulation may be seen after voluntary exercise of 10 seconds or after a tetanic stimulation of 20–50 Hz.

62. A 25-year-old male developed an acute episode of nausea, vomiting, diarrhea, and abdominal pain, followed a few hours later by diplopia, dysarthria, and progressive lower extremity weakness. Neurological examination demonstrated bilateral external ophthalmoplegia, dilated pupils, paraparesis with absent deep tendon reflexes in lower extremities, and normal sensory examination. Nerve conduction study showed decreased compound muscle action potentials of lower extremity muscles. Needle EMG showed small amplitude and short duration of recruited motor unit action potentials under voluntary contraction. Repetitive never stimulation showed a decrement at 3 Hz stimulation and incremental response at 50 Hz stimuli. The most likely diagnosis is

(A) botulism

(B) tetanus

(C) venom poisoning

(D) Lambert-Eaton myasthenic syndrome

(E) organophosphate poisoning

63. Which of the following drugs does NOT exacerbate the neuromuscular blockade in myasthenia gravis?

(A) Magnesium sulfate

(B) Tobramycine

(C) Quinidine

(D) Ciprofloxacin

(E) Acyclovir

64. Which of the following hereditary myasthenic disorders has an autosomal dominant penetrance?

(A) Familial infantile myasthenia

(B) Limb-girdle myasthenia

(C) Benign congenital myasthenic syndrome with facial dysmorphism

(D) Slow channel myasthenic syndrome

(E) Acetylcholine deficiency syndrome

65. Which of the following drugs may cause a necrotizing myopathy?

(A) Lovastatin

(B) Amiodarone

(C) Zidovudine

(D) D penicillamine

(E) Colchicine

Questions 66 through 70
Match each of the following causes of peripheral neuropathies to the most frequent cranial nerve involved in each disease.

(A) Diphtheria

(B) Refsum's disease

(C) Diabetes

(D) Sjögren syndrome neuropathy

(E) Wegener's granulomatosis

66. Glossopharyngeal nerve

67. Vestibulocochlear nerve

68. Oculomotor nerve

69. Trigeminal nerve

70. Facial nerve

71. A predominantly motor neuropathy is seen in cases of

    (A) pyridoxine neuropathy
    (B) paraneoplastic neuropathy
    (C) spinocerebellar degeneration
    (D) dapsone-induced neuropathy
    (E) a deficiency in vitamin E neuropathy

72. Which of the following is NOT true about the safety factor in neuromuscular transmission?

    (A) It is defined by the difference between the membrane potential and the threshold potential for initiating an action potential.
    (B) Postsynaptic folds form a high resistance pathway and increase the action potential threshold.
    (C) The loss of synaptic folds reduces the safety factor.
    (D) Myasthenia gravis, like all neuromuscular transmission disorders, is characterized by a compromise of the safety factor.
    (E) The conduction properties and density of acetylcholine receptors contribute to the safety factor.

73. Which of the following suggests that CD4+ T helper cells have a major role in the pathogenesis of myasthenia gravis?

    (A) Most anti-acetylcholine receptor antibodies in myasthenia gravis patients are high-affinity IgG, and their synthesis requires CD4+ and T helper factors.
    (B) Acetylcholine receptors reactivate CD4+ cells from the blood, and the thymus of myasthenia gravis patients has a T-cell cytotoxic function.

    (C) Thymectomy does not modify the reactivity of blood T-cells against acetylcholine receptors.
    (D) In vitro treatment of CD4+ T-cells from the blood of myasthenia gravis patients with anti CD4+ antibodies increases the reactivity of T-cells to acetylcholine receptors.
    (E) In experimental autoimmune myasthenia gravis, suppression of the synthesis of pathogenic anti-acetylcholine receptor antibodies requires CD4+ cells.

74. Which of the following is true about the role of the thymus in myasthenia gravis?

    (A) Ten percent of patients with myasthenia gravis have follicular hyperplasia of the thymus.
    (B) Acetylcholine receptors are expressed only in the thymus of these patients.
    (C) Thymic myoid cells expressing acetylcholine receptors, or antigenically similar proteins, may act as antigen presenting cells.
    (D) Only myasthenia gravis patients have CD4+ T-cells that react against self-antimuscle acetylcholine receptors; normal patients' CD4+ T-cells do not react to self-antigens.
    (E) Myoid cells are the only thymic cells that express acetylcholine receptor sequences.

75. All of the following are true about the mechanism of action of corticosteroids in the treatment of myasthenia gravis EXCEPT

    (A) reduction of lymphocyte proliferation
    (B) stimulation of antigen processing by macrophages
    (C) alteration of lymphokine function
    (D) redistribution of lymphocytes from circulation
    (E) increasing muscle acetylcholine receptor synthesis

Answers and Explanations

1. **(C)**

2. **(D)**

3. **(A)**

4. **(E)**

5. **(B)**

Explanations 1 through 5

End-plate noise is generated at the end-plate region. It represents normal spontaneous activity, and it manifests as low amplitude, monophasic negative potentials that fire at 20–40 Hz. It has the characteristic of a seashell or hissing sound on EMG. It represents miniature end-plate potentials. It is a normal finding in all individuals when the EMG needle is near the neuromuscular junction. End-plate spikes are another normal waveform that can occur when the needle is near the neuromuscular junction. They are brief irregular spikes with an initial negative deflection for each spike. They have a crackling, buzzing, or sputtering sound on EMG. They are caused by irritation of the terminal axon twig by the EMG needle, resulting in a depolarization of axon twigs, which propagate across the neuromuscular junction to give motor fiber action potentials. Both fibrillation potentials and positive sharp waves are the extracellular recording of a single muscle fiber's electrical activity occurring as a result of membrane instability. They are the electrophysiological markers of loss of functional activity between the motor axon and the muscle membrane. Fibrillation potentials are often described as being a "rain on a tin roof" type of

sound. They are primarily recognized by their regular firing pattern (usually at a rate of 1–10 Hz), their morphology is that of a single motor unit action potential, and they have an initial positive deflection (1–5 milliseconds in duration and typically 10–100 μV in amplitude). Positive sharp waves have a brief initial positivity followed by a long negative phase. They create a dull popping sound. A myotonic discharge is the spontaneous discharge of a muscle fiber in which the amplitude and frequency of the potentials wax and wane. It is characteristically seen in myotonic dystrophy, myotonia congenita, and paramyotonia congenita. *(Preston and Shapiro, 6–10)*

6. **(B)**

7. **(D)**

8. **(A)**

9. **(C)**

Explanations 6 through 9

Complex repetitive discharges occur from depolarization of a single muscle fiber followed by ephaptic spread to adjacent denervated fibers. On EMG, they are recognized as high-frequency, multiserrated repetitive discharges with an abrupt onset and termination and a machine-like sound. They are present in chronic neuropathic and myopathic disorders.

A fasciculation potential is a spontaneous involuntary discharge of an individual motor unit. The source generator of a fasciculation is the motor neuron or its axon. Fasciculations fire slowly, typically 0.5–1 Hz, and irregularly.

Clinically, they are recognized as individual brief twitches that seldom result in significant movement of a joint.

Myokymic discharges are rhythmic, grouped, and repetitive discharges of the same motor unit. Clinically, myokymia is usually recognized as the continuous, involuntary, quivering, rippling, or undulating movement of a muscle. Myokymia is seen in a variety of conditions, including radiculopathy, entrapment neuropathy, and demyelinating neuropathies. In a patient with a history of brachial plexopathy and history of cancer and radiation therapy, the presence of myokymia is a specific, although not necessarily a sensitive, sign supporting the diagnosis of radiation plexitis rather than recurrent neoplastic invasion. Neuromyotonic discharges are high-frequency (150–250 Hz) decremental discharges of a single motor unit that have a characteristic pinging sound on EMG. *(Preston and Shapiro, 11–19)*

10. **(E)** Acute axonal damage in a nerve causes Wallerian degeneration after the first 4–7 days. This is followed by denervation of the distal muscle fibers of the involved motor units. Sprouting of the nearby axons reinnervates these denervated fibers. The number of newly reinnervated fibers may exceed the normal number of fibers in the motor unit. This may lead to an increase in the duration, amplitude, and number of phases. This process takes many weeks to months to occur. In the acute setting, the motor unit action potential morphology remains normal. The only abnormality is decreased numbers of motor unit action potentials in weak muscles due to the initial loss of motor units. *(Preston and Shapiro, 32–33)*

11. **(D)** In myopathies, the number of functioning muscle fibers in a motor unit decreases. Fewer muscle fibers per motor unit results in shorter-duration and smaller-amplitude motor unit action potentials. With dysfunction of the remaining muscle fibers, less synchronous firing results in increased polyphasia. However, the number of functioning motor unit action potentials remains normal. Thus, the recruitment remains normal for the level of activation. Since each motor unit contains fewer muscle fibers,

each unit generates less force. Consequently, more motor unit action potentials, as compared to normal, are needed to generate a level of force equivalent to the premorbid state resulting in early full recruitment. *(Preston and Shapiro, 34–35)*

12. **(B)** In humans, 2 major types of muscle fibers, type 1 and type 2, have been defined on the basis of histochemistry and physiology. Type 1 fibers are high in myoglobin and oxidative enzymes and have many mitochondria, in keeping with their ability to perform tonic contraction; histologically, they are defined by their dark staining for adenosine triphosphatase (ATPase) at pH 4.2 but light staining at pH 9.4. Type 1 fibers are slow-twitch, red fibers. Type 2 fibers are rich in glycolytic enzymes and are involved in rapid phasic contractions. They stain dark for ATPase at pH 9.4 but light at pH 4.2. Type 2 fibers are fast-twitch, white fibers. Since the motor neuron determines fiber types, all fibers of a single unit are of the same type. These fibers are distributed randomly across the muscle, giving rise to the checkerboard pattern of alternating light and dark fibers, as demonstrated especially well with ATPase. Type-specific atrophy is characteristic of some disease states. Type 2 fiber atrophy is a relatively common finding and is associated with inactivity or disuse. This type of "disuse atrophy" may occur after fracture of a limb and application of a plaster cast, in pyramidal tract degeneration, or in neurodegenerative diseases. It may occur also with hyperthyroid myopathy and corticosteroid-induced myopathy. Type 1 fiber atrophy occurs with myotonic muscular dystrophy, centronuclear myopathy, and congenital fiber-type disproportion myopathy. *(Karpali 47–48)*

13. **(C)** Myotonic dystrophy (DM) disease is an autosomal dominant multisystem degenerative disease characterized by myotonia, progressive muscular weakness, gonadal atrophy, cataracts, and cardiac dysrhythmias. The molecular basis of DM is an unstable trinucleotide repeat sequence—cytosine, thymine, and guanidine (CTG)—in the protein kinase-encoding gene (DMK), located at 19q13.3. The normal CTG repeat is between 5 and 30 repeats, whereas in DM the CTG repeat is 50 to several thousands.

The size of the repeats correlates with the anticipation phenomenon as well as with the severity of symptoms. There is an estimated prevalence of 3 to 5 per 100,000 population and an incidence of 1 in 8000 live births, making it the most common adult muscular dystrophy.

The clinical presentation is variable, ranging from a single relatively benign presentation (such as cataracts) that presents in middle age to severe neonatal hypotonia that can lead to death if respiratory support is not provided. The classic presentation of noncongenital DM includes marked weakness in the face, jaw, and neck muscles and milder distal extremity weakness, often perceived earlier than the myotonia. Myotonia can be elicited by a brisk percussion of the thenar muscles causing flexion opposition of the thumb with slow relaxation. In the advanced stage of myotonic dystrophy, the patient may present a characteristic long and thin face with sunken cheeks due to temporal and masseter wasting, and atrophy of the sternocleidomastoid, causing a swan neck and ptosis. Congenital myotonic dystrophy presents a distinctive picture that is different from other myotonic disorders. Facial diplegia, jaw weakness (without concomitant extremity weakness), hypotonia, and weakness of respiratory muscles (with absence of clinical myotonia) are hallmarks. Additionally, 75% of the noncongenital patients and 81% of the congenital patients have cardiac abnormalities, primarily conduction defects, demonstrated on EKG. The heart is prominently involved, and the severity of cardiac symptoms does not correlate with the severity of other symptoms in this disorder.

Central nervous system manifestations may include apathy, inertia, and hypersomnolence. Structural changes in the brain are not common; however, generalized atrophy and ventricular dilatation may be seen. Endocrinological abnormalities have been reported, including hyperinsulinism with reduced insulin receptors, elevated pituitary FSH and LH, testicular atrophy (seen in 60% to 80% of patients), Leydig cell hyperplasia, and reduced testosterone level. (*Goetz, 707–708*)

14. (C) Neurological complications of diphtheria parallel the extent of the primary infection and are multiphasic in onset. Two to 3 weeks after the onset of oropharyngeal inflammation, weakness of the posterior pharynx, larynx, and facial nerves occurs, causing nasal speech. Death may occur from aspiration. Blurred vision, strabismus, and accommodation abnormalities are manifestations of oculomotor and ciliary paralysis and may occur in the fifth week. The peripheral nervous system manifestations of diphtheria include symmetric polyneuropathy that has its onset between 10 days to 3 months after the onset of the disease, with distal weakness that progresses proximally and decreased deep tendon reflexes. Paralysis of the diaphragm can ensue. Complete recovery is likely. Rarely, 2 to 3 weeks after onset of the illness, dysfunction of the vasomotor centers can cause hypotension or cardiac failure.

Diabetic cranial mononeuropathies are caused by peripheral nerve microinfarction, as well as fascicular ischemic lesions within the brain. Diabetic oculomotor cranial mononeuropathies primarily involve the oculomotor nerve and the abducens nerve; the trochlear nerve is uncommonly affected alone. Clinically, the patient may report eye pain or headache followed by a diplopia. In the setting of oculomotor involvement, pupillary sparing is noted in 80% to 90% of cases.

Sarcoidosis may affect virtually any part of the nervous system. Involvement of the facial nerve leading to unilateral facial-nerve palsy is the most commonly recognized symptom, although any cranial nerve can be affected. Unusual combinations of neurological deficits affecting the central nervous system and/or peripheral nerves should raise the clinical suspicion of sarcoidosis.

The neuropathy in porphyria is primarily motor. Weakness begins in the proximal muscles, arms more commonly than legs. Paresis is often focal; cranial nerve involvement may occur, especially in the oculomotor, facial, and vagus nerves.

The possible neurological manifestations of Lyme disease include lymphocytic meningitis with episodic headache and mild neck stiffness, subtle encephalitis with difficulty with mentation, cranial neuropathy (particularly unilateral or bilateral facial palsy), motor or sensory radiculoneuritis, mononeuritis multiplex, cerebellar ataxia, or myelitis. In children, the optic nerve may also be affected because of inflammation or increased intracranial pressure, which may lead to blindness. (*Crimlisk, 319–328; Newman, Rose, and Maier, 1224–1234; Steere, 115–125*)

15. **(A)** Characteristic cranial nerve syndromes associated with diabetes include, in decreasing frequency: monocular palsies of the abducens nerve, the oculomotor nerve, the trochlear nerve. Acute onset, an accompanying headache, and pupillary sparing in oculomotor lesions are typical. Prognosis for near or complete recovery over days to months is excellent. Careful MR imaging has occasionally shown T2 signal changes in the mesencephalon. This, associated with careful postmortem histological examination, suggests that focal vascular injury with secondary demyelination is the most likely mechanism. Facial neuropathy, indistinguishable in clinical presentation and prognosis from Bell's palsy, is reported to be associated with diabetes or impaired glucose tolerance in 12% to 45% of patients. (*Smith, 457–467*)

16. **(E)** The dominant form of X-linked Charcot-Marie-Tooth (CMT) neuropathy accounts for approximately 10% to 15% of the dominant forms of CMT neuropathy cases. It becomes symptomatic in the first decade. The disorder is related to an abnormal marker of the connexin-32 gene, which is a gap junction protein involving intercellular communication. Clinical manifestations include distal muscle weakness and atrophy, areflexia, distal sensory loss, pes cavus, hammertoes, and claw hands deformity. Women are less severely affected than men. Enlarged nerves are infrequent. The recessive form is rare. Spasticity and pyramidal signs may also be present, but mental retardation is only seen when the onset is in infancy. Pathologically, there is primary axonopathy with secondary demyelination.

Charcot-Marie-Tooth neuropathy type 1 (CMT1) is the most common hereditary motor and sensory neuropathy (HMSN). It is an autosomal dominant disorder with onset before the second decade. Family history may be absent in about 20% of cases. There are two main genetic variants of CMT1: CMT1A (75%) and CMT1B (20%).

Up to 90% of CMT1A patients have a tandem DNA duplication on the short arm of chromosome 17. Several laboratories have mapped the human peripheral myelin protein PMP22 gene to chromosome 17p11.2-p12. The duplication leads to an overexpression of the PMP22. Histologically, CMT1A may show small-diameter axons and frequent onion bulbs.

CMT1B is linked to chromosome 1q22-q23, where the gene locus for myelin protein zero (P0) gene is mapped. Histologically, CMT1B biopsies show loss of myelinated fibers, small onion bulbs, and tomaculous formations.

Charcot-Marie-Tooth neuropathy type 2 (CMT2) is also an autosomal dominant condition. It is significantly less common than CMT1 and accounts for one-third of all autosomal dominant CMT. There are three genetic variants: CMT2A, CMT2B, and CMT2C. Electrophysiologically, all CMT2 patients exhibit findings of primary axonal sensorimotor neuropathy. The motor nerve conduction velocities are normal or mildly slowed. Sensorimotor nerve action potential amplitudes are reduced. CMT2A is linked to the short arm of chromosome 1 (1p35-36), while CMT2B is mapped to the long arm of chromosome 3 (3q13-22).

Charcot-Marie-Tooth neuropathy type 3 (CMT3) is a severe neuropathy that begins in infancy or early childhood. Occasionally, infants have neonatal hypotonia and delayed motor milestones. There is proximal and distal limb weakness, significant sensory ataxia, and diffuse areflexia. The peripheral nerves are enlarged and palpable. Skeletal and foot abnormalities are present. Most CMT3 cases are sporadic, and the inheritance is traditionally described as autosomal recessive.

Charcot-Marie-Tooth neuropathy type 4 (CMT4) is rare. It also begins in infancy or childhood. There is a delay in acquiring motor milestones. The distal weakness and atrophy spread to proximal muscles in the second decade. Facial muscles may become weak; there is areflexia; adults become wheelchair-bound. Sensory loss is mild. Skeletal abnormalities are common. Electrophysiologically, nerve conduction velocities are slowed to 15–30 m/sec. This helps differentiate CMT4 from CMT3 and CMT2C, which also begin in childhood. CMT4 is inherited in an autosomal recessive mode. The Tunisian form was mapped to chromosome 8q13-21.1 and is termed CMT4A. (*Murakami 233–235*)

17. **(E)** Involvement of organs or tissues other than muscle may provide helpful clues in making the appropriate diagnosis of myopathy. Cardiac arrhythmias are associated with Kearns-Sayre syndrome, Anderson's syndrome, polymyositis, and Emery-Dreifuss muscular dystrophy. Congestive heart failure may be seen in Duchenne muscular dystrophy, Becker muscular dystrophy, Emery-Dreifuss myopathy, nemaline myopathy, acid maltase deficiency, carnitine deficiency, and polymyositis. Respiratory failure may be the presenting symptom of myotonic dystrophy, centronuclear myopathy, nemaline myopathy, or acid maltase deficiency. Hepatomegaly may be seen in myopathies associated with deficiencies in acid maltase, debranching enzyme, and carnitine. (*Schapira, 184*)

18. **(A)** The pattern of weakness described in this case shows distal arm and proximal leg weakness. The distal arm weakness involves the wrist and ulnar finger flexors. The proximal leg weakness involves the quadriceps, which is a knee extensor. The asymmetry of the weakness and the sparing of the face make this pattern highly suggestive of inclusion body myositis. This pattern may also uncommonly occur in myotonic dystrophy; however, unlike inclusion body myositis, muscle weakness is symmetric. In acid maltase deficiency, the weakness involves the trunk and proximal limbs and the progression is slow, taking years. Nemaline myopathy is mainly seen in infancy and early childhood and is characterized by hypotonia and muscle weakness. Polymyositis has a symmetric proximal limb weakness pattern involving the muscles of the hip, thigh, and shoulders. (*Schapira, 311–317*)

19. **(B)**

20. **(A)**

21. **(C)**

22. **(B)**

Explanations 19 through 22

Myotonia congenita is due to point mutations in the muscle chloride channel gene on chromosome 7q35. There are autosomal dominant and recessive forms that are allelic disorders. The autosomal dominant form is also known as Thomsen's disease, and the autosomal recessive form is known as Becker's myotonia congenita. Both diseases are benign and associated with diffuse muscle hypertrophy and electrical myotonia. Cold increases the myotonia, and sustained exercise improves it (warm-up phenomenon). There is no involvement of the heart or other organs. Thomsen's disease patients are not weak, but Becker's myotonia congenita patients develop limb-girdle weakness and the myotonia is more severe. Myotonia congenita patients do not complain of pain, which is a feature that distinguishes them from proximal myotonic myopathy patients. The membrane defect consists of markedly reduced chloride conductance, resulting in hyperexcitability and after-depolarization, producing involuntary myotonic potentials.

Paramyotonia congenita and hyperkalemic periodic paralysis are due to point mutations in the voltage-dependent sodium channel (SCN4A) gene on chromosome 17q23-25. These are autosomal dominant conditions. All have symptoms beginning in the first decade and continuing throughout life. Paramyotonia congenita is characterized by paradoxical myotonia in that the muscle symptoms increase with repetitive movements. This is often best observed on repeated forced eye-closure: after several attempts the patient cannot open the eyelids. Muscle stiffness is worsened by cold temperature. Hyperkalemic periodic paralysis is characterized by attacks of weakness lasting no more than 1 or 2 hours. Attacks are precipitated by fasting, by rest shortly after exercise (minutes or several hours), ingestion of potassium-rich foods or compounds, and cold. During attacks, patients are areflexic with normal sensation and there is no ocular or respiratory muscle weakness. The serum potassium level may or may not be increased during the attack. Strength is generally normal between attacks, but some patients can have mild interictal limb-girdle weakness. Episodes of weakness are rarely serious enough to require acute therapy; oral carbohydrates or glucose may improve weakness.

Hypokalemic periodic paralysis is due to abnormal muscle membrane excitability arising from mutations in the muscle calcium channel alpha-1 subunit on chromosome 1q31-32. The mutation produces a reduction of the calcium current in the T-tubule. During attacks there is an influx of potassium into muscle cells and the muscles become electrically unexcitable. Patients have an increased sensitivity to the effects of insulin on potassium. Hypokalemic periodic paralysis is an autosomal dominant condition. It is the most frequent form of periodic paralysis and is more common in males, with a reduced female penetrance. Attacks begin by adolescence and are provoked by exercise followed by sleep, stress, alcohol, or meals rich in carbohydrates and sodium. The episodes last from 3 to 24 hours. A vague prodrome of stiffness or heaviness in the legs can occur. Rarely, ocular, bulbar, and respiratory muscles can be involved in severe attacks. *(Schapira, 135–175)*

23. **(C)**

24. **(D)**

25. **(C)**

26. **(D)**

27. **(A)**

28. **(A)**

29. **(C)**

30. **(B)**

31. **(B)**

Explanations 23 through 31

Charcot-Marie-Tooth neuropathy type 1 (CMT1) is the most common hereditary motor and sensory neuropathy (HMSN). It is an autosomal dominant disorder with onset before the second decade. Although family history may not be reported in about 20% of cases, detailed investigations, including clinical and electrophysiological evaluations of asymptomatic family members, improve the yield significantly. In all CMT1 subtypes, 50% to 75% of patients have pes cavus and hammertoes. There is distal muscle weakness and atrophy in the legs. About 65% of cases have distal upper limb involvement. Distal sensory impairment is present but usually asymptomatic. The vibratory sensation is most often diminished. Muscle stretch reflexes are absent in about 50%. Nerve enlargement is present in at least 25% of patients. Electrodiagnostic testing reveals slowing of nerve conduction velocities to less than 75% of lower limit of normal in all nerves. The slowing is present in early childhood. Definite conduction block is characteristically absent. Compound sensory and motor action potential amplitudes are often low in the lower limbs. Needle EMG shows chronic neurogenic motor unit action potentials mainly in the distal muscles. The magnitude of axonal changes is a better prognostic indicator than slowing of nerve conduction velocities.

There are two main genetic variants of CMT1: CMT1A (75%) and CMT1B (20%). The remaining cases are genetically more heterogeneous. Up to 90% of CMT1A patients have tandem DNA duplication on the short arm of chromosome 17 (17p11.2-12), causing an overexpression of PMP22 (peripheral myelin protein), which is a 22-kd membrane glycoprotein localized to the compact portion of the peripheral nerve myelin. Nerve biopsy in CMT1A may show small axonal diameter and onion bulbs. CMT1B is linked to chromosome 1q22-q23, where the gene locus for myelin protein zero (P0) gene is mapped. It is a member of the large family of adhesive molecules and plays a role in the compaction of peripheral nerve myelin. Histologically, CMT1B biopsies show loss of myelinated fibers, small onion bulbs, and tomaculous formations. *(Mendell, 431–436)*

32. **(E)** The dominant form of X-linked Charcot-Marie-Tooth disease (CMTX) becomes manifest in the first decade of life. There is distal muscle weakness and atrophy, distal sensory

loss, and areflexia. Pes cavus and hammertoes are common, and claw-hand deformity may occur in the adult male. Women are mildly affected. Enlarged nerves are infrequent. The recessive form is rare. Spasticity and pyramidal signs are also present, but mental retardation is only seen when the onset is in infancy. Pathologically, there is primary axonopathy with secondary demyelination. The disorder is linked to the marker DXYS1, a marker for the connexin-32 gene. CX32 is a gap junction protein involved in intercellular communication. *(Mendell, 445–447)*

33. **(B)** Multifocal motor neuropathy (MMN) is a demyelinating neuropathy, presumably of autoimmune origin. The arguments in favor of an autoimmune origin are the presence of conduction blocks, as seen in chronic inflammatory demyelinating polyneuropathy (CIDP), the presence of anti-GM1 antibodies, and the effectiveness of immunomodulating therapy. Age at onset is highly variable, with reports of patients in their 20s to as old as 70 years. It is more common in males than females. Patients have gradual, progressive, asymmetric weakness in the distribution of one or more motor nerves. The duration of symptoms at presentation is usually greater than 1 year, and durations of 20 years or more have been reported. Upper extremity involvement is more common than lower extremity involvement, and there is usually a distal predominance.

Thus, the most common presentation is that of a young to middle-aged male with slowly progressive asymmetric hand weakness over several months or years. Atrophy may or may not be present; one hallmark of MMN is weakness out of proportion to the degree of atrophy. Bulbar function and other cranial-innervated muscles are usually spared. Sensory symptoms and signs are absent or minimal. Reflexes vary, but usually are decreased focally in affected areas. MMN lacks the upper motor neuron findings of classical ALS. Features that can help differentiate the two include multifocal demyelination on electrodiagnostic studies in MMN, weakness in the distribution of major motor nerves in MMN, the presence of very high titers of anti-GM1 antibodies in some, but not all, patients with MMN, and the response

of MMN to IVIg or cyclophosphamide. Corticosteroids generally have no effect on MMN, or produce worsening. Plasma exchange has not been effective, and may even worsen the condition. Cyclophosphamide leads to improvement in most patients. Although the effect may last for several months after completion of the course of cyclophosphamide, weakness often recurs after discontinuation of the medication, requiring resumption of treatment. IVIg is effective in most patients with MMN, including some who have been unresponsive to cyclophosphamide. *(Mendell, 192–201)*

34. **(B)** Chronic inflammatory demyelinating polyneuropathy (CIDP) is a clinical diagnosis based on symptoms and signs, electrodiagnostic studies, CSF examination, laboratory tests appropriate to the specific clinical situation, and occasionally nerve biopsy. Four features are used as the basis of diagnosis: clinical, electrodiagnostic, pathologic, and cerebrospinal fluid studies. These are further divided into (A) mandatory, (B) supportive, and (C) exclusionary. While these criteria have been established for research purposes, there is a highly variable spectrum of clinical presentation. Mandatory features are those required for diagnosis and should be present in all definite cases. Supportive features are helpful in clinical diagnosis but do not by themselves make a diagnosis. Exclusionary features strongly suggest alternative diagnoses.

The clinical mandatory features include progressive or relapsing motor and/or sensory dysfunction of more than one limb of a peripheral nerve (developing over at least 2 months), and hypo- or areflexia, usually of all four limbs. The supportive clinical features include large-fiber sensory loss, predominating over small-fiber sensory loss. The exclusionary features include mutilation of hands or feet, retinitis pigmentosa, ichthyosis, appropriate history of drug or toxic exposure (known to cause a similar peripheral neuropathy), or family history of an inherited peripheral neuropathy, the presence of sensory level, and unequivocal sphincter disturbance. The mandatory electrodiagnostic study features include predominance of demyelination in the proximal nerve segments with reduced conduction velocity and prolonged distal latency. The mandatory cerebrospinal fluid studies include cell count <10/mm 3, if HIV-seronegative, or <50/mm 3, if HIV-seropositive and negative VDRL. Elevated protein level in the cerebrospinal fluid is a supportive feature. If nerve biopsy is performed, the mandatory pathological features include unequivocal evidence of demyelination and remyelination. The exclusion pathological features for CIDP include vasculitis, neurofilamentous swollen axons, amyloid deposits, or intracytoplasmic inclusions in Schwann cells or macrophages, indicating adrenoleukodystrophy, metachromatic leukodystrophy, globoid cell leukodystrophy, or other evidence of specific pathology. However, nerve biopsies are not required to make a clinical diagnosis. (*Mendell, 173–191*)

35. (B)

36. (C)

37. (B)

38. (B)

39. (A)

40. (A)

41. (B)

Explanations 35 through 41

Chronic inflammatory demyelinating polyradiculoneuropathy (CIDP) is a chronic disorder of the peripheral nervous system. It may have a relapsing, monophasic, or progressive course and is generally steroid-responsive. Multifocal motor neuropathy (MMN) is characterized by a slowly progressive, asymmetric, and multifocal weakness with atrophy that may mimic motor neuron disease, but demonstrates features of multifocal conduction block and slowing in motor nerves. This condition represents a demyelinating neuropathy, which is generally treatable.

The age of onset of CIDP, as well as MMN, is adults of all ages; CIDP rarely affects children. Male predominance is found in both diseases. Weakness tends to be symmetric in CIDP and asymmetric in MMN, with upper extremities more involved than lower extremities and with distal muscles more involved than proximal muscles. Large-fiber impairment is more common in cases of CIDP, whereas it is minimal or absent in cases of MMN. Reflexes are globally decreased in cases of CIDP, whereas they are focally decreased or absent in cases of MMN. Sensory nerve studies are usually abnormal in case of CIDP, but normal in case of MMN. Motor nerve conduction studies in both MMN and CIDP demonstrate acquired demyelination with conduction block, abnormal temporal dispersion, slowed conduction velocities, prolonged distal latencies, and prolonged F-wave latencies. Low titers of anti-GM1 antibodies may be present in CIDP patients, whereas they are present at high titers in about half of MMN patients. Cerebrospinal fluid protein is usually elevated in cases of CIDP and normal or elevated to <100 mg/dL in cases of MMN. Sensory nerve biopsy in CIDP may show demyelination, axonal degeneration, mononuclear inflammation, and endoneurial edema, whereas it is normal or shows minor abnormalities in cases of MMN. Prednisone, IVIg, and plasma exchange are the usual treatment for CIDP, whereas IVIg and cyclophosphamide are usually used in MMN. (*Mendell, 173–201*)

42. (D) Peripheral neuropathy is a common and debilitating complication of arsenic intoxication. It may present as a distal symmetric axonal sensorimotor polyneuropathy with motor predominance. Neuropathic features begin 5 to 10 days after acute exposure, progressing over several weeks, and often resemble Guillain-Barré syndrome. The neuropathy involves sensory and motor axons. Unlike GBS, neuropathy is only one component of a systemic intoxication, and other features provide important clues that something other than idiopathic GBS explains the neuropathy.

Early systemic symptoms of acute arsenic intoxication include nausea, vomiting, and diarrhea. Initial laboratory findings reflect abnormal liver function and depressed bone marrow, sometimes with pancytopenia and basophilic stippling of red blood cells. Cerebrospinal fluid protein is elevated in most patients with severe arsenic neuropathy. Increased urinary arsenic excretion is an important feature of recent exposure. The half-life of urinary arsenic excretion, after acute exposure, is about 3 weeks, making it a helpful test early after exposure. The magnitude of exposure also can be related to accumulation in hair or nails at a later time. Serial nerve conduction studies in patients with arsenic neuropathy demonstrate evidence of a distal dying-back neuropathy with progressive axonal degeneration (findings confirmed on nerve biopsy).

N-hexane, an organic solvent, is thought to be responsible for the neuropathy seen in glue sniffers. The sensory component is usually more prominent when compared to the motor component. Pure motor neuropathy or mixed neuropathy with motor predominance have been reported with n-hexane exposure. An unusual and characteristic feature of this neuropathy is that the clinical condition frequently continues to deteriorate for some months after exposure ceases. Sufficient exposure to n-hexane produces a dying-back sensorimotor neuropathy characterized by distal weakness, stocking-glove sensory loss, and absent ankle reflexes. In the majority of reports, motor signs predominate, but pure motor neuropathy is unusual and inconsistent with the known sural nerve abnormalities. Nerve conduction studies in asymptomatic n-hexane–exposed individuals may be normal or demonstrate mildly slowed motor conduction velocities. In symptomatic patients, initial findings consist of reduced sensory amplitudes, followed by reduced motor amplitudes and conduction velocities, sometimes to 35% to 40% of the lower limit of normal. The reduced conduction velocity and partial conduction block are explained by secondary myelin changes caused in part by axonal swelling, demonstrated in humans and experimental animals in peripheral and central nerve fibers.

Dapsone produces a neuropathy characterized by weakness and muscle wasting that frequently involves the arms more than the legs. It is one of several toxins associated with motor involvement or motor greater than sensory involvement but no conduction block. Dapsone neuropathy is thought to reflect primary or exclusive axonal degeneration of motor fibers, although controversy exists regarding the presence or absence of sensory involvement.

Neuropathic toxicity of pyridoxine is dose related, either to long-term cumulative exposure or to short-term administration of large doses. Symptoms include unpleasant distal paresthesias and numbness. Associated signs include areflexia, profoundly reduced vibration, and joint position sensations with minimally decreased pinprick sensation. With particularly large doses of pyridoxine, sensory loss may be virtually complete, including facial and mucous membrane areas, with little resolution after removal from exposure. Such profound loss is consistent with a sensory neuronopathy. Sensory nerve conduction studies are the only tests able to localize sensory loss to the periphery, but sensory nerve action potentials persist for up to 10 days after clinical sensory loss is identified.

Neuropathy is the exclusive neurotoxicity associated with nitrofurantoin. Neuropathy develops in a small proportion (<0.5%) of patients receiving nitrofurantoin for extended periods (usually exceeding 1 to 2 months). Neuropathy is most common in elderly patients with abnormal renal function, presumably resulting in high blood levels. The neuropathy is a mixed sensorimotor polyneuropathy. Onset is with distal dysesthesias and sensory loss involving large-fiber modalities. With continued use, motor symptoms, sign development, and sensory loss may be severe. Weakness may be subacute and progress to respiratory failure, superficially resembling GBS. When recognized and nitrofurantoin is discontinued, most patients improve or recover. (*Mendell, 316–330*)

43. **(D)** Polymyalgia rheumatica may be one of the more common causes of muscle pain in adults older than 50 years. One study suggested that the prevalence of the disease is 600/100,000.

The condition affects the older population, with a mean age at onset of 70 years and a female to male incidence ratio of 3 to 1. The disorder is characterized by the indolent onset of myalgia, stiffness, aching, and fatigue predominantly affecting the neck, the shoulder, and hip region. Symptoms are typically worse in the morning, when prominent stiffness occurs. Low-grade fever, depression, anemia, and weight loss can accompany the muscular manifestation. Laboratory evaluation reveals typically normal CK level and high sedimentation rate, often to a value greater than 100 mm per hour. Muscle biopsies are invariably normal. Polymyalgia rheumatica occurs in approximately 50% of patients with giant cell arteritis. Approximately 15% of patients with the diagnosis of polymyalgia rheumatica will develop giant cell arteritis. Although occasional patients with polymyalgia rheumatica respond to nonsteroidal anti-inflammatory drugs, most patients require treatment with corticosteroids, which usually results in dramatic improvement of the myalgia and stiffness. *(Schapira and Griggs, 40–41)*

44. **(E)** Facioscapulohumeral dystrophy is an autosomal dominant disorder. The prevalence is approximately 1 in 20,000. There are two distinctive patterns of progressive muscular weakness involving the face, scapular stabilizer, proximal arm, and peroneal muscles. The first one is a gradually descending autosomal dominant form. The second one is a jump form in which the progressive weakness jumps from the upper body to the peroneal muscles. The age of onset is from infancy to middle age. The initial weakness typically affects the facial muscles, especially the orbicularis oculis and oris. The masseter, temporalis, extraocular, and pharyngeal muscles are usually unaffected. Shoulder weakness is the presenting symptom in more than 82% of symptomatic patients. Involvement of the scapular fixator muscles, the latissimus dorsi, trapezius, rhomboids, and serratus anterior, causes a winging of the scapula, a highly characteristic sign. The scapula is placed more laterally than normal. It moves upward in shoulder abduction. The deltoid muscle is typically not affected. *(Schapira and Griggs, 61–68)*

45. **(A)** Miyoshi myopathy is clinically characterized by autosomal recessive inheritance, and the onset is in early adulthood with preferential gastrocnemius muscle involvement and dystrophic muscle pathology. The gene has been mapped to chromosome 2p13 and has been cloned. The predicted gene product has been named dysferlin. The location and function of dysferlin remain unknown. Mutations are variable and include insertions, deletions, altered splicing, and point mutations. Bethlem myopathy is a rare autosomal myopathy characterized by a slowly progressive limb-girdle weakness from childhood onward with periods of arrest for several decades, and flexion contractures of fingers, elbows, and ankles. The disease has been demonstrated to be due to a type VI collagen gene defect. Emery-Dreifuss muscular dystrophy is an X-linked disorder characterized by a slowly progressive wasting and weakness of the scapulohumeral, anterior tibial, and peroneal muscle groups. Cardiomyopathy with conduction defects is common. The defective gene is mapped to Xq28. Oculopharyngeal muscle dystrophy is an autosomal dominant disease linked to the chromosome 14q11. Nonaka myopathy is linked to chromosome 9p1q1. *(Nonaka, 493–499)*

46. **(A)** Duchenne-type muscular dystrophy is the most common form of dystrophy. It is inherited as an X-linked recessive trait and therefore predominantly affects boys. It is a serious condition with progressive muscle wasting and weakness that causes most affected boys to start using wheelchairs by age 12 and to die in their 20s. The associated gene in Duchenne-type muscular dystrophy produces dystrophin. Histochemical studies on muscle sections without muscular dystrophy indicate that dystrophin is localized at the periphery of muscle fibers. It is a cytoskeletal protein located beneath the sarcolemma. In Duchenne-type dystrophy, there is dystrophin deficit and the majority of fibers fail to stain for dystrophin. *(Emery, 991–995)*

47. **(A)** Myotonic muscle disorders represent a heterogeneous group of clinically similar diseases sharing the feature of myotonia: delayed relaxation of muscle after voluntary contraction (action myotonia) or mechanical stimulation

(percussion myotonia). In classic myotonia, the myotonia improves as muscles warm up, whereas in paradoxical myotonia (paramyotonia) it worsens with repeated muscle contractions. Genetic-linkage studies have now pinpointed the lesions to chromosomal loci encoding specific ion channels and a protein kinase. In sodium channel diseases, the gene defect is located on chromosome 17; these include hyperkalemic periodic paralysis, paramyotonia congenita, and potassium-sensitive myotonia congenita. In protein kinase–related diseases, the gene defect is located on chromosome 19 and includes myotonic dystrophy. In chloride channel diseases, the gene defect is located on chromosome 7 and includes autosomal dominant myotonia congenita (Thomsen myotonia), and autosomal recessive myotonia congenita (Becker's myotonia). *(Ptacek, Johnson, and Griggs, 482–489)*

48. **(A)** Congenital myotonic dystrophy is an autosomal dominant disorder caused by an abnormal unstable expansion of a trinucleotide repeat gene on chromosome 19. The tissues that are commonly involved, in addition to the skeletal muscle, include heart, smooth muscle, lens, brain, and endocrine tissues. The cardinal sign of adult myotonic dystrophy is myotonia. It is absent in cases of congenital myotonic dystrophy and gradually appears during childhood. At birth, there is a frequent history of hydramnios and reduced fetal movements. Neonatal respiratory distress may occur. Other signs of congenital myasthenia include hypotonia, bilateral facial weakness, feeding difficulty, and mental retardation. The gene defect results from an abnormal expansion of the trinucleotide repeat (CTG) of a gene on chromosome 19, which codes for serine/threonine kinase. *(Schapira and Griggs, 118–124)*

49. **(D)** Hyperkalemic periodic paralysis is an autosomal dominant disorder that can occur with or without myotonia or with paramyotonia. It usually begins in the first decade of life. The attack commonly starts in the morning before breakfast, lasts from 15 minutes to an hour, and then spontaneously resolves. Rest often provokes an attack, particularly if preceded by strenuous exercise. Potassium loading usually precipitates an attack. Cold environment, emotional stress, glucocorticoids, and pregnancy provoke or worsen the attacks. The generalized weakness is usually accompanied by a significant increase of serum potassium, up to 5 to 6 mM/L. Sometimes the serum potassium level remains within the upper normal range and rarely reaches a toxic level. The frequency of the attacks is variable, from a few times per year to daily. The gene defect is located on chromosome 17q23 (coding for the subunit of the adult human skeletal muscle sodium channel SCN4A). Preventive therapy consists of frequent meals rich in carbohydrates and low in potassium, avoidance of fasting, strenuous work, and exposure to cold, and continuous use of thiazide diuretics or acetazolamide. Some patients can abort or attenuate attacks by the prompt oral intake of a thiazide diuretic or by inhalation of an adrenergic agent that stimulates the sodium-potassium pump. *(Schapira and Griggs, 143–144)*

50. **(C)**

51. **(B)**

52. **(A)**

53. **(D)**

54. **(G)**

55. **(F)**

56. **(E)**

Explanations 50 through 56

Mitochondria serve several important functions within the cell, the most important of which is the production of ATP by the oxidative phosphorylation system (OXPHOS). The ubiquity of mitochondria suggests that a defect of OXPHOS will affect the function of numerous tissues and implies that mitochondrial OXPHOS decrease will be multisystemic. However, different tissues have varying dependence on OXPHOS for normal function and survival: brain and muscle (heart and skeletal) are highly dependent, and bone and fibroblasts less so. Mitochondria also have their own DNA, inherited through the maternal line since no sperm containing mitochondria enter the ovum, leaving the embryo to develop using only maternal mtDNA. Mutations of mtDNA have now been associated with a large variety of clinical presentations, most of which involve muscle and central nervous system features and are collectively referred to as the "mitochondrial encephalomyopathies."

Large-scale rearrangements of mtDNA, in particular deletions, are found in some 40% of adult patients with mitochondrial disease. Most commonly, the resultant clinical picture is one of chronic progressive external ophthalmoplegia (CPEO), with or without the associated features that make up Kearns-Sayre syndrome (KSS), which are retinitis, ataxia, cardiac conduction block, or elevated cerebrospinal fluid protein. The case described in question 55 shows a symptomatic high-degree atrioventricular heart block, ophthalmoplegia, retinal abnormalities, and cerebellar signs in a young patient. These symptoms are highly suggestive of Kearns-Sayre syndrome. The diagnostic criteria of Kearns-Sayre syndrome include onset before the age of 20 years, CPEO, and a pigmentary retinopathy in association with ataxia, heart block, or raised cerebrospinal fluid protein. A proximal myopathy commonly develops as the disease progresses, and there may also be deafness, strokelike episodes, bulbar symptoms, areflexia, and lactic acidosis. Muscle biopsy may show up to 60% of all fibers lacking COX activity.

The patient described in question 50 died from a progressive necrotizing encephalopathy involving the thalamus, pons, inferior olive, and spinal cord, with sparing of the cortex. These findings are suggestive of Leigh's syndrome, also known as subacute necrotizing encephalopathy. Although it is a multisystemic disorder with hepatic dysfunction and chronic acidosis, the clinical picture is dominated by nervous system involvement, including developmental delay and psychomotor regression, ataxia, optic atrophy, seizures, peripheral neuropathy, and brain stem dysfunction. Serum and CSF lactate and pyruvate are high, and in most patients, the diagnosis is further supported by a characteristic MRI showing midbrain, basal ganglia, and brain stem lucencies with or without cortical changes. Postmortem spongiform degeneration is seen in the brain stem, with marked loss of neuronal cells and vascular proliferation. The cerebral and cerebellar cortices are characteristically spared.

The case described in question 54 has clinical and radiological evidence of recurrent episodes of stroke with headaches and biochemical evidence of lactic acidosis. The most likely diagnosis is mitochondrial encephalomyopathy with lactic acidosis and strokelike episodes. The key features of the disease include strokelike episodes with headache, vomiting, and focal neurological disturbance, lactic acidosis, and biochemical or morphological evidence of mitochondrial dysfunction on muscle biopsy. Other common features include a pigmentary retinopathy, psychomotor deterioration, convulsions, myopathy (87%), deafness, diabetes, and short stature (55%).

The association of cerebellar signs, seizures, and severe myopathy in a 30-year-old male, as described in case 56, is suggestive of myoclonic epilepsy with ragged-red fibers. The major clinical features of the disease are myoclonic epilepsy, usually with tonic-clonic generalized seizures, a progressive cerebellar syndrome, and a myopathy. Deafness is common in both clinically overt cases and in otherwise asymptomatic maternal relatives. Other features may include pes cavus, peripheral neuropathy, optic atrophy, dorsal column loss, heart block, and in severe cases dementia. CPEO, pigmentary retinopathy, and strokelike episodes are said to be typically absent. The onset is commonly in the second or third decade, but cases have been reported from age 3 to 62 years. Early childhood development is often normal, but there may be a history of muscle fatigue, cramps, epilepsy, or developmental delay before the diagnosis becomes clear. In those with clear central nervous system involvement, the disease is usually progressive, although milder cases may remain minimally affected for many years.

A rapid loss of vision in a young healthy man with external ophthalmoplegia and bilateral optic atrophy, as described in question 52, points toward the diagnosis of Leber's hereditary optic neuropathy (LHON). It is recognized as the most common cause of isolated blindness in young men, with an estimated incidence of 1 in 50,000. Maternal inheritance has long been recognized, and it is an obvious target in which to search for mtDNA mutations. Recovery is variable and to some extent may be linked to the underlying mtDNA genotype, but most individuals remain visually handicapped for life.

The association of extraocular ophthalmoplegia with neuromuscular and gastrointestinal symptoms is suggestive of myoneurogastrointestinal encephalopathy (question 51). It is defined by the combination of chronic intestinal pseudo-obstruction with skeletal myopathy, ophthalmoplegia, and peripheral neuropathy. The gastrointestinal motility disturbance manifests as chronic nausea, vomiting, diarrhea, and malabsorption with progressive malnutrition, often leading to death in the third or fourth decade of life. Postmortem changes include a severe visceral neuropathy or scleroderma-like changes. The peripheral sensorimotor neuropathy and skeletal myopathy contribute to muscle weakness and atrophy accompanying the CPEO. Deafness is also common, and there may be cognitive decline due to a leukoencephalopathy. CT or MRI has shown extensive white matter changes in around 50% of the cases described, and electrical studies confirm the presence of a sensorimotor neuropathy with both axonal and demyelinating components. Muscle biopsy shows numerous ragged-red fibers with a partial defect of COX as the most common biochemical finding.

Question 53 reported a 2-year-old female with intractable seizures, hypotonia, and liver dysfunction. These symptoms are consistent with the diagnosis of Alpers disease.

Alpers disease, or progressive neuronal degeneration of childhood with liver disease, is a rare familial disorder of unknown etiology. Typically, onset of symptoms follows normal delivery and early development. Infants most often present with intractable generalized convulsions associated with developmental delay, marked hypotonia, episodes of vomiting, and failure to thrive. There may be signs of liver disease at presentation. Investigations reveal occipital and posterior temporal hypodensities and atrophy on CT scan, very slow activity of very high amplitude spikes interspersed with lower amplitude polyspikes on EEG, absent visual evoked responses, and abnormal liver histology. (*Schapira and Cock, 886–898*)

57. **(C)** Kearns-Sayre syndrome is a mitochondrial disease characterized by a clinical triad: progressive external ophthalmoplegia, retinal degeneration, and onset before the age of 20 years. It is variably associated with cerebellar ataxia, growth failure, sensorineuronal deafness, heart block, and raised CSF protein. Diabetes mellitus, hypoparathyroidism, and growth deficiency may occur. Both ragged-red fibers and COX-negative are present in biopsied muscle. Ninety percent of patients have a large-scale rearrangement of their muscle mitochondrial DNA. (*Schapira and Griggs, 184*)

58. **(A)** Cardiac conduction defects are the frequent features of Kearns-Sayre syndrome, whereas hypertrophic cardiomyopathy has been reported in myoclonic epilepsy, with ragged-red fibers, mitochondrial encephalomyelopathy with lactic acidosis and strokelike episodes, Leigh syndrome, and progressive external ophthalmoplegia. (*Schapira and Griggs, 190–191*)

59. **(C)** The patient described in the vignette has an acute recurrent and reversible exercise intolerance (especially during a brief, intense isometric exercise or less intense but sustained exercise), normal neurological examination, increased CK level in the serum, myoglobinuria, and normal pyruvate and lactate level in the serum. This is highly suggestive of muscle energy deficit. The fuel used by muscle depends on several factors, most importantly the type, intensity, and duration of exercise, but also diet and physical conditioning. At rest, muscle uses predominantly fatty acids, whereas the energy for intense aerobic exercise in dynamic exercise derives from the oxidation of carbohydrate. The energy for maximal force generation in intense isometric exercise derives from anaerobic metabolism, particularly anaerobic glycogenolysis. During submaximal dynamic exercise, the type of fuel used by muscle depends on the relative intensity and duration of exercise. At low intensity, the

initial oxidative fuel is glycogen, with increasing proportions of oxidative energy supplied by blood, glucose, and free fatty acids as exercise duration increases. The type of circulating substrate during mild exercise varies with time. There is a gradual increase in the use of free fatty acids (as exercise duration increases) over glucose until, a few hours into exercise, lipid oxidation becomes the major source of energy. At high intensities of aerobic exercise, the proportion of energy derived from carbohydrate oxidation increases and glycogen become an important fuel. Fatigue appears when the glycogen is exhausted. Hence, the symptoms of patients with glycogenoses are almost invariably related to a strenuous bout of exertion. In contrast, patients with a disorder of lipid metabolism usually have little difficulty with short-term intense exercise.

In this vignette, the observation that venous pyruvate and lactate did not increase after exercise pointed to a failure of the breakdown of glycogen to lactic acid. The administration of epinephrine elicited a normal rise of blood glucose, indicating intact hepatic glycogenolysis and abnormal muscle glycogen metabolism. The most likely diagnosis is myophosphorylase deficiency, or McArdle disease. In typical cases, the cardinal manifestation of the disease is exercise intolerance manifested by myalgia, premature fatigue, and weakness or stiffness of exercising muscles. Muscle necrosis and myoglobinuria after exercise occur in about half of the patients, and about half of these develop acute renal failure. Mild proximal limb weakness is seen in about one-third of patients and is more common in older individuals. The electromyogram may be normal or may show nonspecific myopathic changes. No electrical activity is recorded by needle EMG from maximally shortened muscles during the cramps induced by ischemic exercise. Examination of a muscle biopsy specimen under light microscopy may show subsarcolemmal deposits of glycogen as bulges or blebs at the periphery of the fibers. Accumulation of glycogen, between myofibrils, generally is less marked but may be sufficient to give the fibers a vacuolar appearance.

In phosphofructokinase deficiency, typically, there is intolerance to intense exercise, often accompanied by cramps of exercising muscles, which are relieved by rest. Although a careful history reveals that exercise intolerance is present since childhood, patients usually do not come to medical attention until adolescence, and the diagnosis is established most commonly in young men. Symptoms are more likely to occur with isometric exercise. The exercise intolerance seems to worsen with high carbohydrate intake. The resting serum creatine kinase level is usually increased. The electromyogram may be normal or show myopathic abnormalities. Studies of 31 P-nuclear MR spectroscopy show the accumulation, even with mild exercise, of glycolytic intermediates in the form of phosphorylated monoesters. The accumulation of phosphorylated monoesters with exercise also occurs in other defects of glycolysis, but not in myophosphorylase deficiency.

Another important clinical difference between McArdle disease and phosphofructokinase deficiency is related to the fact that because phosphofructokinase deficiency blocks the metabolism of glucose, the patients experience a substantial drop in exercise capacity in response to glucose infusion or high carbohydrate meals. This response is termed "out of wind" phenomenon and is related to the fact that in phosphofructokinase deficiency the muscle is highly dependent on the availability of fatty acids and ketones for oxidative metabolism. Glucose causes an insulin-mediated inhibition of triglyceride hydrolysis and a fall in blood levels of the fatty acids and ketones necessary for muscle oxidative fuel. Definitive diagnosis requires biochemical documentation of the enzyme defect in muscle or careful measurement of the enzyme activity in erythrocytes to show partial deficiency. (*Schapira and Griggs, 230–233*)

60. **(C)** The cardinal clinical features of myasthenia gravis are fluctuating weakness and abnormal fatigability affecting all voluntary muscles, with a predilection for extraocular, bulbar, and proximal limb muscles. Initial symptoms involve the external ocular muscles in approximately 50% of cases, but bulbar symptoms are present in 16% of cases, and more rarely limb muscles may also be affected initially. Muscle weakness tends to be worse with repeated or prolonged exercise and typically exhibits diurnal fluctuation, worsening toward the evening hours. Within 1 year of onset, the disease remains purely ocular in about 40% of cases, generalized in about 35% of cases, confined to the extremities in about 10% of cases, and bulbar or oculobulbar in about 15% of cases. Within 2 years after onset, myasthenic syndrome remains restricted to the extraocular muscles in about only 14% of the patients whose initial manifestations are only ocular, whereas about 86% of patients develop generalized manifestations. The primary pathogenic event in myasthenia gravis is identified as an antibody-triggered acceleration, internalization, and progressive loss of acetylcholine receptors associated with a complement-mediated degeneration of synaptic folds. The loss of acetylcholine receptors results in decreased postsynaptic sensitivity to acetylcholine. Repetitive stimulation studies are the most commonly used electrophysiologic test of neuromuscular transmission. In myasthenia gravis, the major physiologic defect is the decremental response of the compound muscle action potential to a train of supramaximal stimuli, at a frequency varying from 2 to 3 Hz, of a nerve innervating the affected muscle. The administration of magnesium may depress the neuromuscular conduction and worsen the symptoms of myasthenia gravis. (*Schapira and Griggs, 254–266*)

61. **(D)** Lambert-Eaton myasthenic syndrome is due to an impairment of presynaptic release of acetylcholine at the neuromuscular junction. Presynaptic loss of voltage-gated calcium channels is the suggested primary pathological event in this disease. It is postulated that the calcium channels are the targets of autoantibodies. As a consequence, the influx of calcium into the nerve terminal is impaired, resulting in decreased quantal release of acetylcholine. Repetitive stimulation, which increases the external calcium concentration, promotes calcium entry into the nerve terminal, thus enhancing the acetylcholine release and neuromuscular transmission. In about 92% of patients with Lambert-Eaton myasthenic syndrome, antibodies directed against the P/Q type of voltage-gated calcium channels have been found with or without association to neoplasms. The N type of voltage-gated

calcium channel antibodies are detected in 40% to 49% of all early Lambert-Eaton myasthenic syndromes and in approximately 70% of those associated with malignancies.

In its classic presentation, the syndrome is characterized by weakness and fatigability, mostly affecting the proximal limb muscles, with minimum or moderate extraocular involvement or bulbar symptoms. Onset of symptoms usually occurs in the proximal lower limb muscles, which remain more predominantly involved. Autonomic symptoms and signs are usually prominent, and may include dry mouth and eyes, impotence, orthostatic hypotension, and hyperhidrosis. The reflexes are reduced or absent. Repetitive stimulation studies represent the most specific diagnostic tool. They may show the neurophysiologic characteristic of this presynaptic disorder: initial reduced compound muscle action potential amplitude with postactivation facilitation after voluntary exercise of 10 seconds or tetanic stimulation. There is an incremental response of the amplitude of the first compound muscle action potential of at least 100%. Tetanic stimulation at a rate of 20–50 Hz is more painful than the voluntary exercise and is indicated in cases of absent postactivation facilitation after voluntary activation. (*Schapira and Griggs, 272–274*)

62. **(A)** The case described in this vignette is highly suggestive of botulism intoxication. Botulinum toxin is one of the most potent poisons known. It is produced by the spores of *Clostridium botulinum*. The basic pathophysiology of botulism neurotoxicity relates to its inhibitory effect on acetylcholine release. Individual toxin types differ in their affinity for neuronal tissue, with type A being the most potent, followed by type B. Toxin-induced paralysis of cholinergic nerves involves three basic steps: (a) the binding of exotoxin to external receptors at ganglionic synapses, postganglionic parasympathetic synapses, and neuromuscular junction; (b) the translocated step, during which the toxin molecule or some portion of it passes through the nerve or muscle; and (c) the paralytic step, during which the release of acetylcholine is usually blocked.

Clinical features may include prodromal symptoms with nausea, vomiting, abdominal pain, and diarrhea. Cranial nerve signs appear early, with eye symptoms being the most common. There may be both an internal and external ophthalmoplegia. Rapid involvement of other cranial nerves produces vertigo, deafness, and dysphagia. Swallowing ultimately becomes impossible, and liquids are regurgitated through the nose. The voice often has a nasal quality and may be hoarse. Muscular weakness may appear between the second and fourth day of the illness. At first, the limbs may feel tired and the patient is unable to climb stairs. This weakness may become so severe that moving about or even turning in bed is impossible. Often this muscular involvement is limited to the neck muscles, so that the patient is unable to raise his or her head. Restlessness and agitation may occur; however, consciousness is preserved.

The neurophysiological findings of botulism are similar to the ones observed in Lambert-Eaton myasthenic syndrome. Sensory conduction studies are usually normal. In motor nerve conduction studies, the compound muscle action potential amplitudes are decreased in affected muscles with normal latencies and conduction velocities. Needle EMG may show abnormalities at rest with fibrillations and positive sharp waves. Repetitive stimulation studies may show decrement at slow rates of stimulation and characteristic increment, after a brief exercise or tetanic stimulation, between 20 and 50 Hz. The diagnosis is confirmed by detection of the neurotoxin in the patient serum or feces.

Clostridium tetani produce a powerful exotoxin under the anaerobic conditions of wounds or soil-contaminated injuries. Clinical features involve both the central and the peripheral nervous systems as well as the muscular system. The incubation period is usually from 5 to 25 days but may be as short as a few hours. In most cases, the clinical onset is characterized by a seemingly preferential affinity of the toxin for the facial and bulbar muscles. Premonitory signs may consist of a chill, headache, and restlessness, with pain and erythema at the site of injury. A sensation of tightness in the jaw and a mild stiffness and soreness in the neck are usually noticed within a few hours. Pain between the shoulder blades may also be present. Later, the jaw becomes stiff and tight and trismus results. This muscular

involvement soon spreads to the throat muscles, producing dysphagia, and when the facial muscles are involved, facial asymmetry and a fixed smile result. As the disease progresses, muscular hypertonicity may spread and become generalized, involving the muscles of the trunk and extremities. The rigidity of the back muscles produces an arching of the spine that, together with the retraction of the head, results in opisthotonos. Spasms or tonic contractions occur in any muscle group and may be spontaneous or precipitated by the slightest stimulus, such as noises, touching the patient, or even touching the bed.

Organophosphorus compounds are powerful inhibitors of acetylcholinesterase and pseudocholinesterase. In the human, the former enzyme is found in nervous tissue, specifically in brain and spinal cord myoneural junctions (at pre- and postganglionic parasympathetic synapses and at preganglionic synapses) and in some postganglionic sympathetic nerve endings. Excess acetylcholine causes overstimulation and then depolarization blockade of cholinergic transmission. Two major neurophysiological features of acetylcholinesterase inhibition are repetitive discharges following the compound muscle action potential (CMAP) and the decrement in the CMAP with repetitive stimulation.

Clinically, intoxication may range from latent, asymptomatic poisoning to a life-threatening illness, depending on the level of serum cholinesterase activity. A decrease of 10% to 50% of serum cholinesterase activity may not even be clinically detectable. When levels are moderately depressed (20% normal), sweating, cramps, tingling of the extremities, and mild bulbar weakness with fasciculation may occur. At 10% of serum cholinesterase activity, consciousness becomes depressed, and myosis with no pupillary response to light occurs. The patient may become cyanotic from respiratory weakness, and pooled secretions may obstruct the airway. Central nervous system manifestations include confusion, convulsions, depression of respiratory and circulatory centers, nightmares, headaches, progressive generalized weakness, slurred speech, ataxia, and tremor. Muscarinic manifestations include bradycardia with hypotension, excessive sweating and salivation, miosis and blurring of vision, nausea and vomiting with cramps, and wheezing with bronchial constriction. Nicotinic manifestations include muscular twitching, fasciculation, and cramps. Venom poisoning may rarely cause a disorder of the neuromuscular junction with a curare-like effect.

Lambert-Eaton myasthenic syndrome is diagnosed based on the triad of fatigable weakness predominantly in the proximal limb muscles, reduced or absent reflexes, and autonomic features. Repetitive stimulation studies show an incremental response on titanic stimulation. Antibodies against the P/Q voltage-gated calcium channel may be detected. *(Schapira and Griggs, 272–280)*

63. **(E)** The deleterious effects of aminoglycosides on neuromuscular transmission have been well established for practically all agents of this family of antibiotics, which are contraindicated in patients with myasthenia gravis. Most aminoglycosides, including neomycin and tobramycin, exert their effect through reduction of the number of acetylcholine quanta released at the nerve terminal, after the arrival of the propagated nerve action potential. Other antibiotics have been incriminated in myasthenic exacerbation, including ampicillin, ciprofloxacin, perfloxacin, and norfloxacin. Clindamycin and lincomycin may produce a neuromuscular blockage, not reversible with anticholinesterases but reversible with 3,4 aminopyridine. Quinidine can produce a worsening of weakness in patients with myasthenia gravis, acting at the nerve terminal by inhibiting acetylcholine synthesis or release. Magnesium derivate may worsen myasthenia symptoms by blocking calcium entry into the nerve terminal. *(Schapira and Griggs, 277–278)*

64. **(D)** Congenital myasthenic syndromes (CMS) are heterogeneous disorders arising from presynaptic, synaptic, or postsynaptic defects. In each CMS, the specific defect compromises the safety margin of neuromuscular transmission by one or more mechanisms. The European neuromuscular center classification of congenital myasthenic syndrome classifies congenital myasthenia into three groups: Type I, with autosomal recessive transmission, includes familial infantile

myasthenia, limb-girdle myasthenia, acetylcholinesterase deficiency, acetylcholine receptor deficiency, and benign congenital myasthenic syndrome with facial dysmorphism. Type II, with autosomal dominant transmission, includes slow-channel syndrome. Type III includes sporadic cases. The clues for the diagnosis of a slow-channel myasthenic syndrome consist of selectively severe weakness of the forearm extensor muscles, repetitive compound muscle action potential response to single nerve stimuli that is accentuated by edrophonium, prolonged and biexponentially decaying miniature end-plate current, and end-plate myopathy. The end-plate myopathy, which results from calcium overloading of the postsynaptic region, is evidenced by degeneration of junctional folds with loss of acetylcholine receptors and widening of the synaptic space. *(Engel et al., 140–156; Schapira and Griggs, 279–286)*

65. **(A)** Cholesterol- and lipid-lowering agents are associated with myopathy, occurring in less than 0.5% of patients on monotherapy and increasing in frequency up to 5% with combined lipid-lowering therapy. Patients complain of myalgia and weakness. CK concentration is elevated. Biopsy reveals type II atrophy and myofiber necrosis. The 3-hydroxy-3-methylglutaryl coenzyme A (HMG-CoA) reductase inhibitors (such as lovastatin) and niacin have all been implicated in producing myopathy. The HMG-CoA reductase inhibitors produce rhabdomyolysis as a direct toxic effect on myocytes. Amiodarone may cause a lysosomal-related myopathy. Zidovidine may cause mitochondrial myopathy. D penicillamine may cause inflammatory myopathy. Colchicine may cause antimicrotubular myopathy. *(Schapira and Griggs, 364–366)*

66. **(A)**

67. **(B)**

68. **(C)**

69. **(D)**

70. **(E)**

Explanations 66 through 70

Cranial nerves may be affected in certain diseases that cause peripheral neuropathies. Diphtheritic neuropathy most commonly causes glossopharyngeal nerve palsy or, less commonly, oculomotor cranial nerve palsies. The facial nerve is the most commonly affected cranial nerve in sarcoidosis, but olfactory, oculomotor, and trochlear nerves can also be affected. Diabetic neuropathy may be associated with oculomotor nerve palsy with conservation of the pupillary reflexes. The trochlear, the abducens, and the facial nerves can be affected. Guillain-Barré syndrome may be associated with abducens and facial nerve paralysis, whereas Miller-Fisher syndrome (a variant of Guillain-Barré syndrome) may be associated with oculomotor and trochlear nerve paralysis. Sjögren's syndrome neuropathy may be associated with trigeminal neuropathy. Polyarteritis nodosa may commonly involve the oculomotor and facial nerves, less likely the vestibulocochlear nerve. Wegener's granulomatosis may commonly affect the facial nerve. The trigeminal and facial nerves are the most commonly affected in Lyme disease. The trigeminal and vagus nerves are the most commonly affected cranial nerves in porphyria. The oculomotor nerve is the most commonly affected in syphilis. Primary amyloidosis commonly affects the facial, the trigeminal, and the oculomotor nerves, whereas in Refsum's disease, the olfactory nerve as well as the vestibulocochlear nerve are most commonly affected. *(Rolak, 81)*

71. **(D)** A predominantly sensory type of neuropathy may be seen in cases of pyridoxine or doxorubicin toxicity, sensory variants of acute and chronic demyelinating polyneuropathy, IgM paraproteinemia, paraneoplastic neuropathy, Sjögren's syndrome neuropathy, vitamin E deficiency, abetalipoproteinemia, and spinocerebellar degeneration. A predominantly motor neuropathy is commonly seen in cases of Guillain-Barré syndrome, diphtheric neuropathy, dapsone-induced neuropathy, porphyria, and multifocal motor neuropathy. *(Rolak, 82)*

72. **(C)** A useful concept in understanding neuromuscular transmission is the safety factor. It is defined as the difference between the membrane potential and the threshold potential of initiating an action potential. As long as the threshold potential is reached, the action potential initiates muscle contraction. Several factors contribute to the safety factor: quantal release, acetylcholine receptor conduction properties and density, and cholinesterase activity. Postsynaptic folds form a high-resistance pathway that focuses end-plate current flow on voltage-gated sodium channels concentrated in the depth of the folds. Both these factors reduce the action potential threshold at the end plate and serve to increase the safety factor. All disorders of neuromuscular transmission are characterized by the compromise of the safety factor for neuromuscular transmission. The functional effect of reduced acetylcholine receptors is decreased end-plate potential. If quantal release is lowered (such as in cases of repetitive stimulation or activity), the end-plate potential may fall below the threshold and the muscle action potential will not be generated. *(Schapira, 254)*

73. **(A)** Several lines of evidence suggest that CD4+ T helper cells have a major role in the pathogenesis of myasthenia gravis: (a) Most anti-acetylcholine receptor antibodies in myasthenia gravis patients are high-affinity IgG and their synthesis requires CD4 and T helper factors. (b) Acetylcholine receptors reactive CD4+ cells from the blood, and the thymus of myasthenia gravis patients have a T helper function. (c) Thymectomy decreases the reactivity of blood T-cells against acetylcholine receptors. (d) In vitro treatment of CD4+ T-cells from the blood of myasthenia gravis patients with anti CD4+ antibodies decreases the reactivity of T-cells to acetylcholine receptors. (e) In experimental autoimmune myasthenia gravis, the synthesis of pathogenic anti-acetylcholine receptor antibodies requires CD4+ cells. *(Drachman 1797–1810)*

74. **(C)** Myasthenia gravis (MG) is characterized clinically by muscle weakness, enhanced by physical effort. Although the acetylcholine receptor (AChR) expressed on muscle is the main target of the disease, the thymus has long been known to be involved in the pathogenesis of myasthenia gravis. Most myasthenic patients have thymic abnormalities: 70% of patients have lymphoid follicular hyperplasia, and 10% have

a thymoma. Numerous arguments indicate a relationship between myasthenia gravis, the anti-acetylcholine receptor antibodies, and the thymus: (a) Thymic abnormalities are seen in seropositive patients. (b) Thymectomy has a beneficial effect. (c) Anti-AChR antibody titers are decreased after thymectomy. (d) There is a decreased in vitro production of anti-AChR antibodies from stimulated peripheral blood lymphocytes. (e) There is spontaneous in vitro production of anti-AChR antibodies by thymocytes from a hyperplasic thymus. (f) There is transfer by myasthenia gravis thymic explants of pathogenic parameters in some animal studies. The human thymus may express acetylcholine receptors. Thymic myoid cells may have a role in anti-AChR sensitization. This is supported by their characteristic and unusual microenvironment in myasthenia gravis thymuses with lymphoid follicular hyperplasia. In myasthenia gravis thymuses, but never in normal thymuses, myoid cells, which do not express class II molecules, are in intimate contact with HLA-DR-positive reticulum cells close to, and occasionally inside, germinal centers. These histopathologic findings suggest that the reticulum cells may function as antigen-presenting cells and acetylcholine receptor epitopes. *(Moulian et al., 397–406)*

75. **(B)** Corticosteroids are the mainstay of immunosuppressive treatment of myasthenia gravis. They have numerous effects on the immune system as a whole, leading to a general immunosuppression. The benefit of therapeutic effect for myasthenia gravis appears to be related to (a) reduction of lymphocyte differentiation and proliferation; (b) redistribution of lymphocytes from the circulation into tissues that remove them from the site of immunoreactivity; (c) alteration of lymphokine function, primarily tumor necrosis factor IL-1, and IL-2; (d) inhibition of macrophage function, in particular antigen presentation and processing; and (e) increased acetylcholine receptor synthesis in the muscle. *(Ransohoff, 78)*

REFERENCES

Crimlisk HL. The little imitator-porphyria: a neuropsychiatric disorder. *J Neurol Neurosurg Psychiatry*. 1997;62: 319–328.

Drachman DB. Myasthenia gravis. *N Engl J Med*. 1994; 330:1797–1810.

Emery AE. The muscular dystrophies. *BMJ*. 1998;317: 991–995.

Engel AG, Ohno K, Milone M, Sine SM. Congenital myasthenic syndromes. New insights from molecular genetic and patch-clamp studies. *Ann N Y Acad Sci*. 1998; 841:140–156.

Goetz CG, Papper. EJ, eds. *Textbook of Clinical Neurology*. Philadelphia, PA: WB Saunders; 1999.

Karpati G, Hilton-Jones D, Griggs RC, eds. *Disorders of Voluntary Muscle*. 7th ed. Cambridge, UK: Cambridge University Press, 2001.

Mendell JR, Kissel JT, Cornblath DR, eds. *Diagnosis and Management of Peripheral Nerve Disorders*. Oxford, UK: Oxford University Press; 2001.

Moulian N, Wakkach A, Guyon T, et al. Respective role of thymus and muscle in autoimmune myasthenia gravis. *Ann N Y Acad Sci*. 1998;841:397–406.

Murakami T, Garcia CA, Reiter LT, Lupski JR. Charcot-Marie-Tooth disease and related inherited neuropathies. *Medicine (Baltimore)*. 1996;75:233–250.

Newman LS, Rose CS, Maier LA. Medical progress: sarcoidosis. *N Engl J Med*. 1997;336:1224–1234.

Nonaka I. Distal myopathies. *Curr Opin Neurol*. 1999;12: 493–499.

Preston DC, Shapiro BE, eds. *EMG Waveforms* (video companion to *Electromyography and Neuromuscular Disorders. Clinical-Electrophysiologic Correlations*). Boston, MA: Butterworth-Heinemann; 1998.

Ptacek LJ, Johnson KJ, Griggs RC. Genetics and physiology of the myotonic muscle disorders. *N Engl J Med*. 1993; 328:482–489.

Rolak LA, ed. *Neurology Secrets*. 2nd ed. Philadelphia, PA: Hanley & Belfuls; 1998.

Ransohoff R. Neuroimmunology. *Continuum (NY)*. 2001;7:78.

Saifi GM, Szigeti K, Snipes GJ, Garcia CA, Lupski JR. Molecular mechanisms, diagnosis, and rational approaches to management of and therapy for Charcot-Marie-Tooth disease and related peripheral neuropathies. *J Investing Med*. 2003;51:261–283.

Schapira AH, Cock HR. Mitochondrial myopathies and encephalomyopathies. *Eur J Clin Invest*. 1999;29:886–898.

Schapira AH, Griggs RC, eds. Muscle diseases. Boston, MA: Butterworth-Heinemann; 1999.

Smith BE, Cranial neuropathy in diabetes mellitus. In: Dyck PJ, Thomas PK, eds. *Diabetic Neuropathy*. Philadelphia, PA: WB Saunders; 1999:457–467.

Steere AC. Medical progress: Lyme disease. *N Engl J Med*. 2001;345:115–125.

CHAPTER 6

Behavioral Neurology
Questions

Questions 1 through 4
Link the following.

    (A) Neurofibrillary tangles
    (B) Neuropil threads
    (C) Dystrophic neurites
    (D) Senile plaques

1. Filament-containing neuronal processes around extracellular Aβ amyloid deposition

2. Filamentous accumulation of dendrites

3. Neurofibrillary formation in the cell bodies

4. Filament-containing neuronal processes in the distal axons

Questions 5 through 8
Link each of the following gene locations to the appropriate protein implicated in the pathogenesis of Alzheimer's disease.

    (A) Chromosome 21
    (B) Chromosome 19
    (C) Chromosome 14
    (D) Chromosome 1

5. Presenilin 1

6. Amyloid precursor protein

7. Presenilin 2

8. ApoE glycoprotein

9. Injury to which of the following locations is the most critical in causing memory impairment in Alzheimer's disease?

    (A) Hippocampus
    (B) Amygdala
    (C) Basal forebrain cholinergic system
    (D) Brain stem monoaminergic system
    (E) Neocortex

10. In Alzheimer's disease, the enzyme responsible for the endoproteolytic cleavage of amyloid precursor protein to generate N-terminal of Aβ peptide is

    (A) α secretase
    (B) BACE1
    (C) BACE2
    (D) γ secretase
    (E) none of the above

11. Which of the following is true about the β amyloid peptide?

    (A) The soluble β amyloid peptide is the major constituent of the senile plaque.
    (B) β secretase cleaves the N terminal of amyloid precursor protein.
    (C) P3 deposits are found in patients with Alzheimer's disease.
    (D) Alzheimer's disease patients have a reduced glial reaction compared to normal patients.
    (E) Cox1 expression is increased in Alzheimer's disease.

12. In early stage Alzheimer's disease, neuropsychologic tests show a defect in

    (A) remote memory
    (B) immediate memory
    (C) recent memory
    (D) concrete reasoning
    (E) calculation

13. Positron emission tomography shows that the most severe reduction in cerebral metabolism in case of Alzheimer's disease is located in

    (A) temporal association cortex
    (B) frontal association cortex
    (C) motor cortex
    (D) parietal association cortex
    (E) basal ganglia

14. In Alzheimer's disease, the most common psychiatric symptom is

    (A) depression
    (B) visual hallucination
    (C) auditory hallucination
    (D) delusion
    (E) verbal aggressiveness

15. Posterior cortical atrophy, a dementia syndrome with early prominent visual and visuospatial disturbance, is most frequently seen in

    (A) corticobasal degeneration
    (B) Alzheimer's disease
    (C) Creutzfeldt-Jakob disease
    (D) subcortical gliosis
    (E) Huntington disease

Questions 16 through 21
Link each of the following.

    (A) Frontotemporal dementia
    (B) Alzheimer's disease
    (C) Both
    (D) Neither

16. Hyperorality

17. Impairment in executive function

18. Decreased verbal memory

19. Visuospatial short-term memory

20. Associated with chromosome 4

21. Associated with chromosome 17q21-22

22. Which of the following neurodegenerative diseases is associated with the aggregation of tau isoforms without exon 10?

    (A) Supranuclear palsy
    (B) Corticobasal degeneration
    (C) Alzheimer's disease
    (D) Pick's disease
    (E) Familial frontotemporal dementia

23. Which of the following is a feature of progressive supranuclear palsy?

    (A) Aphasia
    (B) Unilateral dystonia
    (C) Marked slowing of vertical saccades followed by the development of vertical supranuclear gaze palsy
    (D) Hallucinations not related to medications
    (E) Onset of symptoms at the age of 30 years

24. In progressive supranuclear palsy, high-density neurofibrillary tangles are LEAST likely to be seen in

    (A) striatum
    (B) thalamus
    (C) pallidum
    (D) dentate nucleus
    (E) prefrontal cortex

25. Which of the following is true about neurofibrillary tangles?

    (A) Neurofibrillary tangles are more specific to Alzheimer's disease than neuritic plaques.
    (B) They contain reactive astrocytes and microglia.
    (C) Their main location is leptomeningeal and superficial cortical vessels.

(D) Neurofibrillary tangles begin in the transentorhinal cortex, progress to the limbic cortex to reach the neocortical areas.

(E) They are made up of dense granules that react with anti-neurofilament antibodies.

26. Which of the following is true about neurotransmitter disturbance in Alzheimer's disease?

(A) There is a dramatic increase in the level of choline acetyltransferase activity in the nucleus basalis of Meynert.

(B) Acetylcholinesterase activity is reduced.

(C) The number of M1 muscarinic receptors is decreased.

(D) M2 muscarinic and nicotinic receptors are preserved.

(E) The level of GABA activity is increased and correlates with the severity of the disease.

27. Early onset of familial Alzheimer's disease has been associated with

(A) chromosome 21

(B) chromosome 4

(C) chromosome 6

(D) chromosome 12

(E) chromosome 17

28. Early HIV dementia is associated with

(A) impaired retrieval

(B) impaired calculation

(C) impaired attention

(D) impaired language

(E) impaired recognition memory

29. The most characteristic neuropathological feature of HIV dementia is

(A) neurofibrillary tangles

(B) periventricular demyelination

(C) caudate atrophy

(D) multinucleated giant cells

(E) neuritic plaques

Questions 30 through 36
Link the following.

(A) Dementia of the frontal type

(B) Progressive nonfluent aphasia

(C) Both

(D) Neither

30. Phonological paraphasic errors are an early feature.

31. It is a frontotemporal type of dementia.

32. Apathy and lack of motivation and mental flexibility are extremely common.

33. Disproportion between poor executive function and preservation of memory and language functions

34. Atrophy of the left polar temporal lobe

35. Atrophy of the left perisylvian region

36. Atrophy of the orbitomedial cortex

37. Which of the following cognitive functions is the LEAST affected in case of dementia with Lewy bodies?

(A) Memory

(B) Visuospatial function

(C) Executive function

(D) Attention

(E) Construction ability

38. The LEAST supportive of the diagnosis of dementia with Lewy bodies is

(A) progressive cognitive decline

(B) spontaneous parkinsonism

(C) neuroleptic hypersensitivity

(D) auditory hallucination

(E) multiple falls

39. Synuclein aggregates are found in

    (A) Pick's disease
    (B) multiple infarct dementia
    (C) Huntington's disease
    (D) spinocerebellar atrophy
    (E) multiple system atrophy

40. In brain injury, irritability and disinhibition are seen in which of the following areas of the frontal lobe?

    (A) Dorsolateral frontal lobe
    (B) Frontal eye field
    (C) Orbitofrontal area
    (D) Medial frontal area
    (E) Supplementary motor area

Questions 41 through 50
Link the following.

    (A) Implicit memory
    (B) Explicit memory
    (C) Both
    (D) Neither

41. Episodic memory

42. Semantic memory

43. Memory that is recalled unconsciously

44. Medial temporal lobe

45. Memory that needs a deliberate conscious effort

46. Short-term memory

47. Priming

48. Memory of skills and habits

49. Amygdala

50. Cerebellum

Questions 51 through 54
Link each of the following cerebral locations to the appropriate neurological deficit.

    (A) Posterior parietal cortex
    (B) Occipital cortex
    (C) Inferotemporal cortex
    (D) Association area of the frontal cortex

51. Associative visual agnosia

52. Apperceptive visual agnosia

53. Prosopagnosia

54. Source amnesia

Questions 55 through 58
Link each of the following steps in memory processing to the appropriate definition.

    (A) Encoding
    (B) Consolidation
    (C) Storage
    (D) Retrieval

55. Processes that make information more stable for long-term storage

56. Mechanism and sites by which memory is retained over time

57. Processes that permit the recall and use of stored information

58. Processes by which new information are attended to and processed when first encountered

59. Which of the following is true about the hippocampus pathways involved in the storage of explicit memory?

    (A) Projections from the entorhinal cortex to the pyramidal cells of CA3
    (B) Mossy fibers that project to pyramidal cells of CA3
    (C) Pyramidal cell of CA1 projecting to CA3
    (D) Entorhinal cortex cells that project to CA1 cells
    (E) Mossy fibers projecting to the entorhinal cortex cells

60. Which of the following is true about long-term potentiation in mossy fiber pathway?

    (A) GABA is the neurotransmitter used by synaptic terminals of mossy fibers.
    (B) The blockade of NMDA receptors affects long-term potentiation in mossy fibers.
    (C) Long-term potentiation in mossy fibers is dependent on presynaptic calcium.
    (D) Cooperativity is a typical feature of long-term potentiation in mossy fibers.
    (E) Long-term potentiation in mossy fibers requires the concomitant activation of pre and post synaptic cells.

61. Conduction aphasia may result from a lesion located in

    (A) supramarginal gyrus
    (B) internal capsule
    (C) corpus callosum
    (D) angular gyrus
    (E) orbitofrontal areas

62. A patient demonstrating the use of a toothbrush at the level of the chest has

    (A) sensory neglect
    (B) ideomotor apraxia
    (C) motor neglect
    (D) hemispatial neglect
    (E) limb kinetic apraxia

Answers and Explanations

1. **(D)**

2. **(B)**

3. **(A)**

4. **(C)**

Explanations 1 through 4

In Alzheimer's disease, many neurons exhibit fibrillary accumulations in the cytoplasm, including neurofibrillary tangles (NFT; neurofibrillary pathology in cell bodies and proximal dendrites), neuropil threads (filamentous accumulations in dendrites), dystrophic neurites (filament-containing neuronal processes, particularly distal axons/terminals), and senile plaques where the β amyloid peptide is their major constituent. Ultrastructurally, fibrillary inclusions represent intracellular accumulations of straight filaments and paired helical filaments, both are composed principally of hyperphosphorylated isoforms of tau, a low-molecular-weight, microtubule-associated protein. Because hyperphosphorylated tau species bind poorly to microtubules and alter microtubule stability, this biochemical modification could affect other cytoskeletal constituents, intracellular transport, cellular geometry, and/or neuronal viability. *(Price et al., 461–493)*

5. **(C)**

6. **(A)**

7. **(D)**

8. **(B)**

Explanations 5 through 8

The inheritance of one of the following genes may predispose the carrier to an increased risk of Alzheimer's disease:

- Polymorphic variant of the apoE gene on chromosome 19.
- Presenilin 1 gene located on the long arm of chromosome 14.
- Presenilin 2 gene isolated and mapped to chromosome 1.
- Amyloid precursor protein gene linked to chromosome 21. *(Price et al., 461–493)*

9. **(A)** The disease process in Alzheimer's disease selectively damages brain regions and neural circuits critical for cognition and memory, including neurons in the neocortex, hippocampus, amygdala, basal forebrain cholinergic system, and brain stem monoaminergic nuclei. The severity of memory impairments and densities of senile plaques correlates with levels of synaptophysin (a presynaptic vesicle protein) in the hippocampus of individuals with Alzheimer's disease. Alterations in the basal forebrain cholinergic system are also believed to contribute to memory difficulties and to deficits in arousal/attention. *(Price et al., 461–493)*

10. **(B)** Alzheimer's disease is characterized by a progressive deposition of neurofibrillary and Aβ-amyloid tangles in many areas of the brain, particularly the hippocampus and cerebral cortex. Endoproteolytic cleavage of amyloid precursor protein by β and γ secretase generates toxic Aβ peptides. BACE1 and BACE2 are two secretases involved in the generation of amyloid precursor protein. The secretion of Aβ peptide is

abolished in cultures of BACE1 deficient embryonic cortical neurons. BACE1 is the principle neuronal protease required to cleave amyloid precursor protein at +1 and +11 sites that generate the N-terminal of Aβ peptides. *(Cai et al., 233–234)*

11. **(B)** The β amyloid peptide is the major constituent of senile plaques. It is present in a soluble nontoxic form in all human brains. It undergoes conformational changes and becomes relatively insoluble in Alzheimer's disease. Soluble β amyloid peptide is mainly formed by 40 amino acid sequences and may originate from cells of the central nervous system as well as from the peripheral nervous system. The amyloid precursor protein is cleaved in its N and C terminials by β and γ secretases, respectively. P3 fragment, a major component of diffuse plaques, originates from the cleavage of the amyloid precursor protein by an α secretase. P3 deposits are seen in normal aging as well as in Alzheimer's disease patients. P3 deposits in normal aging patients lack abnormal neurites and display a reduced glial reaction compared to P3 deposits in Alzheimer's disease. Cyclooxygenase enzymes 1 and 2, biosynthesis inflammatory mediators, are constitutively expressed and mitogen induced, respectively. Cyclooxygenase 2 level is sensitive to IL-1, IL-2, and TNF pro-inflammatory interleukins. Cyclooxygenase 2 expression, but not 1, increases in case of Alzheimer's disease, especially in neurons that are destined for apoptosis. *(Halliday et al., 1–8)*

12. **(C)** Deficits in recent memory are typically the first symptom of Alzheimer's disease (AD) and may be clinically reported as misplacing objects, repeating questions and statements, and forgetting names. Both verbal and visuospatial memory changes occur. Impairments in visuospatial memory are often experienced as getting lost. Early in the disease, these deficits in memory are primarily for recent information. On examination, AD patients have marked difficulty remembering word lists, stories, and designs.

As the disease progresses, the cognitive impairment becomes more diffuse, with reduced ability to do multiple tasks or carry out complex mental tracking tasks, decreased concentration, difficulty with mental arithmetic, and a decline in abstract reasoning. Remote memory impairments also emerge, with the oldest memories tending to be the most stable. Semantic memory as well as implicit memory become impaired as the disease progresses. *(Kramer and Miller, 447–454)*

13. **(D)** Positron emission tomography (PET) examines regional cerebral metabolic rates for oxygen and glucose and has proved to be an effective means of studying brain functioning in dementia patients. PET studies have consistently found that association cortex, primarily in posterior regions, is most severely affected in Alzheimer's disease. Primary sensory and motor cortices, basal ganglia, thalamus, and cerebellum are relatively spared. The parietal lobe has the largest reductions in metabolism. Patients with mild to moderate Alzheimer's disease have reductions in rate of metabolism that range from 23% to 39% for parietal association cortex, 15% to 30% for temporal association cortex, and 15% to 21% for frontal association cortex. Metabolic rate shows further reductions as the severity of the dementia worsens. *(Kramer and Miller, 447–454)*

14. **(A)** Depression is the most common psychiatric symptom associated with Alzheimer's disease. It occurs in 15% to 20% of Alzheimer's disease patients. As the dementia advances, delusions become a more common symptom. More severely, demented Alzheimer's disease patients may have visual and auditory hallucinations as well as restlessness, irritability, repetitive behavior, disturbed sleep patterns, and verbal aggression. *(Kramer and Miller, 447–454)*

15. **(B)** Pathological studies have shown that the most frequent cause of posterior cortical atrophy is Alzheimer's disease. This syndrome can also be seen in subcortical gliosis and Creutzfeldt-Jakob disease. Careful postmortem study has shown that relative to typical Alzheimer's disease cases, patients who initially present with prominent visual symptoms have higher densities of plaques and tangles in primary and visual association areas and relatively fewer lesions in the prefrontal cortex. *(Kramer and Miller, 447–454)*

16. (A)

17. (C)

18. (C)

19. (B)

20. (D)

21. (A)

Explanations 16 through 21

Frontotemporal dementia (FTD) is characterized by the prominence of behavioral abnormalities such as loss of personal awareness, hyperorality, stereotyped and perseverative behavior, and progressive reduction of speech with conservation of spatial orientation. In Alzheimer's disease, spatial orientation loss is more prominent than in frontotemporal dementia, where inappropriate behavior is more prominent. Informed-based questionnaire as well as other behavioral and neuropsychological tests serve to differentiate frontotemporal dementia from Alzheimer's disease. Free recall does not differ between Alzheimer's disease and frontotemporal dementia patients, but the benefit from semantic cueing and recognition is significantly better in FTD patients, suggesting that FTD patients mainly experience retrieval difficulties, provided that encoding is controlled. Verbal and visuospatial short-term memory are both decreased in Alzheimer's disease, whereas only verbal memory is decreased in FTD. Language comprehension profiles in FTD are mainly characterized by sentence comprehension difficulties caused by impaired processing of grammatical phrase structure as well as a relatively selective impairment in action naming. FTD patients perform better than Alzheimer's disease patients on construction and calculation, and have greater impairment in executive than in memory tasks. FTD has been linked to chromosome 17q21-22 in a population based study. Huntington's disease has been linked to chromosome 4. *(Pasquier and Delacourte, 417–427)*

22. (D) Tau proteins are the basic components of neurofibrillary neuronal inclusions that affect numerous causes of dementia. They stabilize microtubules, which play an important role in intraneuronal transport. They are formed by six isoforms resulting from the translation of exons 2, 3, and 10. Tau proteins may be abnormally phosphorylated and aggregate into neuronal inclusion. These inclusions may be biochemically different from one type of dementia to another type. In Alzheimer's disease, all six tau isoforms (with and without exon 10) are aggregated. This is not specific of Alzheimer's disease; the same pattern of tau aggregation is seen in postencephalitic Parkinsonism, Niemann-Pick type C disease, and Down syndrome. In progressive supranuclear palsy and corticobasal degeneration, there is an aggregation of tau isoforms with exon 10, mainly in the frontal subcortical and cortical areas. They are mainly located in small pyramidal cells and astrocytes of layers II and III of the cerebral cortex. In familial frontotemporal dementia, tau isoforms with exon 10 are aggregated. In Pick disease, there is aggregation of two main tau variants lacking exon 10: Tau 55 and Tau 64. They are found in the frontotemporal areas and involve the small pyramidal cells of neocortical layers II and III, as well as granule cells of the dentate gyrus. *(Pasquier and Delacourte, 417–427)*

23. (C) Progressive supranuclear palsy is characterized by early postural instability, supranuclear vertical gaze palsy, parkinsonism insensitive to levodopa therapy, pseudobulbar palsy, and subcortical dementia. Histological features include degeneration in different areas of the basal ganglia and brain stem. The presence of early instability and multiple falls during the first year of symptom onset, in a patient with parkinsonism, should point to the diagnosis of progressive supranuclear palsy, although early instability may be seen in cases of multiple system atrophy and corticobasal degeneration. Marked slowing of vertical saccades is followed by the development of vertical supranuclear gaze palsy. This distinguishes progressive supranuclear palsy from corticobasal degeneration and multisystem atrophy. In corticobasal degeneration, the saccades may have increased latency but normal speed and are equally affected in the vertical and horizontal plane. In multiple system atrophy, the saccades have normal speed and latency. Frontal lobe signs including apathy, impaired abstract thought, decreased verbal fluency, and imitation behavior are seen early in the course of progressive supranuclear palsy, as well as prominent swallowing and speech difficulties. Red flags against the diagnosis of supranuclear palsy include the presence of aphasia, onset earlier than the age of 40, duration of the disease of more than 20 years, presence of cortical dementia, or cortical sensory or visual deficit, hallucinations not due to medications, and maintained response to levodopa replacement. *(Litvan, 41–48)*

24. **(B)** Progressive supranuclear palsy is characterized on neuropathological examination by neuronal loss, gliosis, and the presence of neurofibrillary tangles and/or neuropil threads in specific areas of the basal ganglia and the brain stem. The NINDS neuropathologic criteria for typical progressive supranuclear palsy are:

    • High density of neurofibrillary tangles and neuropil threads in at least three of the following areas: pallidum, subthalamic nucleus, substantia nigra, or pons.
    • Low to high density of neurofibrillary tangles or neuropil threads in at least three of the following areas: striatum, oculomotor complex, medulla, or dentate nucleus.
    • Clinical history compatible with progressive supranuclear palsy. *(Litvan, 41–48)*

25. **(D)** The pathological characteristics of Alzheimer's disease include neurofibrillary tangles, neuritic plaques, loss of synapses and neurons, granulovacuolar degeneration, amyloid angiopathy, and AMY plaques. Neurofibrillary tangles are formed by paired helical filaments that occupy the cell body and may extend to the dendrites but not to the axon. These filaments are arranged to form a tubule that contains abnormally phosphorylated tau protein. They are preferentially located in large pyramidal neurons, particularly those with long ipsilateral cortical-cortical connections. Neurofibrillary tangles are produced in the transentorhinal cortex in the beginning of the disease and progress to limbic cortical regions to reach the neocortical areas. The pattern of progression of neurofibrillary tangles correlates with the early memory deficit seen in Alzheimer's disease. Neurofibrillary tangles are not specific to Alzheimer's disease; they are seen in progressive supranuclear palsy, postencephalitic Parkinson disease, and subacute sclerosing panencephalitis. Neuritic plaques are more specific to Alzheimer's disease than neurofibrillary tangles and are formed by a central immunoreactive amyloid core surrounded by dystrophic neurons, which contain paired helical filaments, normal glial processes, abnormal organelles, reactive astrocytes, and microglia. Amyloid angiopathy involves leptomeningeal and superficial cortical vessels in Alzheimer patients. Granulovacuolar degeneration involves the pyramidal cell layer of the hippocampus with the presence in the cytoplasm of the pyramidal cell of vacuoles. *(Cummings et al., S2–17)*

26. **(B)** The nucleus basalis of Meynert is affected early in the course of Alzheimer's disease. It is a major source of choline acetyltransferase, which is responsible for the synthesis of acetylcholine. There is a marked and consistent decrease of choline acetyltransferase and acetylcholine synthesis. There is a reduction of the activity of acetylcholinesterase, the enzyme responsible of the degradation of acetylcholine. M1 muscarinic receptors located in the hippocampus and in the upper and lower levels of the cerebral cortex are relatively preserved in Alzheimer's disease compared to M2 muscarinic receptors located in the brain stem and nucleus basalis, which are markedly reduced. Nicotinic receptors, serotonin, norepinephrine, GABA, and somatostatin are also reduced. *(Cummings et al., S2–17)*

27. **(A)** Early onset of familial Alzheimer's disease has been linked to mutations in chromosomes 21, 14, and 1. It is inherited as an autosomal dominant disease. Mutations in chromosome 21 involve the amyloid precursor gene affecting the processing of the amyloid precursor protein. Mutations in chromosome 14 involve the presenilin gene and cause an increase of the production of the amyloid β peptide. Mutations in chromosome 1 involve presenilin 2 gene and also

cause an increase of the production of the amyloid β peptide. Mutations on chromosomes 17, 12, and 6 are considered genetic risk factors in Alzheimer's disease. *(Cummings et al., pp. S2–17)*

28. **(A)** Early symptoms of HIV dementia are subtle and may be confused with psychiatric complaints, the effect of substance abuse or delirium. They are characterized by the prominence of subcortical involvement. These symptoms may include:

    - Memory impairment, both verbal and nonverbal.
    - Impaired manipulation of acquired knowledge.
    - Impaired retrieval, and general slowing of psychomotor speed and thought processes.

    Attention, language, and recognition memory are relatively preserved. *(McArthur et al., 129–150)*

29. **(D)** Multinucleated giant cells are characteristically seen in HIV dementia. Their presence correlates with the degree of dementia and the detection of HIV DNA. *(McArthur et al., 129–150)*

30. **(B)**

31. **(C)**

32. **(A)**

33. **(A)**

34. **(D)**

35. **(B)**

36. **(A)**

Explanations 30 through 36

Progressive nonfluent aphasia, in contrast to the fluent language disorder of semantic dementia, is characterized by a nonfluent, Broca-like aphasia, ultimately leading to a state of mutism. Pathological studies show diffuse left perisylvian atrophy involving both the frontal and temporal lobes. The nonfluent output relates to breakdown in the phonological and grammatic aspects of language. These deficits affect production and comprehension. An early feature is phonological, as opposed to semantic, paraphasic errors. Buccofacial apraxia is also a common feature: patients are unable to perform tasks such as licking lips or blowing out matches on command. In spite of profound language dysfunction, these patients often continue to maintain an independent lifestyle without significant behavioral or social disturbance.

Dementia of the frontal type presents with neuropsychiatric symptoms rather than neuropsychological deficits. Patients become distractible and impulsive, yet lack mental flexibility. Apathy and lack of motivation are extremely common; social skills degenerate, with tactlessness, lack of emotional warmth, and disinhibited behavior. The key feature of dementia of the frontal type on neuropsychological examination is a disproportionately poor performance on tests sensitive for frontal lobe function (executive function) in the absence of a significant memory, language, or visuospatial disorder. The orbitomedial frontal lobes are affected earlier than dorsolateral lobes in dementia of the frontal type. Since classic frontal lobe tasks reflect dorsolateral function rather than orbitomedial pathology, patients with gross behavioral changes may perform normally on these frontal lobe tests for a number of years.

Neuroimaging studies may show left perisylvian atrophy in progressive non fluent aphasia, and orbitomedial frontal lobe atrophy in dementia of the frontal type. *(Nestor and Hodges, 439–446)*

37. **(A)** Dementia with Lewy bodies is characterized by a progressive cognitive decline sufficient to interfere with social or occupational function. Fluctuation of cognitive function as well as well-formed and complex visual hallucinations are common features of the disease. Spontaneous parkinsonism is the final core feature of dementia with Lewy bodies that leads to the diagnosis being considered. In early stages of the disease, there is a distinctive profile that distinguishes dementia with Lewy bodies from other types of dementia, as the trend over time is for the development of global impairment. The typical early profile is one of disproportionate

involvement of attention, executive, and visuospatial domains. Visual deficits affect perceptual, spatial, and constructive abilities, and when matched for degree of dementia, memory function is superior to that seen in Alzheimer's disease. *(Nestor and Hodges, 439–446)*

38. (D) The consensus criteria for antemortem diagnosis of dementia with Lewy bodies are divided into mandatory criteria, core features, supportive criteria, and criteria against the diagnosis. The only mandatory criterion for the diagnosis of dementia with Lewy bodies is progressive cognitive decline that interferes with social and occupational function. The core features for the diagnosis of dementia with Lewy bodies include fluctuating state with significant variations in attention and alertness, spontaneous motor features of parkinsonism, and recurrence of hallucinations, particularly of the visual type. Supportive criteria for the diagnosis include repeated falls, syncope, transient loss of consciousness, neuroleptic hypersensitivity, systematized delusions, and nonvisual hallucinations. Criteria against the diagnosis of dementia with Lewy bodies include the presence of evidence of other physical or neurological illness is sufficient to explain the clinical features. *(Nestor and Hodges, 439–446)*

39. (E) A-synuclein is a 140 amino acid protein of unknown function that is abundantly expressed in the brain, where it is located in presynaptic nerve terminals with little staining of nerve cell bodies and dendrites.

A-synuclein 35-residue was found in the nonamyloid component of Alzheimer's disease plaques. This 35-residue segment is referred to as nonamyloid component (NAC) and α-synuclein as a NAC precursor protein. NAC was the second component, after the Alzheimer-β protein, to be found in extracellular Alzheimer's disease plaques. A-synuclein aggregates are not only found in the Lewy bodies of Parkinson disease, but also in the cortical Lewy bodies of Lewy body dementia and in glial cytoplasmic inclusions throughout the brain in multiple system atrophy. Although α-synuclein deposits occur in several neurodegenerative diseases, it is not a ubiquitous phenomenon after neuronal damage; brains of patients with multi-infarct

dementia have no synuclein inclusions and the tau-positive neuronal inclusion bodies in Pick's disease do not have synuclein associated with them. *(Schulz and Dichgans, 433–439)*

40. (C) The frontal lobe function is characterized by the presence of five parallel, but independent, circuits defined by their distinct major reciprocal subcortical connections. Each circuit involves a frontal lobe area, specific projections to striatal regions, continuation to globus pallidus, return to the thalamus, and then back to the frontal region of origin. There are two motor circuits, one involving the supplementary motor area and the second the frontal eye fields. Three circuits determine cognitive and affective behaviors, initiating in three separate regions of the prefrontal cortex: dorsolateral, lateral orbital, and medial frontal/anterior cingulate. Distinct cognitive and behavioral profiles are associated with lesions in the last three separate circuits. Dorsolateral prefrontal lesions produce deficits in verbal and nonverbal fluency, decreased problem solving and set shifting, and reduced learning and retrieval. Orbitofrontal lesions cause disinhibition and irritability. Medial frontal/anterior cingulate lesions result in apathy and decreased initiative. Damage at any point in each circuit will produce similar deficits. Lesions in the subcortical segments of these anatomical systems often cause mixed syndromes because of the proximity of the subcortical structures involved in the different circuits. The rationale for splitting the frontal lobes into these separate operating systems is supported by parallel anatomical observations. The cortical portions of these systems have different connections with posterior cortical areas. *(Alexander and Stuss, 427–437)*

41. (B)

42. (B)

43. (A)

44. (B)

45. (B)

46. (D)

47. (A)

48. (A)

49. (C)

50. (A)

Explanations 41 through 50

Long-term memory is divided into two types: implicit or nondeclarative memory and explicit or declarative memory. Implicit memory is unconscious memory of how to do something, like in training reflexive motor or perceptual skills, whereas explicit memory refers to factual knowledge of people, places, things, and what these facts means. Explicit memory involves a deliberate, conscious effort to associate multiple pieces of information in a highly flexible way. In contrast, implicit memory is more rigid, tightly connected to the original stimulus conditions under which learning occurred. Explicit memory is further divided into episodic memory, a memory of events and personal experience and semantic memory, a memory for facts.

Priming is a form of nondeclarative memory, in which the recall of words or objects is improved by prior exposure to words or objects. Memory of procedural skills and habits as well as habituation and sensitization are part of the implicit memory and are linked respectively to the striatum and reflex pathways. Classical and operant conditioning are parts of associative learning, which is a part of implicit memory. The emotional response of the classical and operant conditioning involves the amygdala, whereas skeletal musculature response involves the cerebellum. The amygdala is involved in affective aspects of memory which is related to implicit as much as explicit memory. Explicit memory is acquired through a processing in one or more of the three polymodal association cortices (the prefrontal, limbic, and parieto-occipital-temporal cortices) that synthesizes visual, auditory, and somatic information. The association cortices then convey the information in series to the parahippocampal and perirhinal cortices, the entorhinal cortex, the dentate gyrus, the hippocampus, the subiculum, and finally back to the entorhinal cortex. The information is then sent back from the entorhinal cortex to the parahippocampal and perirhinal cortex and finally back to the polymodal association areas of the neocortex. *(Kandell et al., 1128–1132)*

51. (A)

52. (B)

53. (C)

54. (D)

Explanations 51 through 54

Associative visual agnosia results from damage to the posterior parietal cortex. The patient cannot name objects but can identify objects by selecting the correct drawing and can faithfully reproduce detailed drawings of the object. A perceptive visual agnosia is caused by a lesion in the occipital lobe and surrounding region. The patient is unable to draw objects but can identify them if appropriate perceptual cues are available. Prosopagnosia is defined by the inability to recognize familiar faces or learn new faces and is caused by a lesion in the inferotemporal cortex. Source amnesia is caused by damage in the association areas of the frontal lobes. These areas of the cortex are responsible for long-term storage of episodic knowledge. A patient with source amnesia has the tendency to forget how the information was acquired. *(Kandell et al., 1236–1237)*

55. (B)

56. (C)

57. (D)

58. (A)

Explanations 55 through 58

Explicit memory is processed by at least four distinct types of processing: encoding, consolidation, storage, and retrieval. Encoding refers to the processes by which newly learned information is processed when first encountered. The quality of the encoding is critical for the integration and storage of newly acquired information. Consolidation refers to the processes that alter the newly stored and still labile information to make it more stable for long-term storage. It involves the expression of genes and the synthesis of proteins that give structural changes necessary for stable storage of the information. Storage refers to mechanisms and sites by which memory is retained over time. Retrieval refers to processes that permit the recall and use of stored information. *(Kandell et al., 1237)*

59. **(B)** Three major hippocampal pathways are involved in the processing of explicit memory: the perforant pathway, which projects from the entorhinal cortex to the granule cells of the dentate gyrus, the mossy fiber pathway, which contains the axons of the granule cells and runs to the pyramidal cells in the CA3 region of the hippocampus, and the Schaffer collateral pathway, which consists of the excitatory collaterals of the pyramidal cells in the CA3 region and ends on the pyramidal cells of the CA1 region. *(Kandell et al., 1259)*

60. **(C)** The mossy fiber pathway consists of the axons of the granule cells of the dentate gyrus. The mossy fiber terminals release glutamate as a neurotransmitter, which binds to both NMDA and non NMDA receptors. NMDA receptors have a minor role in synaptic plasticity. The blockage of NMDA receptors as well as the postsynaptic influx of calcium has no effect on long term potentiation in mossy fibers pathway. However, the presynaptic calcium influx has been found to play a major role in the mossy fibers long-term potentiation. Cooperativity, the process of activation of several afferent axons together, as well as associativity (the concomitant activation of pre and postsynaptic cells to adequately depolarize the postsynaptic cell) are distinctive features of long-term potentiation in the Schaffer collateral pathway. *(Kandell et al., 1260)*

61. **(A)** Conduction aphasia is characterized by fluent speech with paraphasic errors, with conserved comprehension and impaired repetition. It can be caused by lesions in a variety of locations including the supramarginal gyrus as well as by interruption of fiber tracts lying deep to the sensory cortex in the parietal lobe. *(Saffran, 409–418)*

65. **(B)** Patients with ideomotor apraxia make several types of errors when performing skilled, purposive limb movements. The most common errors in ideomotor apraxia are spatial errors. One type of spatial error involves the failure to position the hand in an appropriate posture (e.g., closed fist posture for drinking from a cup). A second type of spatial error involves the failure to orient the movement toward an imagined object (e.g., demonstrating the use of a toothbrush at the level of the chest). A third type of spatial error involves the failure to coordinate joint movement (e.g., demonstrating a screwdriver by rotating at the shoulder instead of at the elbow). Another common apraxic error involves the patient using a body part as if it is the imagined tool (e.g., extending the finger to represent the blade of the screwdriver instead of positioning the hand around the handle of the screwdriver). Apraxic patients may also make sequencing errors (e.g., demonstrating key use by rotating the wrist, then extending the arm) and timing errors such as failure to coordinate speed with the spatial aspects of the gesture. *(Alexander and Stuss, 427–437; Ochipa and Gonzalez Rothi, 417–478)*

REFERENCES

Alexander MP, Stuss DT. Disorders of frontal lobe functioning. *Semin Neurol.* 2000;20:427–437.

Cai H, Wang Y, McCarthy D, Wen H, Borchelt DR, Price DL, Wong PC. BACE1 is the major β-secretase for generation of Aβ peptides by neurons. *Nat Neurosci.* 2001;4:233–234.

Cummings JL, Vinters HV, Cole GM, Khachaturian ZS. Alzheimer's disease: etiologies, pathophysiology, cognitive reserve, and treatment opportunities. *Neurolog.* 1998;51(S1):S2–S17; discussion S65–S67.

Halliday G, Robinson SR, Shepherd C, Kril J. Alzheimer's disease and inflammation: a review of cellular and therapeutic mechanisms. *Clin Exp Pharmacol Physiol.* 2000;27:1–8.

Kandell ER, Schwartz JH, Jessell TM, eds. *Principles of Neural Science.* 4th ed. New York, NY: McGraw-Hill, 2000.

Kramer JH, Miller BL. Alzheimer's disease and its focal variants. *Semin Neurol.* 2000;20:447–454.

Litvan I. Diagnosis and management of progressive supranuclear palsy. *Semin Neurol.* 2001;21:41–48.

McArthur JC, Sacktor N, Selnes O. Human immunodeficiency virus-associated dementia. *Semin Neurolog.* 1999;19:129–150.

Nestor P, Hodges J. Non-Alzheimer dementias. *Semin Neurol.* 2000;20:439–446.

Ochipa C, Gonzalez Rothi LJ. Limb apraxia. *Semin Neurol.* 2000;20:471–478.

Pasquier F, Delacourte A. Non-Alzheimer degenerative dementias. *Curr Opin Neurol.* 1998;11:417–427.

Price DL, Tanzi RE, Borchelt DR, Sisodia SS. Alzheimer's disease: genetic studies and transgenic models. *Ann Rev Genet.* 1998;32:461–493.

Saffran EM. Aphasia and the relationship of language and brain. *Semin Neurol.* 2000;20:409–418.

Schulz JB, Dichgans J. Molecular pathogenesis of movement disorders: are protein aggregates a common link in neuronal degeneration? *Curr Opin Neurol.* 1999;12: 433–439.

CHAPTER 7

Cerebrovascular Diseases
Questions

Questions 1 through 8
Link each of the following brain stem locations, when affected by an ischemic lesion, to the appropriate signs and symptoms.

- (A) Medial medulla
- (B) Lateral medulla
- (C) Ventral pontine
- (D) Lower dorsal pontine
- (E) Upper dorsal pontine
- (F) Ventral midbrain
- (G) Dorsal midbrain
- (H) Dorsolateral midbrain

1. Ipsilateral tongue deviation with contralateral hemiplegia and loss of position and vibratory sensation

2. Ipsilateral loss of sensation of the face, ipsilateral paresis of the pharynx and vocal cord, ipsilateral Horner syndrome and ataxia, dysphagia and dysarthria, and contralateral loss of pain and temperature on the body

3. Ipsilateral paresis of the lateral rectus and face with contralateral hemiplegia

4. Ipsilateral paresis of horizontal gaze and sometimes face with contralateral hemiplegia

5. Ipsilateral ataxia and weakness of mastication muscles, with contralateral hemiplegia of face and body as well as loss of all sensory modalities

6. Ipsilateral oculomotor paresis with ptosis and dilated pupils, and contralateral hemiplegia including the lower face

7. Ipsilateral paresis with contralateral involuntary movements and hemianesthesia

8. Ipsilateral Horner syndrome and severe tremor with contralateral loss of all sensory modalities

9. Spontaneous dissection of the carotid or vertebral artery in young patients accounts for

- (A) 1% of all ischemic strokes
- (B) 1.5% of all ischemic strokes
- (C) 2% of all ischemic strokes
- (D) 3% of all ischemic strokes
- (E) 10% of all ischemic strokes

10. In case of carotid dissection, the most frequently affected cranial nerve is the

- (A) facial cranial nerve
- (B) glossopharyngeal cranial nerve
- (C) trigeminal cranial nerve
- (D) spinal accessory cranial nerve
- (E) hypoglossal cranial nerve

11. A 27-year-old man with a history of migraine developed a right side headache and right anterolateral cervical pain four days after chiropractic manipulation of the neck. One day after becoming symptomatic, he consulted a neurologist because of a transient right eye blindness that resolved within a few hours. Neurological examination demonstrated right miosis, ptosis, and mild right tongue deviation. The most likely diagnosis is

- (A) vertebral artery dissection
- (B) basilar artery occlusion
- (C) complicated migraine
- (D) carotid artery dissection
- (E) cluster headache

12. The chain of events that produces the abnormalities seen in diffusion weighted magnetic resonance imaging in acute stroke includes all of the following EXCEPT

   (A) an increased apparent diffusion coefficient
   (B) glial and neuronal swelling
   (C) failure of the sodium potassium pump
   (D) intracellular accumulation of sodium
   (E) a reduction in extracellular space

Questions 13 through 16
Link each of the following lacunar stroke syndromes to the appropriate anatomical location.

   (A) Hemichorea-hemiballismus
   (B) Pure motor hemiparesis
   (C) Dysarthria clumsy hand syndrome
   (D) Ataxic hemiparesis

13. Posterior limb of the internal capsule

14. Subthalamic nucleus

15. Corona radiata

16. Basis pontis

17. Which of the following is true about the diagnosis of subarachnoid hemorrhage?

   (A) Subarachnoid hemorrhage may appear isodense to brain parenchyma if the serum hemoglobin level is below 12 g/dl.
   (B) Modern CT scan has 93% sensitivity for the diagnosis of subarachnoid hemorrhage when done in the first 12 hours.
   (C) Standard magnetic resonance imaging (MRI) is more sensitive than CT scan in detecting subarachnoid hemorrhage.
   (D) The presence of xanthochromia in the cerebrospinal fluid in patients with a negative head CT scan is the primary criterion for the diagnosis of subarachnoid hemorrhage.
   (E) Less than 10% of patients with subarachnoid hemorrhage have a cardiac arrhythmia.

18. Which of the following is true about the study comparing aspirin to warfarin in preventing the recurrence of ischemic strokes (WARSS)?

   (A) It was a randomized double-blind multicenter study comparing aspirin to warfarin in preventing the recurrence of cardioembolic strokes.
   (B) The only end point of this study was death from an ischemic stroke.
   (C) Aspirin showed a higher risk of major bleed than warfarin when used for preventing the recurrence of nonembolic ischemic strokes.
   (D) Warfarin was superior to aspirin in preventing the recurrence of nonembolic ischemic strokes.
   (E) Warfarin was equivalent to aspirin in preventing the recurrence of nonembolic ischemic strokes.

19. Currently, the most consistent and important predictor of stroke is

   (A) hypertension
   (B) diabetes
   (C) high serum cholesterol
   (D) smoking
   (E) obesity

20. Which of the following is true about the use of thrombolytics in the treatment of acute ischemic stroke?

   (A) The use of plasminogen activator factor (rt-PA) showed a significant benefit in the first 24 hours.
   (B) For every 100 patients treated with rt-PA, an additional 11 patients have a favorable outcome as compared to 100 patients not treated with rt-PA.
   (C) The administration of rt-PA did not show any benefit on small-vessel disease stroke.
   (D) Within the first 36 hours of rt-PA, significant intracerebral bleed was present in 0.6% of cases and was comparable to the placebo group.
   (E) Administration of rt-PA is contraindicated if the age of the patient is over 75 years.

21. Which of the following is NOT true about serum homocysteine level and the risk of ischemic stroke?

    (A) The relative risk of stroke in patients with an abnormal homocysteine level is 1.8 and depends on the level of homocysteine in the serum.
    (B) Homocysteine has a mitogenic effect on vascular smooth muscle.
    (C) Elevated homocysteine increases the activity of factor XII of coagulation.
    (D) Statine reduces the plasma homocysteine level by 25%.
    (E) The progression of atherosclerotic carotid plaque may be decreased by lowering the homocysteine level.

22. Positron emission tomography studies in ischemic stroke show that in necrotic tissue the blood flow is less than

    (A) 30 ml/100 gr/min
    (B) 24 ml/100 gr/min
    (C) 18 ml/100 gr/min
    (D) 12 ml/100 gr/min
    (E) 6 ml/100 gr/min

23. Which of the following is NOT a risk factor for spontaneous hemorrhage?

    (A) Hypertension
    (B) Ethanol abuse
    (C) Cerebral amyloid angiopathy
    (D) Cholesterol greater than 200 mg/dl
    (E) Mutation of the gene coding for factor XIII of coagulation

24. Which of the following is true about the management of spontaneous intracerebral bleed?

    (A) Since a marked increase of intracerebral pressure is seen in all patients with intracerebral hemorrhage, the early use of hyperventilation or osmotic agents is recommended.
    (B) Corticosteroids may be used in intracerebral bleed if osmotic agents or hyperventilation fail to reduce the intracranial pressure.

    (C) Early surgical evacuation of hematoma from the basal ganglia or pons has a better prognosis than medical treatment.
    (D) Early craniotomy is recommended in cases of cerebellar hematoma.
    (E) Long-term use of antiseizure medications is recommended because most seizures occur after the first 24 hours following formation of the hematoma.

25. The LEAST common presentation of an arteriovenous malformation of the brain is

    (A) intracerebral hemorrhage
    (B) seizure
    (C) headache
    (D) focal neurological deficit without signs of underlying hemorrhage
    (E) progressive neurological deficit without signs of underlying hemorrhage

26. Which of the following MR spectroscopy peaks typically increases in acute ischemic stroke?

    (A) Lactate peak
    (B) Creatine peak
    (C) N acetyl aspartate peak
    (D) Choline peak
    (E) None of the above

Answers and Explanations

1. **(A)**

2. **(B)**

3. **(C)**

4. **(D)**

5. **(E)**

6. **(F)**

7. **(G)**

8. **(H)**

Explanations 1 through 8

The brain stem is formed by three main divisions: the medulla, the pons, and the midbrain. The medulla is the rostral extension of the spinal cord. It contains the inferior olivary nucleus as well as the nucleus of the lower cranial nerves (see Fig. 7-1). The hypoglossal nucleus is located near the ventrolateral portion of the central canal. The nucleus ambiguus (the nucleus of the glossopharyngeal nerve, vagus nerve, and spinal accessory nerves) is located within the medullary reticular formation, ventromedial to the nucleus and spinal tract of the trigeminal nerve.

The dorsal motor nucleus of the vagus is located dorsolaterally to the hypoglossal nucleus. The nucleus of the tractus solitarius (nucleus of the sensory facial, glossopharyngeal, and vagus nerves) lies anterolateral to the motor nucleus of the vagus nerve. Posterolateral to the solitary tract lie the medial and inferior vestibular nuclei, and caudal to them are the dorsal and ventral cochlear nuclei of the vestibulocochlear nerve. The nucleus gracilis and nucleus cuneatus are located in the posterior funiculi of the dorsal medulla and give fibers that decussate in the medial lemniscus.

Medial medullary syndrome (Dejerine syndrome) is caused by an occlusion of the anterior spinal artery or its parent vertebral artery (see Fig. 7-2). The syndrome causes ipsilateral paresis of the tongue, due to damage of the hypoglossal nerve, which deviates toward the lesion; contralateral hemiplegia sparing the face, due to damage of the corticospinal tract; and contralateral loss of position and vibratory sensation, due to damage of the medial lemniscus.

The lateral medullary syndrome (Wallenberg syndrome) may be caused by an occlusion of the vertebral artery or posterior inferior cerebellar artery (see Fig. 7-3). The damage is located in the dorsolateral medulla and inferior cerebellar peduncle. The clinical features of lateral medullary syndrome include ipsilateral loss of pain and temperature of the face, due to damage of the descending spinal tract and nucleus of the trigeminal nerve; ipsilateral paralysis of the palate, pharynx, and vocal cords with dysarthria and dysphagia, due to damage of the nuclei and fibers of the glossopharyngeal and vagus nerves; ipsilateral Horner syndrome, due to damage of the descending sympathetic tract fibers; ipsilateral ataxia and dysmetria, due to damage of the inferior cerebellar peduncle and cerebellum; contralateral loss of pain and temperature of the body, due to damage of the spinothalamic tract; and vertigo, nausea, vomiting, and nystagmus, due to damage of the vestibular nuclei.

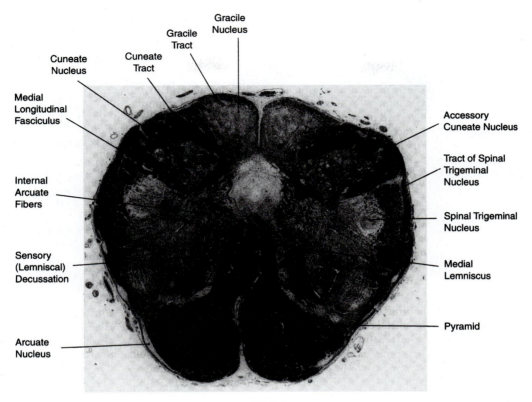

Cuneate
Nucleus

Cuneate
Tract

Gracile
Tract

Gracile
Nucleus

Medial
Longitudinal
Fasciculus

Accessory
Cuneate Nucleus

Tract of Spinal
Trigeminal
Nucleus

Internal
Arcuate
Fibers

Spinal Trigeminal
Nucleus

Sensory
(Lemniscal)
Decussation

Medial
Lemniscus

Pyramid

Arcuate
Nucleus

FIG. 7-1

The pons lies rostral to the medulla (see Fig. 7-4). It has two components: a dorsal part (the tegmentum) and a ventral part (the basis pontis). The tegmentum is largely composed of the pontine reticular formation. Cranial nerve nuclei in the pons include the nucleus of the abducens nerve (located in the dorsomedial pons, dorsolateral to the paramedian pontine reticular formation), the motor nucleus of the facial nerve (situated ventrolaterally), the main motor and sensory nucleus of the trigeminal nerve, the superior and inferior salivatory nuclei, and the lacrimal nucleus. Tracts within the pons include the medial longitudinal fasciculus, the

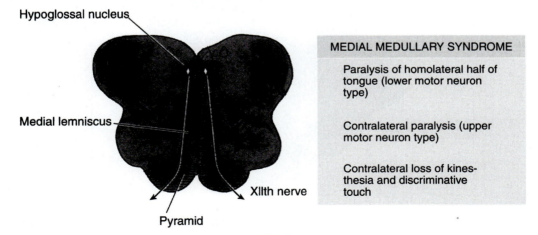

Hypoglossal nucleus

Medial lemniscus

Pyramid

XIIth nerve

MEDIAL MEDULLARY SYNDROME

Paralysis of homolateral half of tongue (lower motor neuron type)

Contralateral paralysis (upper motor neuron type)

Contralateral loss of kines-thesia and discriminative touch

FIG. 7-2

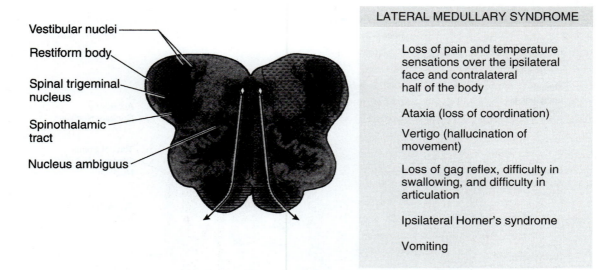

Vestibular nuclei

Restiform body

Spinal trigeminal nucleus

Spinothalamic tract

Nucleus ambiguus

LATERAL MEDULLARY SYNDROME

Loss of pain and temperature sensations over the ipsilateral face and contralateral half of the body

Ataxia (loss of coordination)

Vertigo (hallucination of movement)

Loss of gag reflex, difficulty in swallowing, and difficulty in articulation

Ipsilateral Horner's syndrome

Vomiting

FIG. 7-3

medial lemniscus, the corticospinal, the corticobulbar, the corticopontine, the spinothalamic, the ventral spinocerebellar, the rubrospinal, and the lateral tectospinal tracts.

The basilar artery is the principal source of blood flow to the pons. It gives off three types of branches: the paramedian arteries, the short circumferential arteries, and the long circum-

ferential arteries (which supply the pontine tegmentum and the dorsolateral quadrant of the pons, together with the anterior inferior cerebellar arteries and the superior cerebellar arteries). The ventral pontine syndrome (or Millard Gubler syndrome) is caused by paramedian infarction of the pons (see Fig. 7-5). This results in ipsilateral paresis of the lateral

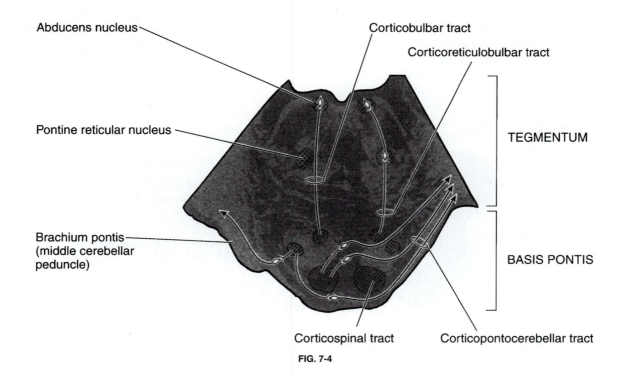

Abducens nucleus

Corticobulbar tract

Corticoreticulobulbar tract

Pontine reticular nucleus

TEGMENTUM

Brachium pontis (middle cerebellar peduncle)

BASIS PONTIS

Corticospinal tract

Corticopontocerebellar tract

FIG. 7-4

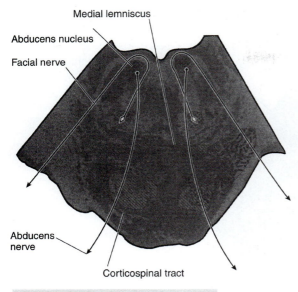

BASAL PONTINE SYNDROME

Ipsilateral paralysis of facial muscle

Ipsilateral paralysis of ocular abduction

Contralateral limb paralysis

FIG. 7-5

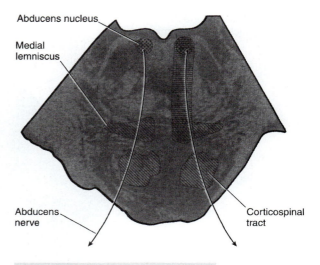

TEGMENTAL PONTINE SYNDROME

Ipsilateral paralysis of lateral gaze

Ipsilateral paralysis of ocular abduction

Contralateral loss of kinesthesia and discriminative touch

Ipsilateral facial muscle paralysis

FIG. 7-6

rectus from damage to the abducens nerve, causing diplopia; in addition, there is ipsilateral paresis of the upper and lower face from damage to the facial cranial nerve and contralateral hemiplegia from damage to the corticospinal tract.

The lower dorsal pontine syndrome (or Foville syndrome) is caused by a lesion in the dorsal tegmentum of the lower pons (see Fig. 7-6). The affected patient may develop ipsilateral paresis of the upper and lower halves of the face from damage to the nucleus or fibers of the facial nerve, and ipsilateral horizontal gaze palsy from damage of the paramedian pontine reticular formation and/or the abducens nerve nucleus. The upper dorsal pontine syndrome is caused by obstruction of the long circumferential branches of the basilar artery, and results in ipsilateral ataxia and coarse intention tremor (the superior and middle cerebellar peduncles). There is also contralateral body sensory loss to all modalities from damage to the medial lemniscus and spinothalamic tract. When the lesion extends to the ventral part of the pons, contralateral

hemiparesis, including the face, occurs from damage to the corticospinal tract.

The midbrain (Fig. 7-7), which is the smallest and the most rostral component of the brain stem, plays an important role in the control of eye movements and coordination of visual and auditory reflexes. The midbrain may be divided into three parts: the tectum, the tegmentum, and the cerebral peduncles. The dorsal tectum contains the corpora quadrigemina, made up of four rounded eminences arranged in pairs, the superior and inferior colliculi. The tegmentum contains ascending and descending tracts, reticular nuclei, and well-delineated nuclear masses. The cerebral peduncles are ventral and contain corticopontine fibers in their medial fifth, corticospinal tract fibers in their middle three-fifths, and temporopontine fibers in their lateral fifth.

The substantia nigra is a pigmented layer possessing melanin granules; it is dorsal to the peduncle and ventral to the red nucleus and is composed of dorsal zona compacta and ventral zona reticulata. The nucleus of the trochlear nerve is located in the ventral part of the central gray matter at the level of the inferior colliculus.

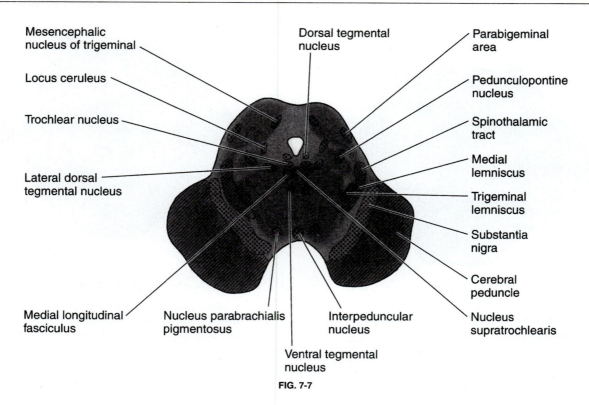

Mesencephalic nucleus of trigeminal

Locus ceruleus

Trochlear nucleus

Lateral dorsal tegmental nucleus

Medial longitudinal fasciculus

Nucleus parabrachialis pigmentosus

Ventral tegmental nucleus

Dorsal tegmental nucleus

Interpeduncular nucleus

Parabigeminal area

Pedunculopontine nucleus

Spinothalamic tract

Medial lemniscus

Trigeminal lemniscus

Substantia nigra

Cerebral peduncle

Nucleus supratrochlearis

FIG. 7-7

The nucleus of the oculomotor nerve lies rostral to the trochlear nucleus beneath the superior colliculus. Mesencephalic tracts include the crus cerebri, the dentatorubrothalamic tract, the medial tegmental tract, the posterior commissure, the median longitudinal fasciculus, the spinothalamic tract, and the median lemniscus. The vascular supply of the midbrain includes the paramedian and circumferential branches of the basilar artery.

Ventral midbrain syndrome (or Weber syndrome) is caused by an occlusion of median and paramedian perforating branches (see Fig. 7-8) and may result in ipsilateral oculomotor paresis, ptosis, and dilated pupils from damage to the fascicle of the third nerve. In addition, there is a contralateral hemiplegia, including the lower face, from damage to the corticospinal tract. Dorsal midbrain syndrome (Moritz-Benedikt syndrome) results from a lesion in the midbrain tegmentum caused by occlusion of the paramedian branches of the basilar or posterior cerebral arteries or both. It results in ipsilateral oculomotor paresis, ptosis, and dilated pupil from damage to the third

nerve. Contralateral involuntary movements also occur, such as intention tremor, ataxia, and chorea, from damage to the red nucleus. There is a contralateral hemiparesis with extension of the lesion ventrally, and contralateral hemianesthesia with extension of the lesion laterally to the spinothalamic tracts and the medial lemniscus. Dorsolateral midbrain syndrome is caused by infarction of the territory of the circumferential arteries and results in: (1) ipsilateral Horner syndrome; (2) ipsilateral severe tremor from damage to the superior cerebellar peduncle; and (3) contralateral loss of all sensory modalities from damage to the spinothalamic and medial lemniscus tracts. (*Afifi, 141–146, 179–186, 227–234; Rolak, 112–121*)

9. **(E)** Spontaneous dissection of the carotid or vertebral artery accounts for about 2% of all ischemic strokes. Its annual incidence in some studies ranges from 2.5% per 100,000 to 3% per 100,000. However, in young and middle-aged populations, it accounts for 10% to 25% of the number of ischemic strokes. Spontaneous dissections of the carotid and vertebral arteries

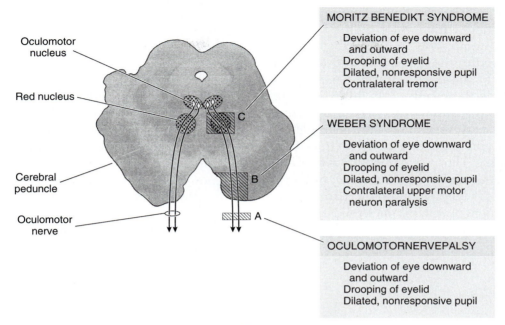

FIG. 7-8

affect all age groups, but there is a distinct peak in the fifth decade of life. Although there is no overall sex-based predilection, women are, on average, about 5 years younger than men at the time of the dissection. *(Schievink, 898–906)*

10. **(E)** Cranial nerves are affected in about 12% of carotid artery dissections. The hypoglossal nerve is the most commonly affected cranial nerve, followed by other lower cranial nerves. The oculomotor nerve, trigeminal nerve, and facial nerve are less affected. *(Schievink, 898–906)*

11. **(D)** The patient described in this vignette has a triad of signs and symptoms that include unilateral headache, unilateral oculosympathetic palsy, and transient monocular blindness (which may be considered in this context as a sign of retinal ischemia). The occurrence of this constellation of signs and symptoms after chiropractic manipulation is highly suggestive of carotid artery dissection. Hyperextension or rotation of the neck may also precipitate carotid dissection. It is estimated that about 1/20,000 of spinal manipulations are associated with a stroke by carotid or vertebral artery dissection.

Unilateral headache develops in two-thirds of patients. It may mimic a migraine headache or a subarachnoid hemorrhage, but most commonly it is a frontotemporal headache with gradual onset, often above the ipsilateral eye. Miosis and ptosis reflect oculosympathetic palsy and are seen in less than 50% of patients with carotid dissection. A cranial nerve lesion is detected in only 12% of cases of carotid artery dissection. The hypoglossal nerve is the most frequently affected cranial nerve. Transient monocular blindness is the most common sign of retinal ischemia seen in patients with spontaneous carotid dissection. Permanent blindness from ischemic optic neuropathy or occlusion of the retinal artery is rare. Symptoms and signs of retinal or cerebral ischemia are reported in 50% to 95% of carotid artery dissections. Ultrasound or magnetic resonance angiography of the carotid artery is useful for an initial assessment, but carotid angiography remains the gold standard. *(Schievink, 898–906)*

12. **(A)** Diffusion-weighted imaging is a technique that permits in vivo measurement of the translational mobility of water along the particular direction of the used diffusion-sensitizing gradient in tissue. The apparent diffusion coefficient that quantifies water mobility is reduced in ischemic tissue. The drop in brain perfusion

caused by an acute ischemic event induces an energy deficit with failure of the sodium/potassium pump. This results in the accumulation of sodium inside the neural and glial cells, which causes an intracellular influx of water inside these cells. This influx of water from the extracellular space into the intracellular space causes swelling of the neuronal and glial cells and reduction of the extracellular volume space. Thus, water mobility is hindered as a consequence of the production of longer diffusion path lengths, and the apparent diffusion coefficient of water is decreased. *(Schievink, 898–906)*

13. **(B)**

14. **(A)**

15. **(D)**

16. **(C)**

Explanations 13 through 16

Lacunar strokes are small infarcts of the noncortical parts of the cerebellum and the brain stem that result from occlusion of penetrating branches of large cerebral arteries, most commonly the middle cerebral, basilar, and posterior cerebral arteries, and less commonly the anterior cerebral and vertebral arteries. The size of a lacunar stroke ranges from 3 mm to 2 cm. Pathologic studies show that the penetrating vessels might be obstructed either by small embolic particles or lipohyalinosis. Signs of lacunar stroke depend on the anatomical location of the ischemic lesion. Hemiballismus is caused by an infarct or hemorrhage in the subthalamic nucleus. Pure motor hemiparesis involves the face, arm, and leg without sensory deficit, aphasia, agnosia, apraxia, or visual field defect. The most frequent location of the lesion is the posterior limb of the internal capsule, and less frequently the corona radiata, pons, and medullary pyramid. Infarction of the basis pontis at the junction of the upper third and inferior two-thirds from obstruction of the paramedian branch of the basilar artery causes dysarthria clumsy hand syndrome. Ataxia hemiparesis results from a lacunar lesion located in the corona radiata, internal capsule, or pons. *(C. Fisher, 871–876; M. Fisher and Bogousslavsky, 108)*

17. **(D)** The typical presentation of subarachnoid hemorrhage includes a sudden onset of severe headache, frequently described as the worst headache in the life of the patient. Nausea, vomiting, transient loss of consciousness, or leg buckling may accompany the headache. Physical examination may show nuchal rigidity, retinal hemorrhages, papilledema, third nerve palsy (in case of posterior communicating artery aneurysm), sixth nerve palsy, bilateral weakness in legs (or abulia in case of aneurysm of the anterior communicating artery), and/or aphasia hemiparesis (or left-sided visual neglect in the case of a middle cerebral artery aneurysm). Arrythmias are a frequent complication of subarachnoid bleeding. Andreoli et al. reported arrhythmias in 91% of patients diagnosed with spontaneous subarachnoid hemorrhage and investigated prospectively with 24-hour Holter monitoring. This study did not demonstrate a correlation between the frequency and severity of cardiac arrhythmias and the neurologic condition, the site and extent of intracranial blood on computed tomography scan, or the location of the ruptured vessel.

CT scan of the head without contrast and with thin cuts through the base of the brain is the first recommended test. In retrospective studies, the sensitivity of modern third-generation CT scanners for detecting subarachnoid hemorrhage is 100% in the first 12 hours and 93% in the first 24 hours. Although magnetic resonance technology is continually advancing and can detect aneurysms, standard magnetic resonance imaging is inferior to CT for the detection of acute subarachnoid hemorrhage. Lumbar puncture should be performed in a patient whose clinical presentation suggests subarachnoid hemorrhage and whose CT scan is negative, equivocal, or technically inadequate. After aneurysmal hemorrhage, erythrocytes invade the subarachnoid space and then gradually lyses to release hemoglobin, which is metabolized to the pigmented molecules oxyhemoglobin (reddish pink) and bilirubin (yellow), resulting in xanthochromia. The presence of xanthochromia is considered by many authors to be the primary criterion for a diagnosis of subarachnoid hemorrhage in patients with negative CT scans, although some authors assert that the presence of erythrocytes, even in the absence of xanthochromia, is more accurate. *(Andreoli et al., 558–564; Edlow and Caplan, 29–36)*

18. **(E)** WARSS was a multicenter, double-blind, randomized trial that compared the effect of warfarin (at a dose adjusted to produce an international normalized ratio of 1.4 to 2.8) and aspirin (325 mg per day) on the combined primary end points of recurrent ischemic stroke or death from any cause within 2 years. The two randomized study groups were similar with respect to baseline risk factors. No significant differences were found between the treatment groups in any of the outcomes measured. The rates of major hemorrhage were low (2.22 per 100 patient-years in the warfarin group and 1.49 per 100 patient-years in the aspirin group). Also, there were no significant treatment-related differences in the frequency of major hemorrhage according to the cause of the initial stroke. The authors concluded that over a 2-year period, there was no difference found between aspirin and warfarin in the rate of major hemorrhage or in the prevention of recurrent ischemic stroke (for a population with noncardioembolic stroke) or death. *(Mohr et al., 1444–1451)*

19. **(A)** Hypertension is reported to be the most consistently powerful predictor of stroke. It is found to be a contributing factor in about 70% of strokes. Hypertension promotes stroke by aggravating atherosclerosis in the aortic arch and cervicocerebral arteries, causing arteriosclerosis and lipohyalinosis in the small-diameter, penetrating end arteries of the cerebrum. For people of all ages and both sexes, higher levels of both systolic and diastolic blood pressure have been associated with an increased incidence of ischemic and hemorrhagic stroke. Treatments for not only severe hypertension, but also mild-to-moderate hypertension, have been associated with a decrease in the incidence of stroke.

Cigarette smoking is also a major cause of both ischemic and hemorrhagic stroke. The relative risk of stroke for smokers, as compared with nonsmokers, is estimated to be close to 1.51. Cigarette smoking may increase the risk of stroke by modifying blood coagulability (increasing blood levels of fibrinogen and other clotting factors, increasing platelet aggregability and hematocrit), modifying the lipid profile of smokers (decreasing the high-density lipoprotein cholesterol level), and promoting atherosclerosis by direct endothelium damage. Tobacco may promote arterial rupture by increasing blood pressure.

Diabetes may increase the risk of stroke independently of hypertension, dyslipoproteinemia, and obesity. Diabetes may increase the risk of stroke by promoting atherogenesis. Obesity, elevated serum cholesterol, and lack of physical activity are also risk factors for stroke. *(Bronner, Kanter, and Manson, 1392–1400)*

20. **(B)** Tissue plasminogen activator (rt-PA) is produced endogenously in physiologic concentrations by endothelial cells. It is relatively fibrin specific. The NINDS trial randomized 624 patients (312 each placebo and intravenous rt-PA) within 3 hours after stroke symptom onset. The trial had two parts: Part 1 (in which 301 patients were enrolled) tested whether rt-PA demonstrated a clinical effect within 24 hours of the onset of stroke (primary end point). Part 2 (in which 333 patients were enrolled) used a global test statistic to assess clinical outcome at 3 months. There was no significant difference between the drug treatment and placebo group in the percentages of patients with neurological improvement at 24 hours. A benefit was observed for the rt-PA group at 3 months for all outcome measures. For every 100 patients treated with rt-PA, an additional 11 to 13 patients will have a favorable outcome as compared with 100 not treated with rt-PA. The benefit did not vary by stroke subtype at baseline, because not only cardioembolic strokes benefited from thrombolytic treatment but also small-vessel ischemic strokes. Symptomatic intracerebral hemorrhage within 36 hours after the onset of stroke occurred in 6.4% of patients given rt-PA but only in 0.6% of patients given placebo ($p < 0.001$). Nevertheless, severe disability and death were higher in the nontreated group. *(Schellinger et al., 1812–1818)*

21. **(D)** A prospective population-based cohort study of patients without a history of stroke, who were followed for a median of 9.9 years, identified homocysteine level as an independent risk factor for stroke. This relative risk increases with the level of homocysteine up to 1.82. Homocysteine may act by inducing endothelial dysfunction and altering the antithrombotic properties of the endothelium with enhancement of the activity of factor XII and factor V. It may also have a mitogenic effect on vascular smooth muscle cells. Statins do not lower homocysteine levels, but dietary folic acid may reduce by approximately 25% the level of homocysteine, and vitamin B_{12} by an additional 7%. It remains unknown whether lowering homocysteine prevents important atherosclerotic vascular events. However, an uncontrolled study has shown that lowering homocysteine, through the combination of folic acid 2.5 mg/day, vitamin B_6 25 mg/day, and vitamin B_{12} 250 µg/day, reduces the progression of atherosclerosis as measured by carotid plaque area. *(Hankey and Eikelboom, 95–102)*

22. **(D)** Positron emission tomography classifies three regions within the disturbed vascular territory. The core zone of ischemia, which usually becomes necrotic, has blood flow below 12 ml/100 gr/min and a cerebral metabolic rate for oxygen ($CMRO_2$) below 60 µmol/100 gr/min. The penumbral region has a flow rate between 12 and 22 ml/100 gr/min (it is a dynamic area where the tissue is still viable but can either become necrotic, or recover; it is characterized by increased oxygen extraction fraction). The third region is an area of hypopofusion (flow >22 ml/100 gr/min), which is not primarily damaged by the lack of blood supply. *(Heiss, Forsting, and Diener, 67–75)*

23. **(D)** Hypertension is the most important risk factor for spontaneous intracerebral hemorrhage. It increases the risk of intracerebral hemorrhage, particularly in untreated people 55 years or younger, or smokers. Excessive use of alcohol also increases the risk of intracerebral hemorrhage by impairing coagulation and directly affecting the integrity of cerebral vessels. Low serum cholesterol (less than 4.1 mmol per liter), especially when associated with hypertension or hypercoagulable status, is a less well-established risk factor for intracerebral hemorrhage. Cerebral amyloid angiopathy, which is characterized by the deposition of (beta)-amyloid protein in the blood vessels of the cerebral cortex and leptomeninges, is another risk factor for intracerebral hemorrhage, particularly in elderly persons with (epsilon)2 and (epsilon)4 alleles of the apolipoprotein E gene. *(Qureshi et al., 1450–1460)*

24. **(D)** Several days after intracerebral hemorrhage, the patient may develop obstructive hydrocephalus from the mass effect caused by the hematoma and the edematous tissue surrounding it. The resulting increased intracranial pressure may subsequently cause central nervous system herniation, which remains the chief secondary cause of death in the first few days after intracerebral hemorrhage. Marked elevation of the intracranial pressure occurs with massive intracerebral hemorrhages because the intracranial volume cannot expand. However, localized intracerebral hemorrhage may occur without significant increase in global intracranial pressure.

The use of hyperventilation and osmotic agents is discouraged in the absence of evidence of critical rise of the intracranial pressure and should be reserved for patients with impending cerebral herniation. This strategy is supported by some experimental studies showing improvement of the blood flow and cerebral metabolism when high intracranial pressure is lowered in cases of intracranial herniation, but no benefit with moderate pressure elevations. Corticosteroids should be avoided, because randomized trials have failed to demonstrate their efficacy in patients with an intracerebral hemorrhage.

Surgical evacuation of a hematoma is indicated to reduce the mass effect. However, there is no sustained benefit from evacuation of basal ganglionic, thalamic, and pontine hemorrhages.

Cerebellar hematomas are unique from a surgical perspective because they can be approached without causing substantial damage to higher cortical or primary motor pathways. Thus early craniotomy is recommended in patients with a cerebellar hematoma that causes compression of the brain stem, because the rate of neurologic deterioration after cerebellar hemorrhage is very high and unpredictable. Most patients with intracerebral bleed do not require long-term antiseizure medications, since most seizures occur at the onset of the hemorrhage or in the first 24 hours. Anticonvulsants can usually be discontinued after the first month in patients who have had no further seizures. Patients who have a seizure more than 2 weeks after the onset of an intracerebral hemorrhage are at higher risk for further seizures and may require long-term prophylactic treatment with anticonvulsants. *(Qureshi et al., 1450–1460)*

25. **(E)** Intracranial hemorrhage is the most common clinical presentation of arteriovenous malformation, with a reported frequency ranging from 30% to 82%. Several factors increase the risk of a first hemorrhage: a small malformation, exclusively deep venous drainage, and high intracranial pressure, resulting in high pressures to the feeding arteries or restriction of venous outflow. Seizures that are not caused by hemorrhage are the initial symptom in 16% to 53% of patients. The majority of seizures are partial or complex partial; grand mal seizures account for 27% to 35% of seizures. Headache is the presenting symptom in 7% to 48% of patients, without distinctive features such as frequency, duration, or severity. Focal neurologic deficits without signs of underlying hemorrhage have been reported in 1% to 40% of patients, and only a few of them (4% to 8%) have well-documented, progressive neurologic deficits. *(Anonymous, 1812–1818)*

26. **(A)** Magnetic resonance spectroscopy (MRS) is a noninvasive in vivo technique that allows the measurement of histochemical cell components. Specific cell types or structures have metabolites that give a change in proton MRS peaks that may reflect a loss of a specific cell component. The methyl resonance of N-acetyl aspartate (NAA) produces a sharp peak at 2.01 ppm. It acts as a specific neuronal marker and reflects neuronal integrity. In cases of acute ischemia, the NAA peak declines, reflecting neuronal loss. Creatine and phosphocreatine have specific MRS signals. They are found in both neurons and glial cells and act as a phosphate transporter system and energy buffer within the cell. In acute ischemic stroke, there is a reduction in the peak of creatine and phosphocreatine, reflecting the disturbance of cellular energy metabolism. The trimethylamine resonance of the choline-containing component is present in 3.2 ppm. It is a marker of cell membrane integrity. Also in acute ischemia, the choline peak may increase, decrease, or remain unchanged. A lactate doublet peak is seen at 1.33 ppm. It is not normally detected within the brain. Its concentration rises when the glycolytic rate exceeds the tissue's capacity to catabolize or remove it from the brain and into the circulation. The presence of lactate may thus represent a perfusion mismatch and it may possibly represent salvageable tissue. *(Saunders, 334–345)*

REFERENCES

Afifi AK, Bergman RA, Ronald A, eds. *Functional Neuranatomy: Text and Atlas.* New York: McGraw-Hill; 1998.

Andreoli A, di Pasquale G, Pinelli G, Grazi P, Tognetti F, Testa C. Subarachnoid hemorrhage: frequency and severity of cardiac arrhythmias: a survey of 70 cases studied in the acute phase. *Stroke* 1987;18:558–564.

Anonymous. Arteriovenous malformations of the brain in adults. *N Engl J Med.* 1999;340:1812–1818.

Bronner L. L., Kanter D. S., Manson J. E. Medical Progress: Primary Prevention of Stroke. *N Engl J Med.* 1995;333:1392–1400.

Edlow JA. Caplan LR. Avoiding pitfalls in the diagnosis of subarachnoid hemorrhage. *N Engl J Med.* 2000;342: 29–36.

Fisher M, Bogousslavsky J, eds. *Current Review of Cerebrovascular Disease.* 4th ed. Philadelphia, PA: Current Medicine; 2001.

Fisher CM. Lacunar strokes and infarcts: a review. *Neurology.* 1982;32:871–876.

Hankey GJ, Eikelboom JW. Homocysteine and stroke. *Curr Opin Neurolog.* 2001;14:95–102.

Heiss WD, Forsting M, Diener HC. Imaging in cerebrovascular disease. *Curr Opin Neurol.* 2001;14:67–75.

Mohr JP, Thompson JLP, Lazar RM, et al. A comparison of warfarin and aspirin for the prevention of recurrent ischemic stroke. *N Engl J Med.* 2001;345:1444–1451.

Qureshi AI. Tuhrim S. Broderick JP. Batjer HH. Hondo H. Hanley DF. Spontaneous intracerebral hemorrhage. *N Engl J Med.* 2001;344:1450–1460.

Rolak LA, ed. *Neurology Secrets.* 2nd ed. Philadelphia, Pa: Hanley & Belfus; 1998.

Saunders, Dawn E. MR spectroscopy in stroke. *Br Med Bull. Stroke.* 2000;56:334–345.

Schellinger PD, Fiebach JB, Mohr A, Ringleb PA, Jansen O, Hacke W. Thrombolytic therapy for ischemic stroke—a review. Part I—Intravenous thrombolysis. *Crit Care Med.* 2001;29:1812–1818.

Schievink WI. Spontaneous dissection of the carotid and vertebral arteries. *N Engl J Med.* 2001;344:898–906.

CHAPTER 8

Infections of the Nervous System
Questions

1. Which of the following pathological features correlates best with the severity of AIDS dementia?

    (A) The number of nodules containing macrophages, lymphocytes, and microglia
    (B) Multinucleated giant cells
    (C) Cortical atrophy
    (D) Neuronal loss
    (E) Macrophage activation

2. A 40-year-old man diagnosed with HIV-associated dementia is able to perform basic activities of self-care but cannot work or maintain the more demanding aspects of daily life. He is able to ambulate. In which stage of HIV-associated dementia (MSK clinical staging system) can the patient be classified?

    (A) Stage 0
    (B) Stage 1
    (C) Stage 2
    (D) Stage 3
    (E) Stage 4

3. Neuropsychological tests in the initial stage of AIDS dementia may show all the following EXCEPT

    (A) selective memory loss for impaired retrieval
    (B) severe attention deficit
    (C) impaired manifestations of acquired knowledge
    (D) general slowing of psychomotor speed
    (E) conservation of language

4. A 35-year-old HIV-positive man consults because of increasing difficulty walking over the last 6 months. He reports slowly increasing stiffness in his lower extremities that slowly became worse. He also noticed increasing urinary frequency and urgency over the last 6 months. On neurological examination, the patient displays mild paraparesis of lower extremities with spasticity and brisk reflexes in the left knee and ankle, and bilateral Babinski sign. Sensory examination showed moderate loss of proprioception in the legs without a sensory level.

    Cerebrospinal fluid analysis shows a protein level of 63 mg/dl, 5 WBC/mm3, 100% lymphocytes, and glucose 50 mg/dl. CSF viral and bacteriologic studies are normal. Vitamin B_{12} level is normal. MRI of the cervical, thoracic, and lumbar spine with gadolinium enhancement is normal. Somatosensory-evoked potentials show a prolongation of the central conduction time. The most likely diagnosis is

    (A) lymphoma
    (B) CMV myelopathy
    (C) AIDS-associated vacuolar myelopathy
    (D) HIV myelitis
    (E) bacterial paraspinal abscess

5. The most common type of peripheral neuropathy in AIDS patients is

    (A) distal symmetric polyneuropathy
    (B) acute inflammatory demyelinating polyneuropathy
    (C) mononeuropathy multiplex
    (D) autonomic neuropathy
    (E) progressive polyradiculopathy

6. Which of the following drugs causes a pure sensory neuropathy as a neurotoxic side effect?

 (A) Stavudine
 (B) Isoniazide
 (C) Vinca alkaloids
 (D) Ethambutol
 (E) Dapsone

7. Which of the following statements is true about progressive multifocal leukoencephalopathy?

 (A) SV 40 virus is the most frequent cause of the disease.
 (B) Approximately 50% of patients with AIDS will develop progressive multifocal leukoencephalopathy during the course of their disease.
 (C) The parieto-occipital region is the site of predilection for progressive multifocal leukoencephalopathy.
 (D) Gait disturbance is the most frequent clinical manifestation of progressive multifocal leukoencephalopathy.
 (E) PCR of the CSF has low specificity for the diagnosis of progressive multifocal leukoencephalopathy.

8. A 31-year-old right-handed man with a history of HIV infection developed headaches and right side weakness, progressing over 1 week. Physical examination demonstrates mild right hemiparesis with increased deep tendon reflexes, right Babinski sign, and a fever of 38.5°C. MRI of the head with contrast shows a single ring-enhanced lesion in the left basal ganglia and internal capsule surrounded by edema. The lesion is hypoactive on thalium-201 SPECT imaging. His CD4 lymphocyte count is 10/μl. Toxoplasmosis gondii serology is positive. The most appropriate approach of treatment for this patient is to

 (A) start corticosteroids alone
 (B) schedule a stereotactic biopsy
 (C) start radiation therapy
 (D) start antitoxoplasmosis therapy without corticosteroids

 (E) start empirical treatment of toxoplasmosis combined with corticosteroids

9. All of the following cerebrospinal fluid features are commonly found in cryptococcal meningitis in HIV patients EXCEPT

 (A) decreased opening pressure
 (B) hypoglycorrhachia
 (C) cryptococcal antigen
 (D) increased protein
 (E) visualization of cryptococcus neoformans organisms on India ink smear

10. The most commonly affected cranial nerve in tuberculosis in non-HIV-infected patients is the

 (A) oculomotor nerve
 (B) abducens nerve
 (C) trochlear nerve
 (D) facial nerve
 (E) vestibulocochlear nerve

11. A 24-year-old man with a history of HIV infection consults because of a chronic headache. Neurological examination is normal. CT scan of the head with contrast shows a ring-enhancing lesion in the left parietal area, which is confirmed by head MRI with gadolinium enhancement. The most appropriate diagnosis or therapeutic approach is to

 (A) proceed to a biopsy to establish the diagnosis
 (B) start the patient on corticosteroids
 (C) start empirical antibiotherapy
 (D) start empirical antitoxoplasmosis treatment
 (E) start the patient on intravenous acyclovir

12. The most frequent presenting symptom of primary central nervous system lymphoma in HIV patients is

 (A) impaired cognition
 (B) seizures
 (C) hemiparesis
 (D) aphasia
 (E) cranial nerve palsy

13. The most common cause of intracranial space occupying mass with contrast enhancing in AIDS patients is

    (A) primary central nervous system lymphoma
    (B) bacterial abscess
    (C) fungal abscess
    (D) toxoplasmosis
    (E) metastatic brain tumor

14. The most frequent abnormal finding on retinal examination in AIDS patients is

    (A) cotton-wool spots
    (B) CMV retinitis
    (C) optic atrophy
    (D) swollen optic nerve
    (E) toxoplasmosis retinitis

15. The most frequently abnormal findings in eastern equine encephalitis are located in the

    (A) brain stem
    (B) cerebellum
    (C) periventricular white matter
    (D) basal ganglia
    (E) meninges

16. Which of the following statements is true about subacute sclerosing panencephalitis?

    (A) It is a slow central nervous system infection with herpes simplex virus.
    (B) The onset of the disease is characterized by a rapid onset of dementia.
    (C) Myoclonic jerks are seen in the second stage of the disease.
    (D) Brain biopsy, if performed in the early stage of the disease, shows a mild inflammation limited to the cortex area.
    (E) The EEG normalizes in the myoclonic phase.

17. The most frequent cause of bacterial meningitis among children aged less than 3 months is

    (A) group B *streptococcus*
    (B) *Listeria monocytogenes*

    (C) *Streptococcus pneumonia*
    (D) *Haemophilus influenzae*
    (E) *Neisseria meningitidis*

18. Which of the following is true about leprosy?

    (A) *Mycobacterium leprae* has a preference for body parts with higher temperature than the core body.
    (B) Loss of light touch is the first manifestation of sensory impairment.
    (C) Peripheral nerve thickening results from bacterial multiplication within the neuron.
    (D) The median nerve is the most frequently affected peripheral nerve in tuberculoid leprosy.
    (E) Impaired cell-mediated immunity causes lepromatous leprosy.

19. Which of the following is true about botulism?

    (A) Toxin production by clostridium botulism colonizing the gut is the most frequent cause of adult botulism.
    (B) Botulism toxin blocks acetylcholine receptors.
    (C) The N-terminal of the heavy chain of botulism toxin governs the internalization of the toxin into the motor neuron.
    (D) Cognition is usually affected in the early stage of the disease.
    (E) Sensory examination is typically altered.

20. Which of the following is true about tetanus?

    (A) Tetanospasmin inhibits glutamate release in the spinal cord.
    (B) Tetanus toxin travels to the anterior horn cells by retrograde axonal transport.
    (C) The heavy chain of tetanus toxin blocks exocytosis.
    (D) Spasms are caused by sympathetic blockade.
    (E) Autonomic dysfunction rarely complicates the course of the disease.

21. The most common cause of viral encephalitis in the United States is

(A) arbovirus
(B) herpes virus
(C) measles virus
(D) mumps virus
(E) enterovirus

22. Repetitive sharp wave complexes over the temporal lobe are commonly seen in

(A) HIV encephalitis
(B) subacute sclerosing panencephalitis
(C) herpes simplex encephalitis
(D) Creutzfeldt-Jakob disease
(E) renal failure

23. The most frequent neurological manifestation of poliovirus infection is

(A) transverse myelitis
(B) paralytic illness
(C) cerebellitis
(D) aseptic meningitis
(E) seizures

Questions 24 through 28
Link each of the following pathogens to the appropriate clinical condition.

(A) *Streptococcus pneumoniae*
(B) *Haemophilus influenzae* type b
(C) *Staphylococcus aureus*
(D) *Acinetobacter calcoaceticus*
(E) *Listeria monocytogenes*

24. Bacterial meningitis in a 40-year-old man with a history of splenectomy

25. Bacterial meningitis in a 56-year-old man with a history of heavy ethanol abuse

26. Bacterial meningitis in a 60-year-old woman with a history of heart transplantation

27. The most common cause of bacterial meningitis in an immunocompetent adult

28. Bacterial meningitis in a 40-year-old man who underwent a ventriculostomy two days ago

29. What is the most appropriate antibiotic therapy for the treatment of hospital-acquired meningitis in a 55-year-old man with severe neutropenia?

(A) Ceftriaxone 2 gr every 12 hours
(B) Vancomycin 0.5 gr every 6 hours and ampicillin 2 gr every 4 hours
(C) Cefotaxime 2 gr every 4 hours and vancomycin 0.5 gr every 6 hours
(D) Vancomycin 0.5 gr every 6 hours and ceftazidine 2 gr every 8 hours
(E) Ampicillin 2 gr every 4 hours and gentamicin 6 mg/kg/day

30. The presence of "owl eye" intranuclear inclusion, with the presence of focal necrosis in the basal ganglia and thalamus, is highly suggestive of

(A) herpes encephalitis
(B) CMV encephalitis
(C) Epstein-Barr meningoencephalitis
(D) varicella-zoster encephalitis
(E) La Crosse virus encephalitis

31. The most frequent cause of viral meningitis is

(A) enterovirus
(B) CMV virus
(C) herpes virus
(D) arbovirus
(E) West Nile virus

32. The most common cause of epidural abscess in immunocompetent patients is

(A) *Klebsiella pneumoniae*
(B) *staphylococcus*
(C) *streptococcus*
(D) fungal infection
(E) *Mycobacterium tuberculosis*

33. The most frequent sign of neurocysticercosis is

(A) seizure
(B) headache

(C) visual disturbance

(D) hemiplegia

(E) ataxia

34. The most common neurological complication of chronic Chagas infection is

(A) seizure

(B) irritability

(C) stupor

(D) dementia

(E) cardioembolic stroke

35. Which of the following HIV complications is the LEAST affected by antiretroviral therapy?

(A) Progressive multifocal leukoencephalopathy

(B) AIDS dementia

(C) Central nervous system toxoplasmosis

(D) Cryptococcal meningitis

(E) CMV polyradiculopathy

36. Hemorrhagic meningitis is caused by the organism leading to

(A) botulism

(B) brucellosis

(C) Q fever

(D) anthrax

(E) Venezuelan equine encephalitis

37. Which of the following statements is true about Creutzfeldt-Jakob disease?

(A) The cerebrospinal fluid opening pressure is usually high.

(B) CSF protein 14-3-3 has a high sensitivity and specificity for patients with the diagnosis of progressive dementia.

(C) CSF fluid protein level is higher than 100 mg/dL.

(D) Brain MRI may show hypersignal in the internal capsule in 80% of cases.

(E) Early in the course of the disease, EEG usually shows triphasic synchronous, sharp-wave complexes.

38. Which of the following statements is true about varicella-zoster virus?

(A) The virus can be cultured from human ganglia during the latent period.

(B) Neurons are the primary site of the latent virus.

(C) The incidence of recurrent Zoster is around 30%.

(D) The abducens cranial nerve is the cranial nerve most commonly affected by varicella-zoster virus.

(E) Facial recovery from Ramsay-Hunt syndrome has a better prognosis for recovery than Bell's palsy.

39. Which of the following is true about fatal insomnia?

(A) Cognitive function is affected early in the course of the disease.

(B) EEG typically shows periodic discharges.

(C) The absence of spongiform changes on neuropathology excludes the diagnosis.

(D) PET scan shows decreased blood flow in the thalamus early in the course of the disease.

(E) Sleep studies are not necessary for the diagnosis of fatal insomnia, as the disease is always clinically obvious.

40. Which of the following is true about Japanese encephalitis?

(A) The disease is limited to the pediatric population.

(B) Ninety percent of patients affected by Japanese encephalitis will recover fully.

(C) The thalamus and basal ganglia are the sites of intense inflammation in affected patients.

(D) Serologic tests in Japanese encephalitis have a low sensitivity and specificity.

(E) A progressive ascending paralysis is the most frequent form of Japanese encephalitis seen in children.

Questions 41 through 44

Link the following:

    (A) Creutzfeldt-Jakob disease

    (B) Gerstmann-Straussler-Scheinker (GSS) disease

    (C) Kuru

    (D) Variant Creutzfeldt-Jakob disease

41. A 40-year-old man developed progressive worsening of anxiety and depressed mood, with auditory and visual hallucinations. Neurological examination demonstrated mild bilateral cerebellar syndrome. His clinical status progressively deteriorated over the next 13 months with decreased cognitive function and chorea followed by myoclonus.

42. A 20-year-old man died after 12 months of progressive cerebellar ataxia without alteration of the cognitive function until the late stage of the disease, when the patient was obtunded.

43. A 60-year-old woman developed progressive onset of fatigue, insomnia, and ill-defined pain over several weeks. This was followed by a progressive mental deterioration and myoclonus. Neurological examination demonstrated cerebellar ataxia, and bilateral pyramidal syndrome. Over the next 3 months, the patient progressed to akinetic mutism and died 5 months after the onset of symptoms.

44. A 40-year-old male died after 4 years of progressive cerebellar ataxia, pyramidal syndrome, and dementia. Postmortem examination showed an abundant prion protein (PrP), amyloid plaques in cerebral and cerebellar cortexes, as well as multicentric prion-protein amyloid plaques.

Answers and Explanations

1. **(E)** Cerebral atrophy involving the fronto-temporal areas is a common finding in patients with HIV dementia. It does not correlate with the severity of the dementia. Multiple microglial nodules containing macrophages, lymphocytes, and microglia may be seen in HIV dementia. They are scattered in the gray and white matter of the brain. They are more common in the white matter, subcortical gray of the thalamus, basal ganglia, and brain stem. They are not specific to HIV dementia and do not correlate with its severity. Other neuropathological findings include neuronal loss, dendritic changes, myelin pallor (which corresponds to changes of the blood-brain barrier), and multinucleated giant cells. The presence of these multinucleated cells correlates with the degree of dementia and the detection of HIV-1 DNA. However, the intensity of macrophage activation does appear to correlate best with the dementia severity. *(Glass et al., 1993, 2230–2237; Glass et al., 1995, 755–762)*

2. **(C)** In 1988, Price et al. developed the following clinical staging of the severity of HIV-associated dementia:

   - Stage 0 corresponds to normal mental and motor function.
   - Stage 0.5 (equivocal subclinical) corresponds to absent, minimal, or equivocal symptoms without impairment of work or capacity to perform activities of daily life. Mild signs such as snout response, slowed ocular, or extremity movements may be present. Gait and strength are normal.
   - Stage 1 (mild severity) corresponds to the ability to perform all but the most demanding activities of daily life, with unequivocal evidence of functional intellectual or motor impairment. The patient can walk without assistance.
   - Stage 2 (moderate severity) corresponds to the ability to perform basic activities of self-care but cannot work or maintain the more demanding aspects of daily life. The patient may ambulate independently.
   - Stage 3 (severe disability) corresponds to major intellectual or motor incapacity.
   - Stage 4 corresponds to the nearly vegetative status. *(Price and Brew, 1079–1083)*

3. **(B)** Neuropsychological testing adds to the neurological evaluation of suspected HIV dementia by virtue of being sensitive to mild or early symptoms of HIV-related cognitive impairment. In addition to quantifying the severity of any cognitive symptoms, it can also provide information regarding the overall pattern of cognitive impairment. Attention, calculation, and language are not usually affected in HIV dementia in its initial stage, fitting with the subcortical pattern of involvement. Impaired memory (verbal and nonverbal), impaired manipulation of acquired knowledge, memory loss selective for impaired retrieval, and deficits in psychomotor speed are characteristic of HIV dementia and are typically more severe than deficits in other cognitive domains. *(McArthur et al., 129–150)*

4. **(C)** The patient described in the vignette demonstrated clinical evidence of an insidiously progressive thoracic or high lumbar myelopathy because of the spastic paraparesis, bladder dysfunction, and corticospinal and posterior columns

signs without a sensory level and normal spinal cord MRI. The differential diagnosis includes:

- CMV myelopathy: it is a rare cause of myelopathy in HIV patients. It usually presents as an acute or subacute radiculo-myelitis involving the lower lumbar, sacral roots, and cauda equina. It is characterized clinically by the acute or subacute development of a flaccid paraplegia and incontinence. The patient in this clinical case did not have signs of radiculopathy and had slow progression of his symptoms, which make the diagnosis of CMV myelopathy unlikely.
- HIV myelitis may appear as an acute or subacute complication of AIDS. It is characterized by features of transverse myelitis with CSF pleocytosis. It is a rare complication of AIDS. It is unlikely to be the diagnosis in this clinical case considering the clinical picture, especially the CSF results.
- AIDS-associated vacuolar myelopathy is a slow progressive disease of the spinal cord. It is prevalent in more than 30% in pathological series, although only a minority of these patients is symptomatic. Pathological features of the disease include the presence of intramyelinic and periaxonal vacuoles in the lateral and posterior columns of the spinal cord. It appears late in the course of the illness. The patient may report erectile or bladder dysfunction and mild paraparesis in the early stage of the disease. Neurological examination typically demonstrates a spastic asymmetric paraparesis, increased deep tendon reflexes in the lower extremities, hyperreflexia, and the absence of a sensory level. MRI may be normal or may show atrophy of the thoracic and cervical spinal cord. CSF examination may show mild pleocytosis or increased protein level. Somatosensory-evoked potential examination may show increased central conduction time. The patient described in the vignette does have signs of AIDS-associated vacuolar myelopathy.
- Other causes of lower extremity weakness in HIV patients, such as syphilis, tuberculosis, cryptococcosis, aspergillosis, vitamin B_{12} or folate deficiency, and lymphoma are unlikely

to be the diagnosis in this case considering the clinical features and the results of ancillary tests. *(DiRocco, 151–155)*

5. **(A)** Distal symmetrical polyneuropathy is the most common form of peripheral neuropathy in HIV-infected patients. The proposed mechanisms of this neuropathy include direct HIV infection, injury from cytokines effect, metabolic abnormalities, or the medications used to control the HIV infection. *(Simpson and Taglia, 769–785)*

6. **(A)** Toxicity from drugs used to treat HIV infection is among the major causes of peripheral neuropathy in these patients. Didanosine, stavudine, and zalcitabine are antiretroviral drugs that may cause a sensory neuropathy. Isoniazid and ethambutol cause sensorimotor neuropathy. Vinca alkaloids and dapsone cause a mixed motor more than a sensory neuropathy. *(Simpson and Taglia, 769–785)*

7. **(C)** Progressive multifocal leukoencephalopathy was initially described on the basis of its distinctive neuropathological features of demyelination, giant astrocytes, and oligodendrocytes with abnormal nuclei. Subsequently, a papovavirus referred to as JC virus was identified in affected oligodendrocytes and astrocytes. JC virus infection typically remains latent until there is impairment of cellular immunity. Approximately 5% of all AIDS patients will develop progressive multifocal leukoencephalopathy. Its clinical manifestations are dependent on the location of the infection. Hemiparesis is the most common clinical manifestation of progressive multifocal leukoencephalopathy in AIDS patients. Other common clinical manifestations are gait disturbance, speech and language disorders, cognitive dysfunction, and cortical blindness. MRI of the head is the most sensitive technique to show the demyelinating lesion involving the white matter in the subcortical U fibers with a predilection for the parieto-occipital areas. The lesions are not typically enhancing, although up to 9% may have peripheral enhancement around the lesion. PCR of the CSF for the diagnosis of progressive

multifocal leukoencephalopathy has high sensitivity and specificity that reaches 100%. The prognosis of progressive multifocal leukoencephalopathy is serious. Death occurs between 1 and 18 months after the onset of symptoms. *(Berger et al., 59–68)*

8. **(D)** In this vignette, the differential diagnosis is of a single brain lesion in an HIV patient with positive toxoplasmosis serology. The main differential diagnoses are toxoplasmosis encephalitis and primary central nervous system lymphoma. Although this patient's head MRI does not present the classic multiple space occupying enhancing lesions of toxoplasmosis encephalitis, the combination of a positive serology of toxoplasmosis, a CD4 count of less than 200/µl, and a decreased thallium-201 SPECT imaging that is more suggestive of toxoplasmosis encephalitis than lymphoma. The recommendations of the American Academy of Neurology Qualified Standards Subcommittee are to institute empirical antibiotic therapy for the presumptive toxoplasmosis and obtain a follow-up imaging study. If the patient shows a clinical and radiological response to the empirical antibiotic therapy, he can be presumed to have central nervous system toxoplasmosis. The patient should be maintained on suppressive antibiotics for life after finishing the induction therapy. If the patient does not show improvement on antibiotics after 2 weeks, he is eligible for stereotactic biopsy. The empirical use of corticosteroids is not recommended for toxoplasmosis treatment. The addition of corticosteroids has not been shown to improve neurological outcome and may interfere with the assessment of a possible primary central nervous system lymphoma. *(Anonymous, 21–26)*

9. **(A)** Cerebrospinal fluid (CSF) abnormalities in cryptococcal meningitis in HIV patients may be subtle. The opening pressure is elevated in two-thirds of cases and may exceed 400 mm H_2O. Mild pleocytosis is seen in 6% to 30% of cases. Hypoglycorrhachia is found in 8% to 76% of cases. Increased protein is observed in 35% to 70% of cases. Visualization of organisms on India ink smear is seen in 72% to 94% of cases. Successful culture of *C. neoformans* in and visualization of cryptococcal antigen in the CSF may be seen in up to 100% of cases. *(Churck and Sande, 794–799)*

10. **(B)** In immunocompetent patients with tuberculosis, cranial nerves are affected in 15% to 40% of cases. The abducens nerve is the most commonly affected, followed in descending order by the oculomotor, trochlear, facial, optic, vestibulocochlear, vagus, accessory, and hypoglossal nerves. *(Lincoln et al., 807–823)*

11. **(D)** The presence of a ring enhancing mass on CT scan of the head of HIV patients should raise the possibility of central nervous system toxoplasmosis. The diagnostic workup should include a toxoplasmosis antibody titer in the serum and the cerebral spinal fluid, and if possible, a thallium SPECT study to rule out a hyperactive lesion (more suggestive of lymphoma). The most appropriate therapeutic approach is to start the patient on antitoxoplasmosis therapy for 2 weeks and to assess the patient clinically and radiologically. In case of improvement, the patient should be maintained on prophylactic antibiotics for life after completion of the induction therapy. If there is no improvement, steriotactic biopsy should be considered. The use of corticosteroids has not been shown to be beneficial for the treatment of central nervous system toxoplasmosis and may delay the diagnosis of primary central nervous system lymphoma. It should be used with caution and rapidly tapered. *(Luft et al., 211–222)*

12. **(A)** The most frequent presenting symptom of central nervous lymphoma is cognitive or mental status impairment. It is seen in 60% of cases. Hemiparesis or aphasia is seen in 35% of cases. Seizures are seen in 15% of cases at presentation. Cranial nerve palsy is seen in only 10% of cases at presentation. *(Baumgartner et al., 206–211)*

13. **(D)** Toxoplasmosis is the most common cause of intracranial space occupying mass in AIDS patients, followed by primary central nervous system lymphoma. Toxoplasmosis lesions are most frequently found in the cerebral cortex,

basal ganglia, and gray-white matter junction. (*Chinn et al., 694–654*)

14. **(A)** The most frequent retinal lesion in AIDS patients is cotton-wool spots, seen in 75% of the cases. It is a buildup of exoplasmic material at the site of a nerve fiber layer infarct. When these spots are coupled with hemorrhage or capillary abnormalities, it is called AIDS retinopathy. Axonal loss in the optic nerve has been estimated at 40% in patients dying from AIDS in the absence of opportunistic infection of the retina. CMV retinitis may affect 25% to 35% of patients with AIDS. Toxoplasmosis retinitis, optic atrophy, and optic edema are less frequently seen. (*Gagliuso et al., 63–86*)

15. **(D)** Eastern equine encephalitis is a life-threatening mosquito-borne arboviral infection found principally along the east and gulf coasts of the United States. Cases have occurred sporadically and in small epidemics. Diagnosing eastern-equine encephalitis is difficult because its symptoms are nonspecific and confirmation requires either specific serologic findings or the isolation of the virus in cerebrospinal fluid or brain tissue. Neuroradiographic abnormalities are common and best visualized by MRI. The abnormal findings include focal lesions in the basal ganglia (found in 71% of patients on MRI and in 56% on CT), thalami (found in 71% on MRI and in 25% on CT), and brain stem (found in 43% on MRI and in 9% on CT). Periventricular white matter changes and cortical lesions as well as meningeal enhancement are less common. (*Deresiewicz et al., 1867–1874*)

16. **(C)** Subacute sclerosing panencephalitis is a slow central nervous system infection caused by measles virus that results in progressive inflammation and sclerosis of the brain. The incidence of the disease in the United States fell from 0.61 case per million, for persons under the age of 20 years, to 0.06 case in 1980, most likely related to measles vaccination. Patients with subacute sclerosing panencephalitis generally have a history of typical measles with full recovery. The symptoms of SSPE follow on average by about 7 years. The clinical course of the disease is divided arbitrarily into 4 stages. Its onset is usu-

ally insidious, marked by subtle changes in behavior and deterioration of school or work, followed by a frank dementia. The appearance of massive repetitive myoclonic jerks marks the onset of stage 2 of the disease. Cerebellar ataxia, dystonia, retinopathy, and optic atrophy may appear. As the disease progresses, the myoclonic jerks tend to disappear, while the dementia progresses to stupor and coma. Death occurs after a mean of 18 months. Brain biopsy in the early stages may show mild inflammation of the meninges and a panencephalitis involving cortical and subcortical gray, as well as white matter. EEG is useful in supporting the diagnosis of SSPE. Early in the course of the disease, it may be normal or show moderate nonspecific slowing. In the myoclonic phase, the EEG shows suppression-burst episodes. Later in the course of the disease, the EEG becomes increasingly disorganized, with high amplitude and random dysrhythmic slowing. (*Garg, 63–70*)

17. **(A)** The likelihood of infection with a specific pathogen in case of bacterial meningitis is related in large part to the age of the patient. Group B streptococcus is the most frequent pathogen among immunocompetent patients aged less than 3 months. *Neisseria meningitidis* is the predominant pathogen among children aged 2 to 18 years, and *streptococcus pneumoniae* is most likely among adults. (*Schuchat et al., 970–976*)

18. **(E)** Leprosy, a primary peripheral nerve and skin infection, is caused by the acid-fast bacterium *Mycobacterium leprae. M. leprae* has a preference for parts of the body with a temperature 7–10°C less than the core body temperature. It has a long incubation period, between 6 months and 40 years. Sensory impairment proceeds in a predictable sequence, with loss of temperature sensation first, followed by pain and then touch. Vibration and proprioception are spared. Impaired cell-mediated immunity causes lepromatous leprosy, a more disseminated infection than the tuberculoid leprosy of patients with conserved cellular immunity. Nerve damage results from bacterial multiplication within Schwann cells or granulomatous damage to the perineurium. The ulnar nerve is the most frequently

affected in case of tuberculoid leprosy. *(Bradley et al., 1332–1334)*

19. **(C)** Botulism is caused by the blockade of peripheral cholinergic transmission by a neurotoxin (secreted by clostridium botulinum). It can be acquired either by contaminated food or by an infected wound spreading the toxin in the bloodstream. Gut colonization by clostridium botulism causes infantile botulism and less commonly adult botulism. Botulinum toxin blocks acetylcholine release from the presynaptic membrane, leading to the paralytic and autonomic symptoms. Botulinum toxin is formed by heavy and light chains. The C-terminal region of the heavy chain binds tightly and specifically to the presynaptic membrane, whereas the N-terminal domain governs internalization of the toxin into the motor neuron, which protects the toxin from neutralizing antibodies. After translocation into the cytosol, the liberated light chain (a zinc endopeptidase) targets various protein-mediating exocytoses, causing irreversible blockade at peripheral cholinergic synapses. The early symptoms of botulism include diplopia, ptosis, dysarthria, and dysphagia. Respiratory muscles, as well as extraocular and limb muscles, are affected symmetrically. Cognitive function is conserved, unless there are metabolic changes from respiratory failure. Sensation is typically normal. Reflexes are decreased or absent. *(Bradley et al., 1384)*

20. **(B)** *Clostridium tetani* secretes tetanospasmin, a neurotoxin that inhibits the release of GABA and glycine (which are inhibitory neurotransmitters) in the brain stem and spinal cord. Tetanus neurotoxin is formed by heavy and light chains linked together by a disulfide bond. The light chain, a zinc endopeptidase, is responsible for blocking exocytosis. Tetanus neurotoxin travels to the anterior horn cells of the spinal cord by retrograde axonal transport, penetrates into the intrasynaptic space, and enters inhibitory neurons. Impaired exocytosis in these spinal inhibitory neurons and in the intermediolateral column of the spinal cord causes muscle contractions and autonomic dysfunction, respectively. The cardinal clinical features of tetanus include muscle rigidity and spasms, which may

be triggered by a sensory stimulus, movement, or emotion. Autonomic dysfunction is frequent in tetanus and includes fever, tachycardia, hypertension, and other signs of sympathetic irritation. *(Bradley et al., 1340–1342)*

21. **(B)** The most common cause of focal viral encephalitis in the United States is herpes simplex virus type 1. Other causes of viral encephalitis are VZV, enterovirus, mumps, measles, and Lacrosse virus. *(Bradley et al., 1358–1359)*

22. **(C)** The EEG in acute viral encephalitis may show patterns suggesting a specific diagnosis. Repetitive sharp-wave complexes over the temporal lobes or periodic lateralized epileptiform discharges are recorded in herpes simplex type 1 encephalitis and in rare cases of infectious mononucleosis encephalitis. Periodic slow-wave complexes occur in subacute sclerosing panencephalitis. Triphasic waves at higher periodic frequency are seen in Creutzfeldt-Jakob disease. *(Bradley et al., 1358)*

23. **(D)** Poliovirus is the agent of acute anterior poliomyelitis. It is one of the most virulent members of the enterovirus group. The virus has a tropism for motor neurons of the spinal cord and brain stem. The most frequent clinical manifestation of poliovirus is aseptic meningitis (seen in 8% of cases). Paralytic illness is seen in 1% of all cases. Other less frequent clinical manifestations include cerebellitis, transverse mellitus, and facial paresis. *(Bradley et al., 1991–1994)*

24. **(B)**

25. **(D)**

26. **(E)**

27. **(A)**

28. **(C)**

Explanations 24 through 28

The most common causative organisms of community-acquired bacterial meningitis are

Streptococcus pneumoniae, and *Neisseria meningitidis*. *Haemophilus influenzae* type b causes meningitis in immunocompromised patients, e.g., postsplenectomy and in chronic lung diseases. *Staphylococcus aureus* causes meningitis following invasive neurosurgical procedure such as ventriculostomy. *Acinetobacter calcoaceticus* and other gram-negative bacilli cause meningitis in alcoholic patients. *Listeria monocytogenes* causes meningitis in immunosuppressed patients, e.g., postorgan transplant. *(Roos, 1–2)*

29. **(D)** Treatment of bacterial meningitis is a medical emergency. The goal is to begin antibiotic therapy within 60 minutes of a patient's arrival in the emergency room. Empiric antimicrobial therapy is initiated in patients with suspected bacterial meningitis before the results of CSF Gram stain and culture are known. *Streptococcus pneumoniae* and *Neisseria meningitidis* are the most common etiological organisms of community-acquired bacterial meningitis. Due to the emergence of penicillin and cephalosporin resistant *S. pneumoniae*, empiric therapy of community-acquired bacterial meningitis should include a third-generation cephalosporin (e.g., ceftriaxone or cefotaxime) or a fourth-generation cephalosporin (cefepime) and vancomycin. Ampicillin and gentamicin should be added to the empiric regimen for coverage of *Listeria monocytogenes* in individuals with impaired cell-mediated immunity due to chronic illness, organ transplantation, pregnancy, AIDS, malignancies, or immunosuppressive therapy. In hospital-acquired meningitis, and particularly meningitis following neurosurgical procedures, staphylococci and gram-negative organisms (including *P. aeruginosa*), are the most common etiological organisms. In these patients, empiric therapy should include a combination of vancomycin and ceftazidime. Ceftazidime should be substituted for ceftriaxone or cefotaxime in neurosurgical patients and in neutropenic patients, as *Pseudomonas aeruginosa* may be the meningeal pathogen, and ceftazidime is the only cephalosporin with sufficient activity against *P. aeruginosa* in the central nervous system. *(Roos, 7–10)*

30. **(B)** Cytomegalovirus (CMV) meningoencephalitis is largely a disease of congenitally infected newborns and immunocompromised individuals, including organ transplant recipients and those with advanced HIV infection. In immunocompromised individuals, infection results predominantly from reactivation of latent virus. It is generally associated with evidence of CMV infection in other organs including the eye, lungs, gastrointestinal tract, or other organs. In individuals infected with AIDS, CMV can produce multifocal CNS disease with involvement of the spinal cord, nerve roots, ventricular and subependymal regions, and both gray and white matter. Infection often shows a predilection for deep gray structures including basal ganglia and thalamus, producing regions of focal necrosis and hemorrhage. Microglial nodules (dense focal aggregates of microglial cells and macrophages) and Cowdry type A intranuclear inclusions are characteristic of CMV, although both are seen in a variety of other infections. "Owl eye" inclusions (large basophilic intranuclear inclusions separated from the nuclear membrane by a thin halo) are virtually diagnostic of CMV infection. *(McCutchan, 747–754)*

31. **(A)** Enteroviruses are responsible for the overwhelming majority (85%–95%) of cases of acute viral meningitis. Less commonly, enteroviruses produce encephalitis or polio-like flaccid paralysis. Most infections occur in the summer and early fall (May–October), although sporadic cases occur all year round. Children are more frequently infected than adults, although infections in older individuals tend to be more severe. *(Rotbart, 971–981)*

32. **(B)** *Staphylococcus aureus* has been traditionally and remains the main pathogen in epidural abscess, accounting for over 60% of the isolates. Other gram positive pathogens that may cause epidural abscess less frequently include *Staphylococcus epidermidis*, streptococci (alpha and beta hemolytic), and anaerobes. Gram-negative pathogens are increasing in frequency (second to *Staphylococcus*), perhaps reflecting an increasing proportion of iatrogenic infections.

Mycobacterium tuberculosis and pathogenic fungi also account for a significant percentage of cases. *(Bradley, 1238–1329)*

33. **(A)** Neurocysticercosis infection is pleomorphic due to individual differences in the number and location of lesions, and in the severity of the host's immune response to the parasites. Seizures are the most common clinical manifestation of the disease, occurring in more than 70% of cases. Indeed, in endemic regions, the presence of adult-onset epilepsy is highly suggestive of neurocysticercosis. Focal neurological signs (pyramidal tract signs, sensory deficits, cerebellar ataxia, signs of brain stem dysfunction, and involuntary movements) occur in 20% to 30% of patients with neurocysticercosis. These manifestations usually follow a subacute or chronic course, making the differential diagnosis with neoplasms or other infections of the CNS difficult on clinical grounds. However, focal signs may occur abruptly in patients who develop a cerebral infarct as a complication of cysticercotic angiitis. Some patients present with intracranial hypertension that may be associated with seizures, focal neurologic signs, or intellectual deterioration. Hydrocephalus is the most common cause of this syndrome. In these cases, clinical manifestations have a subacute onset and a slowly progressive course that may be punctuated by episodes of sudden loss of consciousness related to movements of the head when the cause of hydrocephalus is a fourth ventricle cyst. Intracranial hypertension also occurs in patients with cysticercotic encephalitis, a severe form of the disease resulting from a massive cysticercal infection of the brain parenchyma, inducing an intense immune response from the host. *(Del Brutto, 1392–1393)*

34. **(E)** Acute Chagas disease is usually characterized by an inoculation chagoma in the orbital region (Romaña's sign) and mild constitutional symptoms. However, some children, HIV-infected individuals, and immunosuppressed patients may develop severe encephalitis during the acute phase of the disease. Chagasic encephalitis is characterized by irritability, stupor progressing to coma, seizures, focal neurologic signs (related to granuloma formation),

and a mononuclear pleocytosis in the CSF. Most of these patients die during the acute disease, and survivors are usually left with epilepsy and intellectual impairment. In patients with chronic infection, the most common neurologic complication is a cardioembolic stroke related to the development of cardiac arrhythmias or ventricular aneurysms. The territory of the middle cerebral artery is the most frequently affected, and infarcts may be located in the parietal, frontal and temporal lobes, or in the basal ganglia. The actual prevalence of stroke in Chagas disease is unknown; however, some studies have shown that between 9% and 36% of patients with chagasic cardiomyopathy develop a cerebral infarct. *(Bradley, 1392–1393)*

35. **(B)** Potent antiretroviral therapy may be less effective in preventing HIV-1-associated dementia than other HIV-1-related complications. A study from Australia compared the effect of highly active antiretroviral therapy (HAART) against AIDS dementia complex (ADC) relative to its effect on other initial AIDS-defining illnesses (ADIs). The study demonstrated a proportional increase in ADC, compared with other ADIs. A marked increase in the median CD4 cell count at ADC diagnosis has occurred since the introduction of HAART in Australia. Poor penetration of antiretroviral medication in the central nervous system is suggested by the study as a possible explanation for the modest impact of HAART on ADC. *(Dore et al., 1249–1253)*

36. **(D)** Anthrax meningitis is a rare complication that can occur with any form of anthrax. Meningeal symptoms are usually accompanied by fever, myalgias and vomiting, and less frequently by seizures or delirium. The CSF is typically hemorrhagic and culture for *B. anthracis* is positive. Imaging of the CNS may reveal subarachnoid, intracerebral, or intraventricular hemorrhage with leptomeningeal enhancement, while pathology reveals hemorrhage of the leptomeninges known as "Cardinal's Cap."

Brucellosis is associated with low back pain in 60% of infected people and can be associated with vertebral osteomyelitis, intervertebral disc infection, sacroiliac infection, or paravertebral abscess. The nervous system is involved in approximately 5% of people with brucellosis, and is referred to as neurobrucellosis. Acute neurobrucellosis typically includes symptoms of meningeal irritation, and may be accompanied by seizures or coma. Chronic neurobrucellosis may include meningoencephalitis, demyelination, cranial neuropathy (most often involving the vestibulocochlear nerve), myeloradiculitis, or cerebral arteritis. The CSF examination in neurobrucellosis almost always reveals a moderate elevation of protein and a lymphocytic pleocytosis.

Severe headache is present in most people with symptomatic Q fever, but infection of the nervous system is uncommon. Infection of the CNS usually manifests as an acute aseptic meningitis and/or encephalitis and may be accompanied by cranial nerve palsy, seizures, mental status change, or coma. Examination of the CSF typically reveals a pleocytosis (usually lymphocytic, but can be neutrophilic) in 50% of patients, as well as an elevated protein and negative bacterial culture in nearly all patients. Neuroimaging may reveal hypodense lesions in the subcortical white matter.

Botulism typically presents with bilateral cranial nerve palsies and symmetric descending paralysis. Symptoms often include blurred vision, diplopia, dry mouth and throat, dysphagia, and dysphonia. Sensory deficits do not occur. Deep tendon reflexes may be present or absent. Respiratory failure is a common complication. CSF examination should be normal. Venezuelan equine encephalitis (VEE) causes encephalitis in only 4% of children and less than 1% of adults, and typically occurs after a few days or a week of prodromal illness. CSF examination typically reveals a lymphocytic pleocytosis. (Bradley, 1346)

37. **(B)** Study of the cerebrospinal fluid in Creutzfeldt-Jakob disease shows that it has a normal opening pressure, does not have an increase in cells or abnormal levels of immunoglobulin, and has a normal or mildly elevated protein content. Partial sequencing of these proteins showed that they matched a normal brain protein known as 14-3-3, and a rapid CSF immunoassay for the protein has proved useful in the diagnosis. The sensitivity of the test is 96%

and the specificity is 99%. Elevated levels of this protein are found in the cerebrospinal fluid of patients with viral encephalitis and during the first month after cerebrovascular accidents. Early in the course of the disease, the electroencephalogram may be normal or show nonspecific slowing. Later in the disease, periodic biphasic or triphasic, synchronous, sharp-wave complexes are superimposed on a slow background rhythm in most patients, but these characteristic complexes may disappear as the myoclonus subsides in the terminal phase of the disease. The results of brain imaging are usually normal in the early stages of the disease. Magnetic resonance imaging (MRI) may show hyperintense signals in the basal ganglia on T(2)-weighted images. (Johnson and Gibbs, 1994)

38. **(B)** After it has produced chickenpox, varicella-zoster virus becomes latent in ganglia along the entire neuraxis. The cannot be cultured from human ganglia, although viral DNA was detected by PCR in human trigeminal and thoracic ganglia. Most studies indicate that neurons are the primary, if not exclusive, site of latent virus. Other studies detected the presence of the virus in the perineuronal satellite cells. The incidence of recurrent zoster in immunocompetent patients is less than 5%. The trigeminal nerve is the most common cranial nerve affected by varicella-zoster virus. When the ophthalmic division of the trigeminal nerve is affected, it is frequently accompanied by keratitis, which is a potential cause of blindness if not recognized and treated promptly. When the seventh cranial nerve is involved, there is weakness of all facial muscles on one side, along with rash in the ipsilateral external ear (zoster oticus) or hard palate. Zoster oticus and peripheral facial weakness together constitute the Ramsay-Hunt syndrome. Recovery from facial weakness or paralysis is reported to be less complete than in idiopathic Bell's palsy. Palsies of other cranial nerves occur less frequently. (Gilden et al., 635–645)

39. **(D)** In its most characteristic presentation, fatal insomnia causes an untreatable insomnia that sometimes lasts for weeks or months. The insomnia is followed by dysautonomia,

ataxia, variable pyramidal and extrapyramidal signs, with relative sparing of cognitive function until late in the course. The dysautonomias may include episodic alterations in blood pressure, heart rate, temperature, respiratory rate, and secretions. The EEG shows diffuse slowing rather than periodic discharges. A sleep study is valuable to document a shortening of total sleep time if insomnia is not clinically obvious. Positron emission tomography (PET) shows a reduction in metabolic activity or blood flow to the thalamus relatively early in the disease. The neuropathologic features of fatal insomnia include neuronal loss and astrogliosis within the thalamus, inferior olives and, to a lesser degree, the cerebellum. The lack of spongiform changes does not exclude the diagnosis. The protease-resistant PrP is detectable in the brains of affected patients but is usually present only in small amounts and is often restricted to specific regions such as the thalamus and temporal lobe. *(Mastrianni and Roos, 337–352)*

40. **(C)** Japanese encephalitis (JE) virus is one of the most important causes of viral encephalitis worldwide, with an estimated 50,000 cases and 15,000 deaths annually. The clinical manifestations occur predominantly in children and young adults. Older adults seem to be affected when epidemics occur in new locations. The clinical features include a nonspecific prodromal stage, followed by headaches, nausea, vomiting, behavioral changes, altered state of consciousness, and often seizures. A dull mask-like face with wide staring eyes, tremor, choreoathetosis, head nodding, and rigidity are also found. Approximately one-third of patients die, and 50% of the encephalitis survivors have severe neuropsychiatric sequelae. In addition, Japanese encephalitis virus was recently found to cause acute flaccid paralysis in Vietnamese children. The weakness is usually asymmetric, and the lower extremities are more often affected than the upper. Electrophysiologic studies localized the site of damage to the anterior horn cells. The clinical and pathologic features are therefore similar to those of poliomyelitis. The diagnosis of JE infection is made serologically. The presence of anti-JE virus immunoglobulin M in the CSF has a sensitivity and specificity in excess of

95%. Pathological studies demonstrate that the thalamus, basal ganglia, and midbrain are heavily affected, providing anatomical correlates for the tremor and dystonias that characterize Japanese encephalitis. *(Hinson and Tyor, 369–374; Solomon et al., 405–415)*

41. **(D)**

42. **(C)**

43. **(A)**

44. **(B)**

Explanations 41 through 44

The classic (sporadic) Creutzfeld-Jakob disease is a rapidly progressive, multifocal dementia, usually with myoclonus. Onset usually occurs in the 45 to 75 years age group, with peak onset between 60 and 65 years. Around 70% of those afflicted die less than 6 months after onset of symptoms. Prodromal features occur in approximately one-third of cases and include fatigue, insomnia, depression, weight loss, headaches, general malaise, and ill-defined pain. In addition to mental deterioration and myoclonus, frequent additional neurological features include extrapyramidal signs, cerebellar ataxia, pyramidal signs, and cortical blindness.

Kuru affects both sexes, and onset of disease ranges from age 5 years to over 60 years. The mean clinical duration of illness is 12 months, with a range of 3 months to 3 years; the course tends to be shorter in children. The central clinical feature is progressive cerebellar ataxia. In sharp contrast to Creutzfeld-Jakob disease, dementia is often absent, although in the terminal stages, the faculties of many patients are impaired.

Variant Creutzfeld-Jakob disease has a clinical presentation in which behavioral and psychiatric disturbances predominate, and in some cases there are marked sensory phenomena. Initial referral is often to a psychiatrist, and the most prominent feature is depression, but anxiety, withdrawal, and behavioral changes are also frequent. Other features include delusions, emotional lability, aggression, insomnia, and auditory and visual hallucinations. In most patients, a progressive cerebellar syndrome develops, with gait and limb ataxia. Dementia usually develops later in the clinical course. Myoclonus is seen in most patients, in some cases preceded by chorea. The most remarkable neuropathological feature of variant Creutzfeld-Jakob is the abundant prion protein (PrP) amyloid plaques in the cerebral and cerebellar cortexes. The presence of chronic cerebellar ataxia with pyramidal signs and dementia is highly suggestive of GSS. This diagnosis is supported by the presence of multicentric prion-protein amyloid plaques. *(Collinge, 519–550)*

REFERENCES

Anonymous. Evaluation and management of intracranial mass lesions in AIDS: Report of the Quality Standards Subcommittee of the as American Academy of Neurology. *Neurology.* 1998;50:21–26.

Baumgartner JE, Rachlin JR, Beckstead JH, et al. Primary central nervous system lymphomas: Natural history and response to radiation therapy in 55 patients with acquired immunodeficiency syndrome. *J Neurosurg.* 1990;73:206–211.

Berger JR, Paull L, Lanska D, Whiteman M. Progressive multifocal leukoencephalopathy in patients with HIV infection. *J Neurovirol.* 1998a: 4:59–68.

Bradley WG, Daroff RB, Fenichel GM. *Neurology in Clinical Practice: Principles of Diagnosis and Management.* Oxford, UK: Butterworth-Heinemann; 2000.

Chinn RJS, Wilkinson ID, Hall-Craggs MA, et al: Toxoplasmosis and primary central nervous system lymphoma in HIV infection: Diagnosis with MR spectroscopy. *Radiology.* 1995;197:654–694.

Churck SL, Sande MA. Infection with cryptococcus neoformans in the acquired immunodeficiency syndrome. *N Engl J Med.* 1989;321:794–799.

Collinge J. Prion diseases of human and animals: Their causes and molecular basis. *Annu Rev Neurosci.* 2001;24:519–550.

Del Brutto OH, Sotelo J, Roman GC. *Neurocysticercosis: A Clinical Handbook.* Lisse: Swets & Zeitlinger; 1998.

Deresiewicz RL, Thaler SJ, Hsu L, Zamani AA. Clinical and neuroradiographic manifestations of eastern equine encephalitis. *N Engl J Med.* 1997;336:1867–1874.

Di Rocco A. Diseases of the spinal cord in human immunodeficiency virus infection. [Review] *Sem Neurol.* 1999;19:151–155.

Dore GJ, et al: Changes to AIDS dementia complex in the era of of highly active antiretroviral therapy. *AIDS* 1999. 13:1249–1253.

Gagliuso DJ, Teich SA, Friedman AH, Orellana J. Ocular toxoplasmosis in AIDS patients. *Trans Am Ophtalmol Soc.* 1990;88:63–86.

Garg RK. Subacute sclerosing panencephalitis. *Postgrad Med J.* 2002;78:63–70.

Gilden DH, Kleinschmidt-DeMasters BK, LaGuardia JJ, Mahalingam R, Cohrs RJ. Neurologic complications of the reactivation of varicella-zoster virus. *N Engl J Med.* 2000;342:635–645.

Glass JD, Wesselingh SL, Selnes OA, McArthur JC. Clinical-neuropathologic correlation in HIV-associated dementia. *Neurology.* 1993;43:2230–2237.

Glass JD, Fedor H, Wesselingh SL, McArthur JC. Immunocytochemical quantitation of human immunodeficiency virus in the brain: Correlations with dementia. *Ann Neurol.* 1995;38:755–762.

Hinson VK, Tyor WR. Update on viral encephalitis. *Curr Opin Neurol.* 2001;14:369–374.

Johnson RT, Gibbs CJ Jr. Creutzfeldt-Jakob disease and related transmissible spongiform encephalopathies. *N Engl J Med.* 1998;339:1994–2004.

Lincoln E, Sordillo S, Davies P. Tuberculosis meningitis in children: a review of 167 untreated and 73 treated patients with special reference to early diagnosis. *J Pediatr.* 1960;57:807–823.

Luft BJ, Hafner R, Korzun AH, et al: Toxoplasmosis encephalitis in AIDS. *Clin Infect Dis.* 1992;15:211–222.

Mastrianni JA. Roos RP. The prion diseases. *Sem Neurol.* 2000;20:337–352.

McArthur JC. Sacktor N. Selnes O. Human immunodeficiency virus-associated dementia. *Sem Neurol.* 1999;19:129–150.

McCutchan JA. Cytomegalovirus infections of the nervous system in patients with AIDS. *Clin Infect Dis.* 1995;20:747–754.

Price RW. Brew BJ. The AIDS dementia complex. *J Infect Dis.* 1988;158:1079–1083.

Roos KL. Meningitis. From *Infections of the nervous system.* AAN Courses. 2002.

Rotbart HA. Enteroviral infections of the central nervous system. *Clin Infect Dis* 1995;20:971–981.

Schuchat A, Robinson K, Wenger JD, Harrison LH, Farley M, Reingold AL, Lefkowitz L, Perkins BA. Bacterial meningitis in the United States in 1995. Active Surveillance Team. *N Engl J Med.* 1997;337:970–976.

Simpson DM, Taglia M. Neurological manifestations of HIV-infection. *Ann Intern Med.* 1994;121:769–785.

Solomon T, Dung NM, Kneen R, Gainsborough M, Vaughn DW, Khanh VT. Japanese encephalitis. *J Neurol Neurosurg Psychiatr.* 2000;68:405–415.

CHAPTER 9

Neuroimmunology
Questions

1. Which of the following statements is NOT true about relapsing-remitting multiple sclerosis?

   (A) The female predominance is approximately 2 to 1.
   (B) Slowly-evolving upper-motor-neuron syndrome of the legs is typical of the relapsing-remitting form of multiple sclerosis.
   (C) Body temperature increase may cause exacerbation of symptoms.
   (D The presence of oligoclonal bands increases the risk of recurrence of the disease.
   (E) Women with predominantly sensory symptoms have more favorable prognosis.

2. Which of the following statements is true about the influence of genetic factors in multiple sclerosis?

   (A) The concordance rate of multiple sclerosis in monozygotic twins is equal to the ratio among dizygotic twins.
   (B) The absolute risk of multiple sclerosis in the first degree relative of a patient with multiple sclerosis is not different from the risk in the general population.
   (C) HLA DR2 allele increases the risk of multiple sclerosis.
   (D) The mode of transmission of multiple sclerosis is autosomal recessive.
   (E) HLA DR and DQ polymorphisms are associated with the course and the severity of the disease.

3. Demyelinating lesions in multiple sclerosis are LEAST likely to occur in the

   (A) thalamus
   (B) optic nerve
   (C) cerebellum
   (D) brainstem
   (E) periventricular white matter

4. All of the following are true about the mechanism of action of interferon in multiple sclerosis EXCEPT it

   (A) decreases the antigen presentation.
   (B) increases cytokine production governed by type 2 helper T cells.
   (C) increases the secretion of interferon 10.
   (D) competes with myelin basic protein for presentation on MHC class II molecules.
   (E) decreases the passage of the immune cells across the blood–brain barrier.

5. Which of the following is characteristic of chronic inactive multiple sclerosis plaques?

   (A) Hypercellular infiltrate mainly composed of macrophages, T lymphocytes, and microglia
   (B) Well-demarcated areas of hypocellularity with myelin pallor
   (C) Shadow plaques are seen in the center of the demyelinating lesion
   (D) B lymphocytes tend to concentrate in the periventricular region
   (E) Local precipitation of immunoglobulin and complement in areas of myelin damage

6. Once autoreactive T cells have gained entry into the central nervous system, they invade the extracellular matrix aided by their secretion of

(A) metalloproteinases
(B) adhesion molecules
(C) TNF α
(D) interleukin-6
(E) TNF β

7. Autoreactive T lymphocytes respond to putative multiple sclerosis antigens through formation of a molecular complex involving all of the following EXCEPT

(A) oligodendrocytes
(B) macrophages
(C) T lymphocytes
(D) perivascular monocytes
(E) microglia

8. Which of the following agents has been suggested to cause immunological injury in multiple sclerosis?

(A) HIV virus
(B) herpes virus
(C) E coli
(D) CMV virus
(E) JC virus

9. All of the following are true about axonal injury in multiple sclerosis EXCEPT

(A) Less than 10% of axons are lost in chronically demyelinating cervical spinal cord plaque.
(B) Acute active multiple sclerosis plaque may demonstrate axonal transection.
(C) Axonal loss may underlie the neurological deficit during primary or secondary progressive multiple sclerosis.
(D) The accumulation of amyloid precursor protein identifies damaged axons in actively demyelinating multiple sclerosis.
(E) Acute axonal injury correlates with the number of CD8+ T lymphocytes.

10. Transected axons are identified during the progression of multiple sclerosis as early as

(A) 2 weeks
(B) 1 year
(C) 5 years
(D) 10 years
(E) 20 years

11. All of the following mechanisms contribute to the clinical remission in relapsing remitting multiple sclerosis EXCEPT

(A) resolution of inflammation
(B) redistribution of axolemmal sodium channels
(C) remyelination
(D) accumulation of amyloid precursor proteins
(E) compensatory adaptation of the central nervous system

12. Which of the following is the most likely determinant of disability in multiple sclerosis?

(A) Number of enhancing lesions on T1 MRI with contrast
(B) Number of T2 MRI lesions
(C) Positron emission tomography studies of brain activity
(D) Number of T1 hypodense lesions in the brain
(E) Total white matter axonal status

13. In MR spectroscopy, axonal integrity correlates with which of the following peaks?

(A) Choline
(B) Lactate
(C) N-acetylaspartate
(D) Creatinine
(E) None of the above

14. The decrease in NAA peak on MR spectroscopy in multiple sclerosis is a marker of

(A) axonal regeneration
(B) axonal loss
(C) demyelination

(D) astrocyte activity

(E) oligodendrocyte activity

15. Which of the following is true about neuro-physiologic tests in multiple sclerosis?

(A) EEG studies are abnormal in less than 10% of patients with multiple sclerosis.

(B) In case of cognitive deficit, EEG may show increased β activity in the frontal lobe.

(C) P 300 event related potential latency correlates with the degree of white matter disease.

(D) Evoked potentials are very sensitive in detecting the spatial distribution of multiple sclerosis lesions.

(E) The evaluation of middle latency auditory evoked potential does not affect the sensitivity of brain stem auditory evoked potential.

16. All of the following are associated with unfavorable prognosis in multiple sclerosis EXCEPT

(A) male sex

(B) younger age of onset

(C) motor or cerebellar signs at onset

(D) early disability

(E) incomplete remission after the first attack

17. All of the following drugs may be used in the treatment of spasticity in multiple sclerosis EXCEPT

(A) paroxetine

(B) baclofen

(C) clonidine

(D) cyproheptadine

(E) dantrolene

18. Which of the following antispasticty medications acts as an α2 sympathetic agonist with effects on polysynaptic reflexes?

(A) Tizanidine

(B) Dantrolene

(C) Baclofen

(D) Cyproheptadine

(E) Phenol

19. All of the following drugs are used for improving fatigue in multiple sclerosis patients EXCEPT

(A) carbamazepine

(B) pemoline

(C) amantadine

(D) modafinil

(E) 4-aminopyridine

20. Which of the following myelin sheath proteins is found in the central nervous system as well as in the peripheral nervous system?

(A) Protein zero (P0)

(B) Peripheral myelin protein 22 (Pmp 22)

(C) Myelin basic protein

(D) Proteolipid protein

(E) Oligodendrocyte specific protein

21. Which of the following cytokines is NOT produced by Th2 lymphocytes?

(A) Interleukin-4

(B) Interleukin-5

(C) Interferon γ

(D) Interleukin-10

(E) Interleukin-13

22. Upregulation of interleukin-4 is most likely seen in which phase of experimental autoimmune encephalitis?

(A) Induction

(B) Demyelination

(C) Relapse

(D) Epitope spreading

(E) Remission

23. Which of the following is a proinflammatory cytokine?

(A) IL-4

(B) IL-10

(C) TNF α

(D) IFN β

(E) TGF β

24. Which of the following is the correct combination of a paraneoplastic syndrome and the antineuronal antibody associated with that syndrome?

   (A) Lambert-Eaton myasthenic syndrome
   (B) Myasthenia gravis/Anti-CV2
   (C) Limbic encephalitis/Anti-Ma2
   (D) Peripheral neuropathy/Anti-amphiphysin
   (E) Cerebellar degeneration/Anti-MAG

25. Small cell lung cancer is associated with all of the following paraneoplastic antibodies EXCEPT

   (A) anti-P/Q type VGCC antibody
   (B) anti-Hu antibody
   (C) anti-MAG antibody
   (D) antiamphiphysin antibody
   (E) anti-Ri antibody

Questions 26 through 35
Link each of the following antibodies to the appropriate neurological disorders.

   (A) Anti-P/Q type voltage-gated calcium channels
   (B) Anti-acetylcholine receptors antibody
   (C) Anti-Hu antibody
   (D) Antivoltage-gated potassium channel antibody
   (E) Anti-Yo antibody
   (F) Anti-Ri antibody
   (G) Anti-amphiphysin antibody
   (H) Anti-CV2 antibody
   (I) Anti-Ma2 antibody
   (J) Anti-MAG antibody

26. Myasthenia gravis

27. Neuromyotonia

28. Stiff-man syndrome

29. Small cell lung cancer-related encephalomyelitis

30. Thymoma related sensory neuronopathy

31. Cerebellar degeneration

32. Lambert-Eaton myasthenic syndrome

33. Testicular cancer limbic encephalitis

34. CIDP-like neuropathy

35. Opsoclonus

36. The most frequent cause of anti-Yo antibodies is

   (A) breast cancer
   (B) ovarian cancer
   (C) small cell lung cancer
   (D) bladder cancer
   (E) uterine cancer

37. Anti-Hu antibodies are seen most frequently in

   (A) small cell lung cancer
   (B) breast cancer
   (C) prostate cancer
   (D) neuroblastoma
   (E) sarcoma

38. Opsoclonus associated with ocular motility abnormalities is most commonly associated with

   (A) anti-Ma antibody
   (B) anti-Yo antibody
   (C) anti-Hu antibody
   (D) anti-Ri antibody
   (E) anti-amphiphysin antibody

39. Which of the following antineuronal antibodies is associated with testicular cancer?

   (A) Anti-Tr antibodies
   (B) Anti-acetylcholine receptors antibodies
   (C) Anti-CV2 antibodies
   (D) Amphiphysin antibodies
   (E) Anti-Ma2 antibodies

40. All of the following antineuronal antibodies may be associated with limbic encephalitis EXCEPT

   (A) anti-Hu antibodies
   (B) anti-Ma2 antibodies
   (C) anti-CV2 antibodies

(D) anti-PCA2 antibodies

(E) anti-Yo antibodies

41. A 60-year-old right-handed woman came to the emergency room because of the development of new onset of unsteady gait, dizziness, and double vision progressing over several weeks. Neurological examination showed generalized severe ataxia, more prominent in the trunk, and mild dysarthria. Ocular examination showed opsoclonus ocular flutter and abnormal visual tracking. MRI of the head was normal. Laboratory evaluation showed the presence of antineuronal antibodies. Which of the following is TRUE about the patient condition?

(A) Diffuse loss of pyramidal cells is the pathological hallmark of patient condition.

(B) Anti-Hu antibody is the most likely type of antineuronal antibody found in this patient.

(C) Small cell lung cancer is the most likely malignancy that causes the symptoms of this patient.

(D) Inflammatory infiltrate, involving the tegmentum of the pon and mesencephalon, may be seen with cerebellum degeneration.

(E) Immunosuppressive treatment does not reverse these symptoms.

42. A 50-year-old man developed progressive increase of muscle stiffness, rigidity, lumbar lordosis, and urinary incontinence. If his symptoms are caused by a paraneoplastic syndrome, which of the following is TRUE?

(A) The use of clonazepam does not improve the rigidity.

(B) Small cell lung cancer is the major cause of the syndrome.

(C) Antiamphiphysin antibodies are the major antineuronal antibodies found in the serum of the patient.

(D) Antiglutamic acid decarboxylase (GAD) is found in 70% of patients with similar paraneoplastic condition.

(E) Treatment of the primary tumor does not improve the patient's neurological symptoms.

43. In acute inflammatory demyelinating polyneuropathy, the most frequently detected antigangliosides antibody is

(A) IgG antibody against GM1

(B) antibody against GQ1b

(C) antibody antiglycolipids

(D) antibody anti-EVB

(E) antibody anti-GD1a

44. Which of the following is suggestive of the mechanism of action of intravenous immunoglobulins in the treatment of demyelinating polyneuropathy?

(A) Down regulation of Th2 cytokine production

(B) T cell activation

(C) Complement activation

(D) Immunoglobulin Fab receptor blockade

(E) Stimulation of immunoglobulin production

Questions 45 through 50
Link the following.

(A) Inclusion body myositis

(B) Polymyositis

(C) Dermatomyositis

45. It is the most common inflammatory myopathy after the age of 50 years.

46. Asymmetric muscle involvement.

47. It is associated with the diagnosis of malignancy in 45% of cases.

48. It affects men 3 times more than women.

49. Irregular rimmed vacuoles are present in up to 70% of muscle fibers.

50. Capillary changes represent early and prominent findings on histological examination.

51. Which of the following syndromes has the LEAST likely chance of having a paraneoplastic origin?

    (A) Stiff-man syndrome
    (B) Cerebellar degeneration
    (C) Limbic encephalitis
    (D) Motor neuron disease
    (E) Brain stem encephalitis

52. MRI of the brain is useful in which of the following paraneoplastic syndromes?

    (A) Subacute sensory neuronopathy
    (B) Limbic encephalitis
    (C) Lambert-Eaton myasthenic syndrome
    (D) Stiff-man syndrome
    (E) Brain stem encephalitis

Questions 53 through 59
Link the following.

    (A) Multiple sclerosis
    (B) Postinfectious encephalomyelitis
    (C) Both
    (D) Neither

53. It is commonly monophasic

54. Equal ratio gender incidence

55. Seizure is seen in 50% of cases

56. Optic neuritis

57. Level of consciousness is preserved

58. Periventricular lesions are frequently seen on head MRI

59. CSF examination may show increased number of cells

60. All of the following factors may increase the risk of developing multiple sclerosis after isolated transverse myelitis EXCEPT

    (A) complete transverse myelitis
    (B) symmetric sensory and motor deficit on neurological examination
    (C) abnormal CSF examination
    (D) limited nonconfluent intramedullary lesions on brain MRI
    (E) abnormal multimodality evoked potentials

Answers and Explanations

1. **(B)** In relapsing-remitting multiple sclerosis, the type of multiple sclerosis present in 80% of patients, symptoms and signs typically progress over a period of several days, stabilize, and then often improve spontaneously, or in response to corticosteroids, within weeks. Relapsing-remitting multiple sclerosis typically begins in the second or third decade of life and has a female predominance of approximately 2 to 1. The tendency for corticosteroids to speed recovery from relapses often diminishes with time. Persistent signs of central nervous system dysfunction may develop after a relapse, and the disease may progress between relapses. Twenty percent of affected patients have primary progressive multiple sclerosis, which is characterized by a gradually progressive clinical course and a similar incidence among men and women. Relapsing-remitting multiple sclerosis typically starts with sensory disturbances, unilateral optic neuritis, diplopia (internuclear ophthalmoplegia), Lhermitte's sign, limb weakness, clumsiness, gait ataxia, and neurogenic bladder and bowel symptoms. Many patients describe fatigue that worsens in the afternoon and is accompanied by physiologic increases in body temperature. Prominent cortical signs (aphasia, apraxia, recurrent seizures, visual-field loss, and early dementia) and extrapyramidal phenomena only (chorea and rigidity) rarely dominate the clinical picture.

Patients who have primary progressive multiple sclerosis often present with a slowly evolving upper-motor-neuron syndrome of the legs. Typically, this variant worsens gradually, and quadriparesis, cognitive decline, visual loss, brain stem and cerebellar syndromes, bowel, bladder, and sexual dysfunction may develop. The diagnosis is based on established clinical and, when necessary, laboratory criteria. Advances in cerebrospinal fluid analysis and MRI, in particular, have simplified the diagnostic process. The relapsing forms are considered clinically definite when neurological dysfunction becomes disseminated in space and time. Studies of the natural history of the disease have provided important prognostic information. Ten percent of patients do well for more than 20 years and are thus considered to have benign multiple sclerosis. Approximately 70% will have secondary progression. Frequent relapses in the first 2 years, progressive course from the onset, male sex, early permanent motor or cerebellar findings, and presence of oligoclonal bands in the cerebrospinal fluid are associated with the more severe course of the disease. Women and patients with predominantly sensory symptoms and optic neuritis have a more favorable prognosis. *(Noseworthy et al., 938–952)*

2. **(C)** Evidence that genetic factors have a substantial effect on susceptibility to multiple sclerosis is unequivocal. The concordance rate of 31% among monozygotic twins is approximately 6 times the rate among dizygotic twins (5%). The absolute risk of the disease in a first-degree relative of a patient with multiple sclerosis is less than 5%; however, the risk in such relatives is 20 to 40 times the risk in the general population. HLA-DR2 allele substantially increases the risk of multiple sclerosis. The magnitude of the relative risk depends on the frequency of the HLA-DR2 allele in the general population. The mode of transmission of genetic susceptibility to multiple sclerosis is complex.

Most cases are sporadic, despite the clear excess risk among the relatives of patients. Investigators have used the usual genetic approaches to identify genes associated with an increased risk of multiple sclerosis. HLA-DR and DQ polymorphisms are not associated with the course and severity of multiple sclerosis despite their substantial contribution to disease susceptibility. *(Noseworthy et al., 938–952)*

3. **(A)** The pathological hallmark of chronic multiple sclerosis is the demyelinated plaque, which consists of a well-demarcated hypocellular area characterized by the loss of myelin, relative preservation of axons, and formation of astrocytic scars. Lesions have a predilection for the optic nerves, periventricular white matter, brain stem, cerebellum, and spinal cord white matter; and they often surround one or several medium-sized vessels. Although the lesions are usually round or oval, they often have finger-like extensions along the path of small- or medium-sized blood vessels (Dawson's fingers). Inflammatory cells are typically perivascular in location, but they may diffusely infiltrate the parenchyma. The composition of the inflammatory infiltrate varies, depending on the stage of demyelination. In general, it is composed of lymphocytes and macrophages; the latter predominate in active lesions. *(Noseworthy et al., 938–952)*

4. **(D)** Interferon beta-1a and glatiramer acetate reduce the frequency of relapses of multiple sclerosis. Interferon beta-1a may delay the progression of disability in patients with minor disability who have a relapsing form of multiple sclerosis. The specific mechanisms of action of these agents in multiple sclerosis are incompletely understood. The interferons reduce the proliferation of T cells and the production of tumor necrosis factor α, decrease antigen presentation, alter cytokine production to favor ones governed by type 2 helper T (Th2) cells, increase the secretion of interleukin-10, and reduce the passage of immune cells across the blood–brain barrier by means of their effects on adhesion molecules, chemokines, and proteases. Glatiramer acetate may promote the proliferation of Th2 cytokines, compete with myelin

basic protein for presentation on MHC class II molecules, alter the function of macrophages, and induce antigen-specific suppressor T cells. *(Noseworthy et al., 938–952)*

5. **(B)** Multiple sclerosis plaques may be characterized as active or inactive. The presence in macrophages of activation markers and specific myelin degradation products is suggestive of active plaque. Macrophages are numerous in active lesions, which are hypercellular and contain patchy infiltrates of autoreactive T cells and antigen-nonspecific monocytes. Macrophages and lymphocytes form prominent perivascular cuffs and invade the parenchyma, whereas plasma cells and B cells tend to concentrate in the perivascular region only. Most lymphocytes within plaques are T cells, including both CD4+ (helper) and CD8+ (cytotoxic) cells. The CD4+ cells can be functionally divided into Th1 (which secrete proinflammatory cytokines, such as tumor necrosis factor-α and γ-interferon) or Th2 (which secrete antiinflammatory cytokines such as interleukins [IL]-4,-5,-6).

Chronic plaques display well-demarcated areas of hypocellularity with myelin pallor or loss. There are varying degrees of axonal loss, usually most obvious in the center of the lesion. There is typically a persistent but minor inflammatory response, with only a few scattered perivascular lymphocytes present, although plasma cells may occasionally be prominent. Shadow plaques are circumscribed regions where axons maintain uniformly thin myelin sheaths. They may occur within acute plaques or at the edge of chronic ones. These plaques represent areas of remyelination and are macroscopic evidence that the CNS white matter possesses the means for self-repair. Shadow plaques are seen in conjunction with actively demyelinating lesions that retain viable oligodendrocytes in the plaque center. *(Wingerchuk et al., 263–281)*

6. **(A)** An intact blood–brain barrier allows limited passage of T lymphocytes that may not have antigen specificity. This may be initiated by the interaction of adhesion molecules expressed on the surface of lymphocytes with complementary integrins present on the endothelium,

resulting in T cell rolling and adherence to the luminal surface. Examples of such molecules include vascular cell adhesion molecule (VCAM) and intercellular adhesion molecule (ICAM). After crossing the blood–brain barrier, activated T cells invade the extracellular matrix, aided by their secretion of matrix metalloproteinases, which degrade myelin components as well as type IV collagen matrix and regulate cytokine production. *(Wingerchuk et al., 263–281)*

7. **(A)** Autoreactive T cells respond to putative multiple sclerosis autoantigens presented by antigenpresenting cells (APC) through formation of a trimolecular complex involving perivascular monocytes, microglia and macrophages, parenc-hymal lymphocytes, and possibly astrocytes. These cells express MHC molecules. There are two principal types of MHC molecules: class I (includes HLA-A, -B, and -C) and class II (includes HLA-DR, -DP, and -DQ). These molecules bind peptide antigens as part of the processing they require for presentation to different T lymphocytes. Lymphocytes of the CD4+ type recognize antigens in conjunction with MHC class II molecules; whereas, CD8+ lymphocytes recognize antigens in the context of MHC class I molecules. The trimolecular complex is completed by interaction with the T cell receptor.

Multiple sclerosis seems primarily to be a disease involving immune responses to antigens presented by class II molecules, although class I mechanisms are receiving increased attention. The interaction between a CD4+ T lymphocyte and an APC results in antigen-specific signaling; however, T cell activation requires the presence of co-stimulatory molecules. Co-stimulatory molecules CD28 and CTLA-4 are present on the T cell surface. These molecules interact with their ligands B7-1 and B7-2 to promote activation; when absent, the T cell-APC interaction results in T cell apoptosis and limitation of the immune response. When the co-stimulatory molecules and their respective ligands are present, intracellular signaling pathways involving phosphorylation-dependent enzymes and second messenger systems activate secretory and proliferative mechanisms within the T lymphocyte. *(Wingerchuk et al., 263–281)*

8. **(B)** Dysregulation of the immune system may contribute to the initiation or propagation of a pathological state in multiple sclerosis (MS) by autoreactive T cells. The causative autoantigen(s) in MS is still not known; however, the leading candidates are myelin protein constituents. The role of other myelin components is less well studied. Molecular mimicry has been hypothesized to explain immunological injury in autoimmune diseases. Under this schema, antigens present in or originating from an exogenous pathogen activate T cells. These cells then induce CNS demyelination by recognizing cross-reactive myelin antigens. This explanation has been used to implicate Herpes virus in MS pathogenesis, although a latent viral infection, rather than mimicry, could also potentially result in demyelination and oligodendroglial loss. The T cell receptor normally maintains an extremely high level of cross-reactivity, probably to balance the requirement to recognize nonself antigens and to reduce the possibility of loss of self-tolerance. The concept of molecular mimicry remains speculative. *(Wingerchuk et al., 263–281)*

9. **(A)** It has long been recognized that axons are relatively, but not absolutely, spared in multiple sclerosis (MS), especially early in the disease. Recent pathological and noninvasive radiological studies have focused attention on how early in the disease axons may be injured or lost, the possible contribution of axonal injury to clinical disability, and the development of progressive MS. Not surprisingly, axonal density is reduced in chronic plaques. Whereas estimates of axonal number and density are challenged by the variable presence of edema, myelin loss, atrophy, and inflammatory cell infiltrates, between 50% and 80% of axons may be lost in chronically demyelinated cervical spinal cord plaques. The accumulation of β-amyloid precursor protein identifies damaged axons in actively demyelinating MS lesions. Acute, active MS plaques may also demonstrate axonal transection, swelling, formation of terminal spheroids, and regenerative sprouting.

Others have confirmed early axonal loss in the early inflammatory phases of the disease, even in the absence of demonstrable primary demyelination. Axonal loss is irreversible and probably underlies the worsening neurological deficits that accrue in the primary and secondary progressive forms of the disease; clinical progression correlates with brain atrophy in both of these forms of MS. The mechanisms of axonal injury are largely unknown. In particular, it is not clear whether inflammatory effects may damage axons directly or whether they operate primarily through a pathway that includes demyelination. Recently, it was found that acute axonal injury correlates with the number of macrophages and CD8+ T lymphocytes within plaques but not with TNF-α or nitric oxide synthase expression. This suggests that axonal injury is not solely due to demyelination. Glutamate-driven excitotoxic mechanisms may be operative as well. *(Wingerchuk et al., 263–281)*

10. **(A)** Histopathologic studies of multiple sclerosis (MS) brains have demonstrated axonal injury in lesions undergoing inflammatory demyelination. Axonal ovoids (which are characteristic of newly transected axons) and extensive accumulation of the amyloid precursor protein (APP) have been reported in active lesions and at the border of chronic active lesions. APP is detected immunohistochemically only in axons with impaired axonal transport. This result indicates not only axonal dysfunction within inflammatory MS lesions, but also suggests that many of the axons are transected. Importantly, these changes are observed in patients with a short duration of disease. A morphological investigation quantified axonal ovoids in MS brains with disease durations from 2 weeks to 27 years. The results of the study not only confirm that axonal transection is abundant during the early stages of the disease, but also demonstrate that the density of transected axons correlates with inflammatory activity in the lesions. Because APP accumulation correlated with number of macrophages and CD8+ T lymphocytes, but not with expression of putative mediators of demyelination such as tumor necrosis factor-α and inducible nitric oxide synthase, it is suggested that axonal damage in MS lesions might not be directly proportional to demyelinating activity. *(Bjartmar and Trapp, 271–278; Trapp et al., 278–285)*

11. **(D)** Four mechanisms may contribute to clinical remission in multiple sclerosis: resolution of the inflammation, redistribution of axolemmal sodium channels, remyelination, and compensatory adaptation of the CNS. *(Bjartmar and Trapp, 271–278)*

12. **(E)** The correlation between clinical disability and atrophy, as revealed by MRI of the cerebellum, spinal cord, and cerebrum, in multiple sclerosis (MS) has been interpreted as a reflection of axonal loss. In secondary progressive multiple sclerosis (SP-MS), cervical spinal cord atrophy averages 25% to 30%. In a group of RR-MS patients with mild-to-moderate disability followed over 2 years, brain atrophy increased yearly. Axonal loss is a conceivable contributor to atrophy in MS, although demyelination and reduced axon diameter may also decrease tissue volume. Axonal pathology and loss is not restricted to MS lesions, as all axons will undergo Wallerian degeneration distal to the site of axonal transection of the MS lesion.

Axonal loss in normal-appearing white matter (NAWM) has been quantified in a number of recent autopsy studies. Axonal density was reported to be reduced by 19% to 42% in the lateral corticospinal tract of MS patients with lower limb weakness. Axonal loss was investigated in NAWM from cervical spinal cords of patients with SP-MS. The average reduction in axonal density in these samples was as much as 57%. As NAWM constitutes the greatest proportion of white matter in MS patients and as levels of the neuron-specific marker N-acetyl aspartate (NAA) in NAWM show a strong correlation with disability, the possibility has been raised that total white matter axonal status may be a more precise determinant of disease progression than the presence and characteristics of individual lesions. *(Bjartmar and Trapp, 271–278)*

13. **(C)** The clinical importance of axonal degeneration in MS suggests that neuronal markers could be useful for noninvasive monitoring of disease progression and efficiency of therapy in these patients. In this respect, measurement of NAA by proton magnetic resonance spectroscopy

(MRS) is a promising tool. NAA appears relatively specific for neurons and neuronal processes in vivo, although expression by oligodendrocyte progenitors and oligodendrocytes in vitro has been reported. Reduced levels of NAA, as determined by MRS, have been demonstrated in a number of neurodegenerative disorders, including MS. At acute stages of MS, reduced NAA occurs primarily in lesions, is partly reversible, and correlates with reversible functional impairment. Over time, NAA appears to decrease irreversibly in normal-appearing white matter (NAWM), indicating that axonal loss or damage occurs outside MS lesions. Reduced white matter NAA correlates with increased disability over time.

These results demonstrate a side-to-side correlation between NAA levels, motor impairment, and conduction times, conforming with the view that axonal pathology in NAWM is a likely determinant of disease progression in MS. In theory, reduced NAA in MS tissue could reflect multiple mechanisms, including reversible neuronal/axonal damage due to inflammatory demyelination, altered neuronal metabolism related to activity, axonal atrophy, or axonal loss. In order to differentiate between these possibilities, NAA is measured by high-performance liquid chromatography at autopsy in MS spinal cord white matter, and correlated with axonal loss as determined by immunohistochemistry. NAA is significantly reduced in chronic inactive MS lesions compared with MS nonlesion and control white matter, and the reduction correlates with total axonal volume and axonal density. These results demonstrate that reduced NAA levels in inactive lesions correspond to substantial axonal loss, and support axonal loss as a major cause of decreased white matter NAA in secondary progressive MS. *(Bjartmar and Trapp, 271–278)*

14. **(B)** The measurement of N-acetyl aspartate (NAA) by proton MR spectroscopy, as a neuronal marker, is a valuable tool for assessing the progression of multiple sclerosis (MS). Reduced NAA occurs in MS lesions and becomes irreversible as the disease progresses. In theory, reduced NAA in MS tissue could reflect multiple mechanisms, including reversible neuronal/axonal damage due to inflammatory demyelination, altered neuronal metabolism related to activity, axonal atrophy, or axonal loss. In order to differentiate between these possibilities, Bjartmar et al. studied the NAA levels, by high-performance liquid chromatography at autopsy, in MS spinal cord white matter. They found a correlation between the NAA level and the axonal loss as determined by immunohistochemistry. NAA was significantly reduced in chronic inactive MS lesions, compared with MS white matter without lesion and control white matter. The reduction in NAA concentration was found to correlate with total axonal volume and axonal density. These results demonstrate that reduced NAA levels in inactive lesions correspond to substantial axonal loss. *(Bjartmar and Trapp, 271–278)*

15. **(C)** In the early phases of MS, evoked potentials (EP) are used to detect subclinical involvement of the sensory and motor pathways or to objectify vague symptoms. Previous studies indicated that in isolated syndromes, approximately one-third of patients have subclinical involvement of sensory pathways revealed by EP, mostly by visual-evoked potentials (VEP) and somatosensory-evoked potentials (SEP). In a study of 112 patients with isolated optic neuritis, 34.1% of patients had abnormal extravisual EP; however, the contribution of neurophysiological techniques in demonstrating spatial dissemination of the lesions was quite poor: only 4% of patients with abnormal extravisual EP had normal brain MRI.

The major limiting factor on the usefulness of EP in detecting subclinical involvement is that the presence of a lesion is revealed only if it affects pathways explored by neurophysiological investigations. Moreover, a significant proportion of the fibers must be affected to produce recordable modifications of evoked responses. The evaluation of middle latency auditory-evoked potentials, complemented with brain stem auditory-evoked potentials (BAEP), in a group of 30 clinically definite MS patients, increased the sensitivity of the test from 60% to

83%, suggesting that the validation of middle latency auditory-evoked potentials could establish criteria for a more comprehensive evaluation of the auditory system.

The EEG, which is the expression of multiple neuronal network interactions affected by white matter damage, may be used as an indicator of the global status of such interactions. Spectral analysis of the EEG revealed abnormalities in 40% to 79% of MS patients; the main changes were an increase of slow frequencies and decrease of the alpha band, which is related to cognitive dysfunctions. Event-related potentials (ERP) are brain waves related to stimulus processing. P300, the most widely studied ERP, is a positive wave recorded over the scalp when subjects discriminate stimuli differing in some physical dimension. It is thought to represent a closure of the evaluation process stimulus, and its latency has been proposed as an indicator of information processing speed. This process is electively affected in MS, and P300 latency is increased in MS patients. The increase in P300 latency is correlated with cognitive impairment and with the degree of white matter involvement. *(Leocani and Comi, 255–261)*

16. **(B)** Factors associated with unfavorable prognosis in multiple sclerosis include:

- Male sex
- Older age at onset
- Motor or cerebellar signs at onset
- Short interval between initial and second attack
- High relapse rate in early years
- Incomplete remission after first relapses
- Early disability
- High lesion load detected by early magnetic resonance imaging of the brain *(Polman and Uitdehaag, 490–494)*

17. **(A)** Approximately 55% of patients with multiple sclerosis have detectable spasticity. Spasticity is defined as increased resistance to passive range of motion of the limb, which can be associated with exaggerated withdrawal to noxious stimuli, spasms, clonus, and hyperreflexia. Spasticity can interfere with volitional movement, can cause pain, and can disrupt sleep or activities of daily living. The first line of treatment of spasticity involves simple physical measures including stretching, use of reciprocal motion exercises, such as exercycling, and, for some patients, passive standing in a standing frame.

When these measures fail, orally administered pharmacologic agents may be necessary and, in most cases, are sufficient to manage the negative manifestations of increased muscle tone. The classically used medications include baclofen, benzodiazepines, and dantrolene sodium. The first two drugs can cause drowsiness, and all three can increase fatigue and weakness. Careful dose titration is therefore critical. The dose of baclofen, a gamma-aminobutyric acid agonist, should be titrated slowly because patients with multiple sclerosis may be more sensitive than other patients to the side effects of drowsiness and weakness. If the response to baclofen is insufficient or if this drug causes intolerable side effects, diazepam or dantrolene may be substituted or added. For patients with fatigue or drowsiness from baclofen, diazepam may exacerbate these symptoms.

Use of diazepam should be avoided in those patients with a tendency toward depression or a history of substance abuse. Dantrolene can then be used but may cause weakness because of its direct muscle effect of preventing excitation-contraction coupling. If use of dantrolene is continued, liver function should be monitored at least every 3 months; liver toxicity can occur in rare instances. If the usual antispasticity medications fail or are contraindicated, various other medications can be tried. Clonidine hydrochloride or cyproheptadine hydrochloride (Periactin), serotonin, acetylcholine, and histamine antagonist, have been reported to reduce MS-related spasticity. Selective botulinum toxin injections are also used. *(Stolp-Smith et al., pp. 1184–1196)*

18. **(A)** Tizanidine is a centrally acting α2-sympathetic agonist pharmacologically similar to clonidine, with effects on polysynaptic reflex arcs. Tizanidine has been shown to reduce spasticity in several placebo-controlled clinical trials and has had efficacy similar to baclofen. Muscle weakness occurs less frequently with tizanidine

than with baclofen. The most common side effects are drowsiness, dry mouth, and orthostatic hypotension. Liver function abnormalities rarely occur. *(Stolp-Smith et al., 1184–1196)*

19. **(A)** Fatigue is a common problem for patients with multiple sclerosis (MS). Pharmacological therapy may be helpful when other medical problems that may cause fatigue, such as anemia or hypothyroidism, are excluded. Amantadine hydrochloride is the most widely used medication for MS-related fatigue. The mechanism of action in multiple sclerosis is unknown, but the drug has central dopaminergic activity that may be relevant. Pemoline, also used for MS-related fatigue, has had a response rate of approximately 50% in some studies.

In a prospective open label study, modafanil was found to significantly improve fatigue and sleepiness in patients with MS. Unlike the higher dose regimen required in narcolepsy, a low-dose regimen of modafinil was found to be effective and well tolerated by MS patients. Potassium channel blocking agents, such as 4-aminopyridine and 3,4-diaminopyridine, may also prove to be effective for MS-related fatigue. With use of these agents, the major toxic effect is the occasional occurrence of generalized tonic-clonic seizures at high serum levels of these drugs. Patients may experience increased fatigue and a decline in neurologic function due to warm environments (Uhthoff's phenomenon). Thus, remaining in a cool environment can enhance function. *(Stolp-Smith et al., 1184–1196; Zifko et al., 983–987)*

20. **(C)** The central nervous system and the peripheral nervous system myelin sheaths contain distinct sets of proteins, but myelin basic protein is found in the myelin sheath of both of them. In the peripheral nervous system, the compact myelin contains protein 0 (P0), peripheral myelin protein (PMP22), and myelin basic protein (MBP); whereas in the noncompact, myelin contains E-cadherin, myelin-associated glycoprotein (MAG), and connexin 32 (Cx32). In the central nervous system, myelin contains proteolipid protein (PLP), oligodendrocyte specific protein (OSP), myelin-oligodendrocyte basic protein, and myelin basic protein. *(Arroyo and Scherer, pp. 1–18)*

21. **(C)** As CD4+ lymphocyte responses develop in response to immune stimulation, T cell populations become divided toward the production of Th1 or inflammatory cytokines, versus Th2 or regulatory cytokines. The paradigmatic Th1 cytokine is interferon γ, interleukin-4 being the defining Th2 cytokine. IL-12 is implicated in driving responses toward Th1 cytokine patterns: IFN γ, IL-2, GM-CSF, IL-12 itself, and the B cells and macrophage cytokines. IL-4 implicated in Th2 cytokine patterns switch: IL-3, IL-5, IL-10, and IL-13. *(Ransohoff et al., 13–14)*

22. **(E)** Experimental autoimmune encephalitis may pursue a relapsing remitting course. The remission may be caused by natural termination of T cell response through apoptosis or action of regulatory cytokines, including up regulation of Th2 cytokines such as interleukin-4. *(Ransohoff et al., 24)*

23. **(C)** Proinflammatory cytokines include IL-1α,β, IL-2, IL-3, IL-6 (Which has pro and anti-inflammatory proprieties), IL-12, TNF-α, IFNγ, LTα, G-CSF, and GM-CSF. Anti-inflammatory cytokines include IL-4, IL-10, IL-13, IFN-β, and TGF-β. *(Ransohoff et al., 37)*

24. **(C)** A new family of paraneoplastic antigens (the Ma proteins) has recently been identified. There are at least 5 Ma proteins, the best characterized being Ma1 and Ma2. The expression of these proteins is highly restricted to neurons and spermatogenic cells of the testis. The anti-Ta (anti-Ma2) antibodies are present in the serum and spinal fluid of patients with paraneoplastic limbic and brain stem encephalitis associated with testicular cancer. These antibodies recognize epitopes, mainly contained in Ma2 (40-kd neuronal protein). Limbic encephalitis is frequently associated with small cell lung cancer (SCLC) and is characterized clinically by subacute confusion, amnesia, and psychiatric symptoms. Magnetic resonance imaging usually reveals increased signal in the medial temporal lobes on T2-weighted images and cerebrospinal fluid may show a mild lymphocytic pleocytosis. Limbic encephalitis can occur as an isolated syndrome or as part of a multifocal disorder associated with cerebellar, brain stem, spinal cord,

and dorsal root ganglion involvement. The largest study of paraneoplastic limbic encephalitis revealed that anti-Hu antibodies only occurred in 50% of the patients who had an associated SCLC. The antibody positive patients are more likely to have involvement of other areas of the nervous system and to die from the neurological disorder rather than progression of the cancer. (*Dalmau and Posner, pp. 405–408; Rees, pp. 633–637*)

25. **(C)** Small cell lung carcinoma is by far the tumor most commonly associated with paraneoplastic encephalomyelitis (PEM). Nearly all patients display signs and symptoms of multifocal involvement of the central nervous system (CNS) and dorsal root ganglia. The most common clinical manifestation of PEM is a disabling subacute sensory neuronopathy (SSN). A high percentage of patients with PEM/SSN have polyclonal IgG anti-Hu antibodies. These antibodies produce diffuse staining of the nuclei and to a lesser degree cytoplasm of all neurons in human brain, spinal cord, dorsal root ganglia, and autonomic ganglia.

Ninety percent of patients with paraneoplastic cerebellar degeneration (PCD) have small cell lung carcinoma, Hodgkin's lymphoma, or carcinomas of the breast, ovary, or female genital tract. Patients typically have a subacute onset and progression of pancerebellar dysfunction. In addition to the cerebellar deficits, many patients show symptoms or signs of multifocal PEM, including lethargy, cognitive deterioration, bulbar palsy, and limb weakness.

The most prevalent autoantibodies in patients with PCD are high-titer and polyclonal IgG anti-Purkinje cell antibodies (also called anti-Yo antibodies). Anti-Ri antibodies are seen in paraneoplastic opsoclonus. Small cell lung cancer and breast carcinoma together account for approximately 70% of adults with paraneoplastic opsoclonus. Anti-amphiphysin antibodies have been detected in the serum and CSF of a few patients with small cell lung cancer and PEM mainly manifesting as SSN without rigidity.

Lambert-Eaton myasthenic syndrome (LEMS) occurs in around 2 of every 1,000 cancer patients and is characterized by limb weakness, usually of the lower limbs, and is commonly associated with autonomic dysfunction. The deep tendon reflexes are reduced but show facilitation after exercise. Sixty percent of all cases are associated with underlying malignancy and in 40% the LEMS occurs as an autoimmune condition in its own right. Nonparaneoplastic cases of LEMS occur more commonly in middle-aged women. When cancer is identified, it is usually small cell lung cancer, although cancer of the prostate or cervix has been described. Antibodies against- voltage gated calcium channels are present in most patients. Anti-MAG (myelin-associated glycoprotein) antibodies have been seen in Waldenström's macroglobulinemia and are associated with peripheral neuropathy. Immunoglobulin M antibodies seem to have a higher pathogenicity for polyneuropathy than immunoglobulin G or immunoglobulin A antibodies. (*Dropcho, 246–261*)

26. **(B)**

27. **(D)**

28. **(G)**

29. **(C)**

30. **(H)**

31. **(E)**

32. **(A)**

33. **(I)**

34. **(J)**

35. **(F)**

Explanations 26 through 35

Lambert-Eaton myasthenic syndrome is seen in small lung cell cancer and is associated with the synthesis of anti-P/Q type voltage-gated calcium channel antibodies, whereas myasthenia gravis syndrome is seen in thymoma and is associated with the production of antiacetylcholine receptor antibodies. Antivoltage-gated potassium channel antibodies are associated with neuromyotonia and are seen in thymoma or small cell lung cancer. Anti-Hu antibodies may cause encepha-lomyelitis or sensory neuronopathy and are associated with small cell lung cancer, whereas anti-Yo antibodies may cause cerebellar degeneration and are associated with breast or ovarian cancers. Anti-Ri antibodies are seen in breast, small cell lung, and bladder cancers and are associated with opsoclonus, myoclonus, and ataxia. Anti-amphiphysin antibodies are seen in breast or small cell lung cancers and are associated with stiff-man syndrome or encepha-lomyelitis. Anti-CV2 is seen in thymoma or small cell lung cancers causing sensory neuronopathy or encephalomyelitis. Limbic or brain stem encephalitis may be seen with testicular cancer and are associated with the synthesis of anti-Ma2 antibodies. Anti-Tr antibodies are seen in Hodgkin's lymphoma, causing cerebellar degeneration, whereas anti-MAG antibodies are seen in Waldenström's macroglobulinemia causing symmetric sensory or sensory motor neuropathy that may be progressive and may simulate chronic inflammatory demyelinating polyneuropathy. *(Ransohoff et al., 94–104; Ropper and Gorson, 1601–1605)*

36. **(B)** Anti-Yo antibodies are markers of paraneoplastic cerebellar degeneration. The associated tumors include ovarian cancer (60%) and other gynecologic tumors (5%), breast cancer (30%), and other cancers (5% lung and bladder). Low titers of anti-Yo antibodies may also be detected in less than 5% of patients with ovarian cancer without neurological symptoms. The target antigen of the anti-Yo antibodies are several 34- and 62-KD protein expressed predominantly in the cytoplasm of Purkinje cells of the cerebellum, and to a lesser degree in neurons of the molecular layer and large neurons in the brain stem. *(Ransohoff et al., 102)*

37. **(A)** The anti-Hu antibodies are markers of paraneoplastic encephalomyelitis, sensory neuronopathy, and autonomic dysfunction. The detection of these antibodies in patients with focal symptoms, such as limbic encephalopathy or cerebellar dysfunction, indicates that although these areas are the main targets of the immune response, the neuropathologic substrate is a more diffuse encephalomyelitis. Since in 80% of patients with anti-Hu associated syndrome the causal tumor is a small cell lung cancer, a chest CT scan is mandatory for patients with anti-Hu antibodies and a yet undiagnosed cancer. Rarely, other tumors have been identified to be associated with anti-Hu antibodies, including breast cancer, prostate cancer, neuroblastoma, and small cell cancer of unknown origin. The target antigens of the anti-Hu antibodies are a family of neuronal specific RNA-binding proteins expressed predominantly in the nuclei of neurons of the central and peripheral nervous system. *(Ransohoff et al., 102)*

38. **(D)** Anti-Ri antibodies are associated with paraneoplastic cerebellar and brain stem encephalopathy characterized by opsoclonus and other abnormalities of ocular motility. The most commonly associated tumor is breast cancer. The Anti-Ri antibodies react with neuronal proteins located in the nuclei of neurons in the central nervous system but not in the peripheral nervous system. *(Ransohoff et al., 103)*

39. **(E)** Anti-Ma and anti-Ma2 antibodies are markers of paraneoplastic syndromes involving the limbic region, brain stem, and cerebellum. The target antigens are a family of brain-cancer-testicular proteins that include Ma1, Ma2, and several other uncharacterized members. These proteins are highly homologous to each other and are encoded by different genes. Ma1 is expressed in brain and testis, while Ma2 is only expressed in the brain. Antibodies that react with both Ma1 and Ma2 are called anti-Ma. Anti-Ma antibodies are associated predominantly with brain stem and cerebellar dysfunction, and several types of cancer, including lung, breast, colon, and parotid glands. Antibodies that react only with Ma2 are called anti-Ma2 or anti-Ta. The detection of anti-Ma2 antibodies is usually associated with limbic and brain stem encephalitis; 80% of these patients have germ cell tumors and 20% have other tumors including lung and breast cancers. Anti-CV2 antibodies are associated with paraneoplastic cerebellar degeneration and encephalomyelitis. The causal tumors are small cell lung cancer and

thymoma. The target antigen of anti CV2 antibodies is a set of 62- to 66-Kd proteins expressed in neurons and oligodendrocytes. The detection of anti-amphiphysin in patients with neurological symptoms of unknown cause is suggestive of paraneoplastic origin. Anti-amphiphysin antibodies may be seen in breast cancer and small cell lung cancer. Amphiphysin is a major antigen associated with paraneoplastic stiff-man syndrome, although some patients develop paraneoplastic encephalomyelitis and sensory neuronopathy. Anti-Tr antibodies are associated with paraneoplastic cerebellar degeneration and Hodgkin's lymphoma. In adult brain, the Tr antigen is expressed predominantly in the Purkinje cell cytoplasm and dendrites. Anti-acetylcholine receptors antibodies are associated with thymoma. *(Ransohoff et al., 103)*

40. **(E)** Paraneoplastic-limbic encephalitis is a disorder characterized by the subacute development of depression, irritability, seizures, and short-term memory loss. Symptoms usually precede or lead to the diagnosis of the primary tumor. Typical MRI findings of paraneoplastic-limbic encephalitis include uni- or bilateral mesial temporal lobe abnormalities that are best seen on T2-weighted images.

    The tumor most frequently involved is lung cancer. Other tumors include germ-cell tumors of the testis, breast cancer, thymoma, and immature teratoma of the ovary. Antineuronal antibodies associated with limbic encephalitis include anti-Hu, anti-Ma2, anti-CV2, and anti-PCA2 antibodies. Pathological findings include perivascular and interstitial inflammatory infiltrates, neuronal loss, and microglial proliferation that predominate in the limbic system. Neurological symptoms usually develop over days or weeks, and stabilize leaving the patient with severe short-term memory loss. In contrast to other paraneoplastic diseases of the central nervous system, this disorder may improve with treatment of the tumor. *(Ransohoff et al., 107)*

41. **(D)** The patient described in this vignette has symptoms of cerebellar and mesencephalic dysfunction. The presence of antineuronal antibodies is suggestive of paraneoplastic syndrome affecting the brain stem and the cerebellum. Anti-

neuronal antibodies associated with paraneoplastic cerebellar dysfunction include anti-Ri, anti-Tr, anti-Yo, anti-Ma, anti-CV2, anti-GluR1α, and anti-PCA2 antibodies. A number of clinical-immunology correlates have been suggested for some of these antibodies.

The patient in this clinical case has distinctive clinical findings suggestive of an association with anti-Ri antibodies. Up to 75% of patients with anti-Ri antibodies have opsoclonus, ocular flutter, and dysmetria; the latter two developing when the opsoclonus subsides. Patients may also develop nystagmus and abnormal visual tracking. Ataxia predominates in the trunk and may cause severe gait difficulty and multiple falls. Treatment of the primary tumor, which is usually a breast cancer, or the use of immune suppression may result in neurologic improvement. Pathological examination may show perivascular and interstitial inflammatory infiltrates, involving the tegmentum of the pons and mesencephalon with extensive degeneration of cerebellar Purkinje cells.

Patients with paraneoplastic cerebellar degeneration and anti-Yo antibodies generally present with progressive disabling cerebellar syndrome over a few days or weeks. The most frequent cause of this syndrome is ovarian and other gynecological cancers, followed by breast cancer. Treatment of the primary tumor rarely improves the cerebellar symptoms. Cerebellar syndrome associated with anti-Hu antibodies is generally caused by a small cell lung cancer. Treatment of the tumor may improve the symptoms. Hodgkin's lymphoma may cause the production of anti-Tr antibodies leading to cerebellar degeneration in relatively young patients. Improvement of symptoms may result from treatment of the lymphoma. *(Ransohoff et al., 107–109)*

42. **(C)** The patient described in this vignette has symptoms highly suggestive of stiff-man syndrome with sphincter dysfunction. The syndrome may be idiopathic or a paraneoplastic manifestation of breast colon and Hodgkin's lymphoma. When the syndrome is not associated with a cancer, the major autoantigen is GAD and around 70% of patients develop diabetes. When the syndrome is caused by paraneoplastic

manifestation of a cancer, antiamphiphysin antibodies are often found in the serum and the cerebrospinal fluid of affected patients. The use of clonazepam or diazepam may improve the rigidity. Some authors include the improvement of rigidity with the use of diazepam as the diagnostic criteria to maintain stiff-man syndrome as the diagnosis of such rigidity. The treatment of the primary tumor, as well as the use of steroids, may cause definitive improvement of the stiff-man syndrome. *(Ransohoff et al., 113)*

43. **(A)** The improvement of symptoms of acute inflammatory demyelinating polyneuropathy (AIDP) by plasmapheresis, the presence of circulating antibodies directed against peripheral nerve antigens, and the deposition of immunoglobulins and complements in the myelinated fibers are highly suggestive of humoral factors involved in the pathogenesis of this polyneuropathy. Several circulating antibodies against myelin have been found in patients with AIDP. The anti-GM1 antibody is the most frequent antiganglioside antibody detected in serum of patients with AIDP. Some authors reported increased titers of anti-GD1a in the axonal form of AIDP. The anti-GM1β antibody has been reported in the motor form of AIDP as well as in acute motor axonal polyneuropathy. Anti-GQ1β antibodies are invariably associated with the Miller Fisher variant of AIDP. Antiglycolipide antibodies have been associated with AIDP, including antibodies against *campylobacter jejuni, mycoplasma pneumoniae, haemophilus influenzae,* cytomegalovirus, and Epstein virus. *(Ransohoff et al., 126)*

44. **(A)** The therapeutic effect of intravenous immunoglobulin on demyelinating polyneuropathy has been established. The suggested mechanisms are down regulation of Th2 cytokine production, immunoglobulin Fc receptors blockade, inhibition of T cell activation, nonspecific binding of activated complement, and anti-idiopathic suppression of autoantibodies. *(Ransohoff et al., 128)*

45. **(A)**

46. **(A)**

47. **(C)**

48. **(A)**

49. **(A)**

50. **(C)**

Explanations 45 through 50

Inclusion body myositis (IBM) is the most common inflammatory myopathy after the age of 50 years. It is characterized by an insidious onset of asymmetric weakness involving the quadriceps, volar forearm muscles, and ankle dorsiflexors. Up to 25% of patients with inclusion body myositis have an associated autoimmune disease, but there is no increased association with malignancy or lung and heart abnormalities. IBM affects men three times more than women, whereas nonparaneoplastic varieties of dermatomyositis and polymyositis affect women twice as often as men. Paraneoplastic dermatomyositis, however, is slightly more frequent in men than women. Polymyositis is associated with the diagnosis of malignancy in up to 28% of patients; dermatomyositis is associated with malignancy in up to 45% of cases. In IBM, pathological examination shows irregular rimmed vacuoles in up to 70% of muscle fibers. Eosinophilic inclusions are found in the cytoplasm and nuclei, and CD8+ T-cell endomysial infiltrate may be seen in the muscle fibers. In dermatomyositis, pathological findings are characterized by perivascular and perifascicular infiltrates, predominantly formed by B lymphocytes, macro-phages, and CD4+ T cells. Early and prominent capillary changes in dermatomyositis suggest the importance of humoral factors in the pathogenesis of the disease. *(Ransohoff et al., 135–138)*

51. **(D)** Paraneoplastic stiff-man syndrome is associated with the production of antiamphiphysin antibodies and is seen in Hodgkin's disease as well as in breast and colon cancers. Paraneoplastic-limbic encephalitis is associated with the synthesis of anti-Hu, anti-MA-2, anti-CV2, and anti-PCA2 antibodies and is seen in small cell lung cancer and germ cell tumor of testis. Brain stem encephalitis may be seen in testis cancer,

whereas cerebellar degeneration is associated with anti-Yo antibodies and is seen in breast and ovarian cancers. Motor neuron syndrome is rarely reported to be associated with malignancies. *(Ransohoff et al., 94–113)*

52. **(B)** Limbic encephalitis is the most consistent paraneoplastic disorder associated with MRI abnormalities. On T2-weighted images, abnormal signals may be seen in the mesiotemporal lobes, unilaterally or bilaterally. On T1 sequences, the temporal limbic regions may be hypo-intense and atrophic and may sometimes enhance with contrast injection. *(Ransohoff et al., 106–107)*

53. **(B)**

54. **(B)**

55. **(B)**

56. **(C)**

57. **(A)**

58. **(A)**

59. **(C)**

Explanations 53 through 59

Postinfectious encephalomyelitis is an acute disseminated encephalomyelitis that is a monophasic polyregional syndrome, temporally related to an infection or vaccination and is most common in children. Compared to multiple sclerosis, patients with postinfectious encephalomyelitis have a monophasic course and 70% of them reported a precipitating event in the weeks preceding the acute phase, whereas in multiple sclerosis the time course of the disease is multiphasic and preceding events are uncommon. Multiple sclerosis most commonly affects young adults with female predominance, whereas postinfectious encephalomyelitis affects children with equal gender ratio.

Clinically, postinfectious encephalomyelitis has an abrupt onset. Bilateral optic neuritis is more commonly seen than unilateral optic neuritis, seizures are seen in 50% of patients and the level of consciousness is frequently affected.

Complete transverse myelitis with areflexia is seen more in postinfectious encephalomyelitis, compared to the incomplete transverse myelitis more frequently seen in multiple sclerosis. The disease onset of multiple sclerosis has a subacute pattern, seizures are seen in less than 5% of cases, the level of consciousness is generally conserved, and optic neuritis occurs unilaterally rather than bilaterally. Head MRI commonly shows a conservation of the periventricular area in postinfectious encephalomyelitis, whereas in multiple sclerosis periventricular area is frequently affected. Increased cell count may be seen in both postinfectious encephalomyelitis and multiple sclerosis, whereas oligoclonal bands are more seen in multiple sclerosis. *(Burks and Johnson, 91)*

60. **(A)** Transverse myelitis may be a clinical isolated syndrome where the affected patient has an increased risk of developing multiple sclerosis. Certain features of transverse myelitis are helpful to predict the likelihood of multiple sclerosis. Complete transverse myelitis carries a risk lower than 14% of developing multiple sclerosis, whereas incomplete transverse myelitis carries a risk of developing multiple sclerosis that approximates 70%. Other features that increase the risk of developing multiple sclerosis after transverse myelitis include asymmetric sensory or motor findings, abnormal CSF or brain MRI findings, spinal MRI showing limited nonconfluent intramedullary lesions, and abnormal multimodality-evoked potential. *(Burks and Johnson, 93)*

REFERENCES

Arroyo EJ, Scherer SS. On the molecular architecture of myelinated fibers. *Histochem Cell Biol.* 2000;113:1–18.

Bjartmar C, Trapp BD. Axonal and neuronal degeneration in multiple sclerosis: mechanisms and functional consequences. *Curr Opin Neurol.* 2001;14:271–278.

Burks JS, Johnson KP. *Multiple Sclerosis: Diagnosis, Medical Management, and Rehabilitation.* New York, NY: Demo Medical, 2000.

Dalmau JO, Posner JB. Paraneoplastic syndromes. *Arch Neurol.* 1999;56:405–408.

Dropcho EJ. Principles of paraneoplastic syndromes. *Ann N Y Acad Sci.* 1998;841:246–261.

Leocani L. Comi G. Neurophysiological investigations in multiple sclerosis. *Curr Opin Neurol.* 2000;13:255–261.

Noseworthy JH, Lucchinetti C, Rodriguez M, Weinshenker BG. Multiple sclerosis. *N Engl J Med.* 2000; 343:938–952.

Polman CH, Uitdehaag BM. Drug treatment of multiple sclerosis. *BMJ.* 2000;321:490–494.

Ransohoff R, Neuroimmunology. *Continuum.* 2003:7.

Rees J. Paraneoplastic syndromes. *Curr Opin Neurol.* 1998; 11:633–637.

Ropper AH, Gorson KC. Neuropathies associated with paraproteinemia. *N Engl J Med.* 1998;38:1601–1605.

Stolp-Smith KA, Carter JL, Rohe DE, Knowland DP 3rd. Management of impairment, disability, and handicap due to multiple sclerosis. *Mayo Clin Proc.* 1997;72: 1184–1196.

Trapp BD, Peterson J, Ransohoff RM, et al. Axonal transection in the lesions of multiple sclerosis. *N Engl J Med.* 1998;338:278–285.

Wingerchuk DM, Lucchinetti CF, Noseworthy JH. Multiple sclerosis: Current pathophysiological concepts. *Lab Invest.* 2001;81:263–281.

Zifko UA, Rupp M, Schwarz S, Zipko HT, Maida EM. Modafinil in treatment of fatigue in multiple sclerosis. Results of an open-label study. *J Neurol.* 2002;249: 983–987.

CHAPTER 10

Neuropharmacology and Neurochemistry
Questions

1. All of the following substances are amino acids or biogenic amine neurotransmitters EXCEPT

   (A) dopamine
   (B) acetylcholine
   (C) histamine
   (D) glycine
   (E) epinephrine

Questions 2 through 11
Link each of the following drugs to the appropriate site of action at the cholinergic synapse and its effect on acetylcholine metabolism.

   (A) Atropine
   (B) Physostigmine
   (C) Hemicolinium-3
   (D) Botulinum toxin
   (E) β-bungarotoxin
   (F) Curare
   (G) Soman
   (H) Dimethylphenyl piperazinium
   (I) Oxotemorine
   (J) Vesamicol

2. It blocks the transport of acetylcholine into vesicles.

3. It promotes release of acetylcholine from vesicles.

4. It blocks the release of acetylcholine from vesicles.

5. It blocks postsynaptic nicotinic cholinergic receptors.

6. It is a nicotinic agonist.

7. It is a muscarinic receptor antagonist.

8. It is a presynaptic muscarinic agonist.

9. It is a reversible acetylcholinesterase inhibitor.

10. It is an irreversible acetylcholinesterase inhibitor.

11. It is a competitive inhibitor of choline uptake.

12. The rate limiting step for the synthesis of dopamine is

   (A) tyrosine hydroxylase
   (B) aromatic amino acid decarboxylase
   (C) pteridine reductase
   (D) dopamine β-hydroxylase
   (E) phenylethanolamine-N-methyl transferase

13. Serotonin is derived from

   (A) histidine
   (B) tryptophan
   (C) dopamine
   (D) tyrosine
   (E) glutamate

14. Ligand-gated channel opening for acetylcholine depends on all the following EXCEPT

   (A) the value of the membrane potential
   (B) the probability that the channel is open
   (C) the conduction of each open channel
   (D) the driving force that acts on ions
   (E) the total number of end-plate channels

Questions 15 through 24
Link each of the following drugs to the appropriate site of action at gamma-aminobutyric acid synapse, receptors, and metabolism steps.

(A) Allylglycine
(B) Flumazenil
(C) Phenobarbital
(D) Diazepam
(E) Picrotoxin
(F) Gabaculine
(G) Muscimol
(H) Nipecotic acid
(I) Baclofen
(J) Phaclofen

15. It blocks the action of GABA at postsynaptic receptors.

16. GABA A agonist at postsynaptic receptors.

17. GABA transaminase inhibitor.

18. It inhibits glutamic acid decarboxylase.

19. It increases the frequency of GABA A receptor opening.

20. It prolongs the duration of opening of the GABA A receptors.

21. It reverses the action of benzodiazepine agonists and has no pharmacological effect when administrated alone.

22. GABA B receptors agonist.

23. GABA B receptors antagonist.

24. GABA uptake inhibitor.

25. Which of the following statements is true about the molecular mechanism of cocaine addiction?

(A) Methadone is a powerful medication against cocaine addiction.
(B) Cocaine, by blocking the dopamine reuptake transporter, increases the postsynaptic concentration of dopamine.

(C) Dopamine transporter system is not necessary for the mechanism of cocaine addiction.
(D) D1 dopamine agonists stimulate cocaine-seeking behavior.
(E) D2 receptor agonists may decrease episodes of craving for cocaine.

Questions 26 through 31
Link each of the antiepileptic drugs with its side effect.

(A) A 10-year-old boy was treated with ethosuximide for several months because of absence seizures.
(B) A 45-year-old man was treated with phenytoin for several years because of a seizure disorder.
(C) A 25-year-old man, diagnosed with primary generalized seizures, was recently switched to valproic acid. His valproic acid level is 50 m(G)ml.
(D) A 55-year-old man was started on primidone for the treatment of an essential tremor.
(E) A 60-year-old man was started on phenobarbital 4 months ago, after undergoing brain surgery for astrocytoma.
(F) A 35-year-old woman, with a history of complex partial seizure on carbamazepine, consulted because of chronic headache and blurred vision.

26. Hyponatremia

27. Megaloblastic anemia

28. Acute pancreatitis

29. Fatigue

30. Impotence

31. Ataxia

32. Which of the following drugs decrease the serum level of carbamazepine?

(A) Phenytoin
(B) Valproic acid

(C) Verapamil

(D) Erythromycin

(E) Isoniazid

33. Phenytoin may reach a toxic level in the serum of patient a using _____ at the same time.

(A) valproic acid

(B) ethosuximide

(C) cyclosporine

(D) cimetidine

(E) prednisone

34. Which of the following antiepileptic drugs may have its concentration increased by the concomitant administration of aspirin?

(A) Phenobarbital

(B) Valproic acid

(C) Carbamazepine

(D) Lamotrigine

(E) Primidone

Questions 35 through 42
Link each of the following sites of neuronal norepinephrine metabolism to the appropriate drug

(A) Tyrosine hydroxylase inhibitor

(B) Norepinephrine storage depletion

(C) Release of norepinephrine

(D) Presynaptic α2 adrenergic autoreceptor stimulator

(E) Postsynaptic α adrenergic receptor blocker

(F) Norepinephrine reuptake inhibitor

(G) Monoamine oxidase (MAO) inhibitor

(H) Catechol-O-methyl transferase inhibitor

35. Pargyline

36. Amphetamine

37. Phentolamine

38. Tropolone

39. α methyltyrosine

40. Clonidine

41. Desipramine

42. Reserpine

43. D1 dopamine receptors exceed the number of D2 dopamine receptors as well as the number of other types of dopamine receptors in the

(A) Substantia nigra

(B) Caudate nucleus

(C) Hippocampus

(D) Amygdala

(E) Ventral tegmental area

44. For a patient with seizures and acute porphyria, the most appropriate antiepileptic drug is

(A) felbamate

(B) topiramate

(C) lamotrigine

(D) tiagabine

(E) gabapentin

45. The mechanism of action of cocaine in the central nervous system is

(A) inhibition of tyrosine hydroxylase

(B) inhibition of the storage of dopamine

(C) inhibition of dopamine reuptake

(D) inhibition of monoamine oxidase

(E) inhibition of catechol-O-methyltransferase

Questions 46 through 53
Link the following.

(A) D1 dopamine receptors

(B) D2 dopamine receptors

(C) Both

(D) Neither

46. Stimulation of adenylate cyclase.

47. Enhancement of potassium conductance.

48. The number of dopamine receptors increases in case of tardive dyskinesia.

49. Postmortem studies showed an increased number of dopamine receptors in schizophrenic patients.

50. It has the highest affinity to quinpirol.

51. It has the highest affinity to clozapine.

52. Bromocriptine is an agonist.

53. Sulpiride is an antagonist.

54. Which of the following is true about amyloid precursor protein (APP)?

   (A) The dominant isoform of APP contains the protease inhibitor region.
   (B) APP undergoes a fast axonal transport to the synaptic region to interact with the extracellular matrix.
   (C) APP α secretase is associated with the amyloidogenic form of APP.
   (D) β secretases cleave the C terminal of APP and do not participate in the amyloidogenic process.
   (E) Normal cellular metabolism does not synthesize the A β region of APP.

55. Compared to the nigrostriatal system, the mesoprefrontal dopamine system is characterized by

   (A) the presence of dopamine autoreceptors
   (B) lack of biochemical tolerance development following chronic antipsychotic drug administration
   (C) greater increase in the responsiveness to dopamine agonists
   (D) a lower turnover rate of transmitter dopamine
   (E) a lower rate of physiological activity

56. Which of the following is true about the serotoninergic receptors?

   (A) 5-HTA2 A receptors are densely located in the raphe nuclei.
   (B) The activation of 5-HT1 receptors induces an increase of adenylate cyclase.

   (C) The inhibition effect of serotonin in the central nervous system is mediated by 5-HT1 receptors.
   (D) 5-HT2 receptor activation induces the opening of potassium channels.
   (E) 5-HT3 receptors mediate fast excitation that requires a coupling to G protein.

57. The most serious side effect of clozapine is

   (A) tardive dyskinesia
   (B) neuroleptic malignant syndrome
   (C) acute dystonia
   (D) agranulocytosis
   (E) akathisia

58. Which of the following is true about the pharmacological properties of clozapine?

   (A) It has a higher affinity to D2 than to D1 dopamine receptors.
   (B) It has a potent D4 dopamine receptor blocker.
   (C) It inhibits c-fos expression.
   (D) It has serotonin agonist activity.
   (E) It activates the same dopaminergic neurons stimulated by haloperidol.

59. What is the mechanism of action of buspirone?

   (A) It interacts with 5-HT1A receptors.
   (B) It inhibits serotonin reuptake.
   (C) It interacts with 5-HT2 receptors.
   (D) It blocks histamine reuptake.
   (E) It is a potent D1 dopamine receptor antagonist.

60. Which of the following drugs does NOT increase the level of lithium when both are administrated concomitantly?

   (A) Ibuprofen
   (B) Furosemide
   (C) Aspirin
   (D) Lisinopril
   (E) None of the above

Answers and Explanations

1. **(B)** A substrate is accepted as a neurotransmitter when it is present in the presynaptic terminal, synthesized by neurons, and released in amounts sufficient to exert an effect on the postsynaptic neurons or effector organ, mimics its endogenous action when given exogenously and has a specific mechanism for removing it from the site of action. Biogenic amine neurotransmitters include dopamine, norepinephrine, epinephrine, serotonin, and histamine. Amino acid neurotransmitters include χ-aminobutyric acid, glycine, and glutamate. Acetylcholine is the only accepted low-molecular weight amine transmitter substance that is not an amino acid or derived directly from one. *(Kandell et al., 280)*

2. **(J)**

3. **(E)**

4. **(D)**

5. **(F)**

6. **(H)**

7. **(A)**

8. **(I)**

9. **(B)**

10. **(G)**

11. **(C)**

Explanations 2 through 11

Acetylcholine is synthesized from the combination of Acetyl CoA and choline in a reaction catalyzed by a choline acetyltransferase. Acetylcholine is then transported in vesicles into the cholinergic synapse. This transport can be blocked by vesamicol. The release of acetylcholine in the cholinergic synapse is promoted by β-bungarotoxin and inhibited by botulinum toxin and magnesium. The action of acetylcholine in the synapses depends on the type of receptors found in the synapses. Cholinergic receptors fall into two categories:

- Muscarinic receptors that exhibit a slow response time are coupled to G proteins and are linked to phosphoinositide hydrolysis or cyclic AMP as a second messenger. Presynaptic or postsynaptic muscarinic receptors are blocked by atropine. Oxotremorine is a presynaptic muscarinic agonist that inhibits the evoked release of acetylcholine.
- Nicotinic receptors are blocked by curare and hexamethonium, whereas dimethylphenyl piperazinium acts as a postsynaptic nicotinic receptors antagonist.

Acetylcholine is deactivated in the cholinergic synapse when it is hydrolyzed into choline and acetate by acetylcholinesterase, which may be inhibited reversibly or irreversibly by, respectively, physostigmine or soman. Choline reuptake, for further acetylcholine synthesis, may be inhibited by a competitive blocker such as hemicolinium-3. *(Cooper et al., 201–221)*

12. **(A)** Dopamine is synthesized from the essential amino acid tyrosine pathway involving 5 enzymes. The first enzyme is tyrosine hydroxylase. It is an oxidase that converts tyrosine to L-DOPA. It is the rate-limiting step of dopamine

synthesis and requires reduced pteridine as a cofactor, which is generated from pteridine by a pteridine reductase. L-DOPA decarboxylase produces dopamine after decarboxylation of L-DOPA. Dopamine is converted to norepinephrine by dopamine β-hydroxylase. Norepinephrine is methylated to epinephrine by phenylethanolamine-N-methyl transferase. *(Kandell et al., 282–283)*

13. **(B)** Serotonin is derived from the hydroxylation of tryptophan by a tryptophan hydroxylase followed by decarboxylation of hydroxytryptophan by a 5-hydroxytryptophan decarboxylase. *(Kandell et al., 283–284)*

14. **(A)** The stimulation of a motor nerve releases acetylcholine into the synaptic cleft, where it diffuses to bind, and activates acetylcholine receptors. The activation of postsynaptic acetylcholine produces a rapid increase in the end-plate current. After deactivation of acetylcholine, the random closure of the opened channels causes the end-plate current to decay smoothly. The end-plate current depends on the number of acetylcholine channels available for activation. The probability that a channel is open depends on the concentration of acetylcholine at the channel, the conduction of each open channel, and the driving force that acts on the ions. As the postsynaptic acetylcholine receptor channels open by the binding of acetylcholine, not by change in voltage, the value of the membrane potential does not influence the end-plate current. *(Kandell et al., 190)*

15. **(E)**

16. **(G)**

17. **(F)**

18. **(A)**

19. **(D)**

20. **(C)**

21. **(B)**

22. **(I)**

23. **(J)**

24. **(H)**

Explanations 15 through 24

GABA is formed by the decarboxylation of glutamic acid by a glutamic acid decarboxylase, an enzyme located in the central nervous system and the retina. Allyglycine is an inhibitor of glutamic acid decarboxylase. GABA is metabolized by transamination by GABA-transaminase yielding succinic semialdehyde and regenerating glutamate. GABA receptors fall into 2 major types: GABA A and GABA B. Presynaptic and postsynaptic GABA receptors cause a shift in membrane permeability to chloride primarily, when coupled with GABA. This change in chloride permeability results in hyperpolarization of the receptive neurons in case of postsynaptic inhibition or depolarization in case of presynaptic inhibition.

The GABA A receptor-associated channels predominantly conduct chloride ions. Since the equilibrium potential of chloride is close to the resting potential of most neurons, an increase of the permeability of chlorides decreases the depolarization effect of an excitatory input, resulting in the depression of excitability.

Diazepam is a benzodiazepine that acts by increasing the frequency of opening of the chloride channels without altering either their conduction or their duration of opening; however, phenobarbital, which is a barbiturate, prolongs the duration of chloride channel opening by slightly decreasing the opening frequency. Flumazenil is a benzodiazepine agonist as it binds to the same site of action of benzodiazepine in GABA A receptors. Flumazenil, when administrated alone, has no pharmacological effect. However, when administrated with a benzodiazepine, it reverses its effect.

Muscimol is a direct postsynaptic GABA agonist that passes the blood-brain barrier and is active after systemic administration. Muscimol interacts directly with GABA A receptors causing their activation. Indirect GABA agonists act to facilitate GABA-ergic transmission by increasing the amount of GABA that reaches the receptors or by altering the interaction between the receptor and GABA. GABA transaminase inhibitors, such as gabaculine, or GABA uptake inhibitors, such as nipecotic acid, are indirect GABA agonists, as the availability of the neurotransmitter to the GABA receptor is increased. GABA receptors can be antagonized either directly or indirectly. Bicuculline acts as a direct competitive GABA A antagonist at the receptor level, whereas picrotoxine acts as a noncompetitive antagonist by blocking GABA A activated inophores.

GABA B receptors are not linked to a chloride channel. Presynaptic GABA B receptors are linked through GTP sensitive proteins to a calcium or potassium channel. The inhibitory effect of GABA B receptor activation is probably mediated through either an increase in potassium conductance or a decrease in calcium conductance. GABA B receptor activation with baclofen decreases calcium conductance and GABA release. Postsynaptic GABA B receptors are indirectly coupled to a potassium channel via G proteins mediating late inhibitory postsynaptic potentials. Phaclofen is an antagonist of GABA B receptors. *(Cooper et al., 126–150)*

25. **(B)** The dopamine-reuptake transporter controls the levels of dopamine in the synapse by rapidly carrying the neurotransmitter back into nerve terminals after its release. Cocaine, which binds strongly to the dopamine-reuptake transporter, blocks dopamine reuptake after normal neuronal activity and increases its level at the synapses, producing the characteristic cocaine euphoria. Animal studies show that the effect of dopamine is dependent on the type of dopamine synaptic receptors with which it interacts. D1-receptor agonists suppress cocaine-seeking behavior and may diminish episodes of intense craving for cocaine, whereas D2 receptor agonists may increase the cocaine-seeking behavior. Neutralization of the dopamine-reuptake transporter inhibits the psychostimulatory effect of cocaine. Methadone is an active medication against chronic addiction to heroin, whereas naloxone is the treatment of heroin overdose. *(Leshner, 128–129)*

26. **(F)**

27. **(B)**

28. **(C)**

29. **(E)**

30. **(D)**

31. **(A)**

Explanations 26 through 31

Antiepilepsy medication side effects can be divided into two categories: dose-related and idiosyncratic.

Ethosuximide is the drug of choice for the treatment of uncomplicated absence seizures. It acts by reducing low-threshold, transient, and voltage-dependent calcium conductance in thalamic neurons. Its dose-dependent side effects include nausea, vomiting, abdominal pain, agitation, headaches, lethargy, drowsiness, dizziness, and ataxia. Idiosyncratic reactions to ethosuximide are rare and include rash, erythema multiforme, Stevens-Johnson syndrome agranulocytosis, and aplastic anemia.

Phenytoin is effective for the treatment of partial and tonic-clonic seizures. It appears to act by inducing voltage and use-dependent blockade of sodium channels. Its dose-dependent side effects include nausea, vomiting, ataxia, nystagmus, depression drowsiness, paradoxical increase of seizures, gum hypertrophy, and megaloblastic anemia. Its idiosyncratic effects are hepatotoxic effects, teratogenicity, acne, Stevens-Johnson syndrome, lupus-like syndrome, coarsening of facial features, hirsutism, and Dupuytren's contracture.

Valproic acid is effective in patients with all types of seizures, and especially in those with idiopathic generalized epilepsy. The drug may act by limiting sustained repetitive neuronal firing through inhibition of frequency dependent blockade of voltage-dependent sodium channels. It may also increase brain GABA concentrations. Dose-related side effects to valproic acid are tremor, weight gain, alopecia, peripheral edema nausea, and vomiting.

Idiosyncratic reactions to valproic acid are acute pancreatitis, hepatotoxicity, encephalopathy, thrombocytopenia, and teratogenicity.

Phenobarbital is as effective as phenytoin in abolishing partial and generalized tonic-clonic seizures. At the cellular level, it prolongs inhibitory postsynaptic potentials by increasing the mean chloride-channel opening time and hence the duration of γ-aminobutyric acid-induced bursts of neuronal activity. Its dose-related side effects include decreased cognition, fatigue, lethargy and depression in adults, irritability, distractability, hyperkinesia, and insomnia in children. Its idiosyncratic reactions are maculopapular rash, toxic epidermal necrosis, hepatotoxicity, arthritis, teratogenicity, and Dupuytren's contracture.

Primidone is metabolized to phenobarbital and another active metabolite, phenylethylmalonamide. The efficacy of primidone is similar to that of phenobarbital, but primidone is less well tolerated. Its dose-dependent side effects are fatigue, lethargy, depression, psychosis, decreased libido, and impotence. Its idiosyncratic side effects include rash, thrombocytopenia, lupus-like syndrome, agranulocytosis, and teratogenicity.

Carbamazepine is effective for the treatment of partial and generalized tonic-clonic seizures but is not effective, and may even be deleterious, in patients with absence or myoclonic seizures. The drug acts by preventing repetitive firing of action potentials in depolarized neurons through voltage- and use-dependent blockade of sodium channels. Its dose-dependent side effects are hyponatremia, by its antidiuretic hormone-like effect, neutropenia, nausea, drowsiness, headache, dizziness, and diplopia. Idiosyncratic reactions include morbilliform rash in about 10% of cases, erythema multiforme and Stevens-Johnson syndrome, agranulocytosis, aplastic anemia hepatotoxicity, and teratogenicity. *(Brodie and Dichter, 168–175)*

32. **(A)** Carbamazepine induces hepatic enzymes to accelerate the hepatic metabolism of other lipid soluble drugs, such as oral contraceptive pills. In addition to inducing its own metabolism, carbamazepine not only accelerates the metabolism of valproic acid, ethosuximide, corticosteroids, anticoagulants, antipsychotic drugs, and cyclosporine, but also decreases their serum levels and the potency of their therapeutic effects. However, the metabolism of carbamazepine is inhibited by the administration of phenytoin, which paradoxically induces the metabolism of carbamazepine. Thus, adding phenytoin decreases plasma carbamazepine concentrations by about a third, whereas adding carbamazepine to phenytoin increases plasma phenytoin concentrations by a similar amount. Cimetidine, propoxyphene, diltiazem, erythromycin, isoniazid, and verapamil may inhibit the metabolism of carbamazepine to the point that the drug may reach a toxic level. *(Brodie and Dichter, 168–175)*

33. **(D)** Phenytoin may increase the hepatic oxidation of lipid-soluble drugs including carbamazepine, valproic acid, ethosuximide, anticoagulants, corticosteroids, and cyclosporine. Drugs that inhibit the metabolism of phenytoin include allopurinol, amiodarone, cimetidine, imipramine, and some sulfonamides. This inhibition of the metabolism of phenytoin may bring the drug concentration to a toxic level. *(Brodie and Dichter, 168–175)*

34. **(B)** Aspirin displaces valproic acid from its binding sites on plasma proteins and inhibits its metabolism. *(Brodie and Dichter, 168–175; Goulden et al., 1392–1394)*

35. **(G)**

36. **(C)**

37. **(E)**

38. **(H)**

39. **(A)**

40. **(D)**

41. **(F)**

42. **(B)**

Explanations 35 through 42

Catecholamines are synthesized from tyrosine in the brain, chromaffin cells, and sympathetic ganglia. Tyrosine is metabolized in norepinephrine in the peripheral nervous system, or in dopamine, norepinephrine, or epinephrine in the brain. Tyrosine hydroxylase is the first enzyme in the biosynthesis pathway of norepinephrine allowing the conversion of tyrosine to DOPA. It requires molecular Fe^{++}, oxygen, and tetrahydropteridine as cofactors. Since it is the rate limiting step in the synthesis of norepinephrine in the brain as well as in the peripheral nervous system, pharmacological blockade at this stage would reduce norepinephrine synthesis.

α-methyltyrosine is an amino acid analogue that competitively inhibits tyrosine hydroxylase. Dihydropteridine reductase is indirectly related to norepinephrine synthesis and intimately linked to tyrosine hydroxylase as it reduces the quinonoid dihydropterin that has been oxidized during the hydroxylation of tyrosine to DOPA. The substitution of dihydropteridine with its analogue is an effective inhibitor of dihydropteridine reductase.

L DOPA is decarboxylated to dopamine by L DOPA decarboxylase. Dopamine is then hydroxylated by dopamine hydroxylase to give norepinephrine. The chelation of copper, which is a cofactor of dopamine hydroxylase, is an effective inhibitor of norepinephrine production. Norepinephrine is stored in granules in the sympathetic nerve endings as well as in the central nervous system. Reserpine interferes with the storage of norepinephrine causing irreversible long-lasting depletion of the storage of norepinephrine, whereas tetrabenazine inhibits the storage of norepinephrine for a shorter period of time and does not appear to be reversible. The release of norepinephrine from storage granules is calcium dependent. Amphetamines may cause an increase in the release of norepinephrine. In the central nervous system, norepinephrine interacts with either the α2 presynaptic receptors to decrease adenyl cyclase activity via coupling to G protein, or with postsynaptic receptors to stimulate phospholipase C action.

Clonidine is a potent stimulator of α2 presynaptic receptors whereas phenotolamine is an effective adrenergic postsynaptic α receptor blocking agent. The action of norepinephrine is ended by its reuptake into the presynaptic terminal. This reuptake may be inhibited by desipramine. Norepinephrine is degraded by monoamine oxidase (MAO) when it presents in a free state within the presynaptic terminal. It is inhibited by pargyline. Outside the presynaptic neuron, norepinephrine is inactivated by catechol-O-methyl transferase (COMT). Tropolone is an inhibitor of COMT. *(Cooper et al., 236–258, 284)*

43. **(D)** D1 dopamine receptors are densely expressed in the amygdala, whereas D2 dopamine receptors as well as D3, D4, and D5 dopamine receptors have low levels of expression. D1 and D2 dopamine receptors are highly expressed in the caudate nucleus, putamen, nucleus accumbens, and olfactory tubercle. D1 dopamine receptors are not expressed in substantia nigra, ventral tegmental area, and zona inserta. *(Cooper et al., 327)*

44. **(E)** Among the drugs mentioned in this question, gabapentin is the only drug that has no liver metabolism as it is entirely eliminated by the kidney. Because of these pharmacological characteristics, gabapentin may be the drug of choice in treating patients with seizure and acute intermittent porphyria. *(Bourgeois, 1181–1183)*

45. **(C)** Mesolimbic dopamine neurons are involved in the reinforcing properties of a variety of abused drugs such as cocaine. It acts by blocking dopamine reuptake and inducing dopamine release. *(Cooper et al., 304)*

46. **(A)**

47. **(B)**

48. **(C)**

49. **(B)**

50. **(D)**

51. (D)

52. (B)

53. (B)

Explanations 46 through 53

Dopamine receptors are classified on the basis of a positive coupling between the receptor and the adenylate cyclase activity, mainly into D1 and D2 receptors. When activated, D1 dopamine receptors increase adenylate cyclase activity, whereas the activation of D2 receptors inhibits adenylate cyclase activity, enhances potassium conductance, and inhibits calcium entry through voltage sensitive calcium channels. The development of molecular biology divides D2 receptor into four subtypes and D1 receptors into two subtypes. D2 receptor subtypes are D2 short, D2 long, D3, and D4. D1 receptor subtypes include D1 and D5. D5 receptors have more affinity to dopamine than D1 receptors, which is the only difference between the two dopamine receptors. D4 receptors have the highest affinity to clozapine, an atypical neuroleptic, whereas D3 receptors have the highest affinity to the dopamine agonist quinpirol. Bromocriptine is a D2 receptor agonist, whereas sulpiride is a D2 antagonist. The expression of dopamine receptors has been observed to change in disease states. In schizophrenia, postmortem studies showed a consistent elevation of D2 receptors of the brain, whereas D1 receptors remain unchanged, even in tissue obtained from patients without neuroleptic treatment. In Parkinson disease, there is an increase in the expression of both D1 and D2 dopamine receptors. The chronic administration of dopamine antagonist, such as neuroleptic drugs, may increase the expression of dopamine receptors in the striatum. The development of tardive dyskinesia, after a chronic use of neuroleptic may be explained by a supersensitivity of dopamine receptors that have been chronically blocked. *(Cooper et al., 317–326)*

54. (B) The major characteristic of Alzheimer's disease is the deposition of A β protein in the microvasculature. This protein is derived from amyloid precursor protein (APP) that is encoded by a single gene on chromosome 21. APP has the structure of a transmembrane receptor with an N extracellular segment and a C intracellular segment. The dominant isoform of APP does not contain a protease inhibitor region. It undergoes fast axonal transport to the synaptic region to interact with the extracellular matrix. APP may undergo a nonamyloidogenic metabolism by cleavage of the A β region (which includes the first 28 extracellular and the following 11–15 transmembrane amino acids), by an α secretase, or by cleavage of the A β sequence by a β secretase in the N-terminal sequence or a χ secretase in the C-terminal region. The production of A β protein is thought to be a minor part of the normal processing of APP. *(Blennow and Cowburn, 77–86)*

55. (B) The mesoprefrontal dopamine system is a part of the mesotelencephalic dopamine system, which also includes the mesocingulate dopamine system. The mesotelencephalic dopamine system lacks neuron autoreceptors (in contrast to other dopamine neurons possessing autoreceptors such as the mesopiriform, mesolimbic, and nigrostriatal dopamine systems), which may explain some biochemical, physiological, and pharmacological characteristics of these midbrain neurons. Compared to dopamine systems possessing autoreceptors, the mesoprefrontal dopamine cells have a higher rate of firing and more bursting, a higher turnover rate and metabolism of transmitter dopamine, a lessened response to dopamine agonists and antagonists, and a lack of biochemical tolerance following chronic drug administration. *(Cooper et al., 335–336)*

56. (C) Radioligand binding studies identified numerous subtypes of serotonin receptors in the brain. 5-HTA1 receptors have a high density in the raphe nuclei and the hippocampus. When activated they hyperpolarize the cell membrane via G protein by opening potassium channels, inhibiting adenylate cyclase, or closing calcium channels. 5-HTA2 receptors are highly concentrated in layer IV of the cortex and the hippocampus. When activated, they depolarize the membrane and activate phospholipase C. 5-HT3 receptors are ligand-gated ion channel receptors.

They mediate fast excitation through ligand-gated cationic ion channels that do not require coupling with G proteins or a second messenger. *(Cooper et al., 371, 374, 384)*

57. **(D)** Agranulocytosis is the most serious side effect of clozapine use. It occurs in 0.25% to 1% of treated patients with peak incidence in the first 4 to 18 weeks of treatment. Other side effects include increased risk of grand mal seizure, sedation, hypersalivation, and weight gain. Clozapine has a very low incidence of acute or chronic motor side effects. *(Enna and Coyle, 36–38)*

58. **(B)** Clozapine modifies the action of a number of neurotransmitter systems. It is an antagonist of both D1 and D2 dopamine receptors in the brain with higher affinity for D1 than D2 dopamine receptors. Its highest affinity is for the D4 receptor. Also, it has a serotonin receptor antagonism, especially 5HT2a, an anticholinergic and histaminergic action. Clozapine induces depolarization blockade in A 10 dopamine neurons and activates c-fos expression, a marker of cellular activity in the nucleus accumbens, ventral striatum, anterior cingulated, and medial prefrontal cortex. In contrast, haloperidol activates c-fos expression in regions that receive projection from A9 dopamine neurons. *(Enna and Coyle, 74–75)*

59. **(A)** Buspirone is an effective treatment of generalized anxiety. It belongs to the azapirones class of drug, which has a high affinity to 5 HT1A receptors. Buspirone may act as a partial agonist at 5 HT1A receptors at postsynaptic sites, potentially in the hippocampus and prefrontal cortex. *(Enna and Coyle, 74–75)*

60. **(C)** The coadministration of lithium with diuretics and angiotensin-converting enzymes may increase lithium serum levels by promoting sodium loss and consequently a decrease in lithium excretion. Nonsteroidal antiinflamatory medications, except for aspirin, may also increase lithium serum levels. *(Enna and Coyle, 126–127)*

REFERENCES

Blennow K, Cowburn RF. The neurochemistry of Alzheimer's disease. *Acta Neurologica Scandinavica. Supplementum.* 168:77–86, 1996.

Brodie MJ, Dichter MA. Antiepileptic drugs. *N Engl J Med.* 334(3):168–75, 1996 Jan 18.

Cooper JR, Bloom FE, Roth RH. *The Biochemical Basis of Neuropharmacology.* New York: Oxford University Press. 1996.

Enna SJ Coyle JT. *Pharmacological Management of Neurological and Psychiatric Disorders.* New York: McGraw-Hill; 1998.

Goulden KJ, Dooley JM, Camfield PR, Fraser AD. Clinical valproate toxicity induced by acetylsalicylic acid. *Neurology* 1987;37:1392–1394.

Kandell ER, Schwartz JH, Jessell TM. *Principles of Neural Science.* 4th ed. New York: McGraw-Hill;2000.

Leshner AI. Molecular mechanisms of cocaine addiction. *N Engl J Med.* 1996;335:128–129.

CHAPTER 11

Neurogenetics
Questions

Questions 1 through 3
Link each of the following cases to the corresponding congenital myasthenic syndromes.

(A) A 4-year-old boy consulted because of fatigue on exertion. The patient has a history of recurrent apneic episodes triggered by fever or vomiting. Neurological examination discloses mild asymmetric ptosis. Test for acetylcholine receptor antibodies is negative. EMG studies show decremental response at 10 Hz stimulation but absence of decremental response at 2 Hz in rested muscle.

(B) A 3-year-old boy was brought in by his mother because of moderate generalized weakness. He was born after 38 weeks gestation. He had a history of weak fetal movements in utero. He was hypotonic from birth with weak suck, lid ptosis, and delayed motor milestones. Neurological examination demonstrates generalized hypotonia, weakness with severe limitation of ocular movement and ptosis, and sluggish pupillary light reflexes. Test for acetylcholine receptor antibodies is negative. The patient shows no response to the edrophonium test. EMG studies show repetitive compound muscle action potential in response to single nerve stimulation.

(C) A 16-year-old boy developed diplopia and weakness, exacerbated by effort. Neurological examination demonstrates mild lid ptosis, limitation of vertical and horizontal eye movements, and generalized weakness predominantly in the wrist, finger extensors, and cervical muscles. EMG studies show a repetitive compound muscle action potential in response to single nerve stimulation with decremental responses on 2 Hz stimulation, which is reversed with neostigmine administration. A younger brother and a maternal uncle have similar symptoms.

1. End-plate acetylcholine esterase deficiency

2. Slow-channel congenital myasthenic syndrome

3. Congenital myasthenic syndrome with episodic apnea

Questions 4 through 8
Link the following neurocutaneous syndromes to the correct inheritance pattern.

(A) Autosomal dominant
(B) Autosomal recessive
(C) X-linked inheritance
(D) Sporadic inheritance

4. Lesch-Nyhan syndrome

5. Neurofibromatosis type I

6. Sturge-Weber syndrome

7. Tuberous sclerosis

8. Ataxia-telangiectasia

9. Which of the following is the major criterion for the diagnosis of tuberous sclerosis?

   (A) Subependymal giant cell astrocytoma
   (B) Vestibular schwannoma
   (C) Meningioma
   (D) Optic glioma
   (E) Neurofibroma

10. Which of the following is NOT a criterion for neurofibromatosis type I?

   (A) Optic glioma
   (B) Bilateral auditory nerve schwannoma
   (C) Two or more Lisch nodules
   (D) Six or more "café au lait" lesions
   (E) A first-degree relative with neurofibromatosis type I

11. The primary mechanism leading to cerebral infarction in patients with hereditary hemorrhagic telangiectasia is

   (A) cerebral abscess
   (B) embolism from pulmonary arteriovenous fistula
   (C) cerebral aneurysm
   (D) cerebral telangiectasia
   (E) cerebral angioma

12. Sturge-Weber disease is transmitted as a

   (A) sporadic pattern
   (B) autosomal dominant pattern
   (C) chromosomal deletion
   (D) X-linked transmission
   (E) mitochondrial transmission

Questions 13 through 24
Link the following.

   (A) Neurofibromatosis type I
   (B) Neurofibromatosis type II
   (C) Both
   (D) Neither

13. Autosomal dominant disorder

14. Neurofibrimin

15. Merlin

16. It is linked to chromosome X

17. It is linked to chromosome 22

18. Subcutaneous neurofibroma

19. Lisch nodule

20. Moyamoya syndrome

21. Bilateral vestibular schwannomas

22. Systemic hypertension

23. Optic nerve glioma

24. High risk of severe mental retardation

Questions 25 through 31
Link each of the following leukodystrophies to the appropriate genetic or molecular deficit.

   (A) X-linked adrenoleukodystrophy
   (B) Alexander's disease
   (C) Canavan's disease
   (D) Cerebrotendinous xanthomatosis
   (E) Globoid leukodystrophy
   (F) Metachromatic leukodystrophy
   (G) Pelizaeus-Merzbacher disease

25. Accumulation of very long fatty acid chains

26. Sterol 27 hydroxylase

27. Glial fibrillary acidic protein

28. Galactocerebroside deficit

29. Asparto-acylase deficiency

30. Arylsulfatase deficiency

31. Abnormal proteolipid protein

32. Which of the following trinucleotide repeat expansion diseases is a type I disorder (i.e., occurs in the frame within the coding region)?

   (A) Myotonic dystrophy
   (B) Kennedy's disease

(C) Fragile X syndrome

(D) Friedreich ataxia

(E) Progressive myoclonic epilepsy type I

33. Which of the following types of frontotemporal dementia is linked to tau gene mutation on chromosome 17?

(A) Semantic dementia

(B) Corticobasal degeneration

(C) Frontotemporal dementia with motor neuron disease

(D) Pick disease

(E) Dementia with parkinsonism

Questions 34 through 36
Link each of the following disorders to its molecular abnormality.

(A) Ataxia with selective vitamin E deficiency

(B) Ataxia telangiectasia

(C) Friedreich ataxia

34. Chromosome 9q

35. Tocopherol transport protein gene mutation

36. Chromosome 11q

37. Which of the following spinocerebellar atrophies has a benign course and normal life span?

(A) Spinocerebellar atrophy type 3

(B) Spinocerebellar atrophy type 4

(C) Spinocerebellar atrophy type 1

(D) Spinocerebellar atrophy type 6

(E) Spinocerebellar atrophy type 7

38. All of the following progressive ataxias are related to GAC repeats EXCEPT

(A) spinocerebellar ataxia type 8

(B) spinocerebellar ataxia type 7

(C) dentatorubral-pallidoluysian atrophy (DRLPA)

(D) spinocerebellar ataxia type 6

(E) spinocerebellar ataxia type 3

Questions 39 through 43
Link each of the following proteins of triplet repeats to the corresponding chromosome.

(A) Huntingtin

(B) Myotonin

(C) Atrophin

(D) Ataxin 3

(E) Androgen receptor

39. Chromosome 12

40. Chromosome X

41. Chromosome 19

42. Chromosome 4

43. Chromosome 14

44. The genetic phenomenon responsible for the clinical heterogeneity of mitochondrial diseases is

(A) sporadic mutation

(B) chromosome deletion

(C) anticipation

(D) heteroplasmy

(E) mitotic instability

Questions 45 through 52
Link the following.

(A) Autosomal dominant

(B) Autosomal recessive

(C) X-linked inheritance

(D) Mitochondrial inheritance

45. Myotonic dystrophy

46. Wilson disease

47. Metachromatic leukodystrophy

48. Tuberous sclerosis

49. Adrenoleukodystrophy

50. Neurofibromatosis

51. Fabry lipid storage disease

52. Myoclonic epilepsy with ragged-red fibers

Answers and Explanations

1. **(B)**

2. **(C)**

3. **(A)**

Explanations 1 through 3

End-plate acetylcholine esterase deficiency causes a congenital myasthenic syndrome characterized by delayed pupillary light reflexes, refractoriness to cholinesterase inhibitors, and repetitive compound muscle action potential. The illness is caused by the absence of acetylcholine esterase in the synaptic space. The neuromuscular transmission is compromised by the reduced size of the nerve terminals, with their encasement by Schwann cells reducing the number of releasable acetylcholine quanta. The cholinergic overactivity may induce the Schwann cells to encase the nerve terminals, thus protecting the end plate from overexposure to acetylcholine. The absence of acetylcholine esterase in the synaptic terminals results in an overexpression of acetylcholine, causing a prolongation of the synaptic potentials beyond the refractory period of the muscle fiber, which triggers repetitive compound muscle fiber action potentials. The progression of the disease is attributed to an end-plate myopathy from cholinergic overactivity.

The molecular basis of the disease involves a recessive mutation in COLQ, a triple stranded collagenic tail of the acetylcholinesterase enzyme. Typical clinical manifestations of the disease are described in case B. The diagnosis is confirmed by muscle biopsy that demonstrates absence of acetylcholine esterase from end plates.

Case A has the characteristic features of congenital myasthenic syndrome with episodic apnea: recurrent apneic episodes triggered by fever or vomiting, mild ptosis, absence of decremental response on 2 Hz stimulation and the presence of decremental response on 10 Hz stimulation. Muscle biopsy confirms the diagnosis by showing end-plate acetylcholine receptor deficiency without postsynaptic structural abnormalities. The abnormality involves a presynaptic defect. There is a marked decrease in the number of acetylcholine quanta released by the nerve impulse due to a defect in the synthesis or axonal transport of vesicle precursors from the anterior horn cell to the nerve terminal.

Case C has features that point to slow channel congenital myasthenic syndrome: selective involvement of wrist and finger extensors, possible dominant inheritance, repetitive compound muscle action potentials with decremental response on 2 Hz stimulation repaired by neostigmine administration. An end-plate myopathy is caused by prolonged opening episodes of acetylcholine receptors during activity and spontaneous opening of acetylcholine receptors at rest. *(Conneally et al., 9–23)*

4. **(C)**

5. **(A)**

6. **(D)**

7. **(A)**

8. **(B)**

Explanations 4 through 8

Neurofibromatosis type I is an autosomal dominant disorder characterized by dermatological and neurological features. Cutaneous features include "café au lait" spots, axillary freckling, neurofibroma, Lisch nodules of the iris, and plexiform neurofibromas. Neurological features include learning disability, cognitive impairment, and neuraxis tumors. Lesch-Nyhan disease has X-linked inheritance and is characterized by self-mutilation of digits and lips. Its neurological features include mental retardation and dystonia. Sturge-Weber disease has sporadic inheritance. Epilepsy, mental retardation, and focal deficits comprise the neurological features. Epilepsy, mental retardation, autism, and giant cell astrocytoma complicate tuberous sclerosis, a neurocutaneous disease with autosomal dominant transmission. Ataxia-telangiectasia is an autosomal recessive disease characterized by ataxia, intention tremor, abnormal saccades, and decreased deep tendon reflexes. *(Roach, 591–620)*

9. **(A)** Tuberous sclerosis complex (TSC) arises from abnormal cellular differentiation, proliferation, and neuronal migration. It affects the brain (cortical and subcortical tubers, subependymal nodules, and giant cell astrocytomas), kidney, skin (hypomelanotic macules, shagreen patches, facial angiofibromas, and periungual fibromas), eye (retinal hamartomas), heart, and to a lesser extent other organs. The Tuberous Sclerosis Complex Consensus Conference divided the criteria for diagnosis of tuberous sclerosis into major and minor features. The major features include cortical tuber, subependymal nodule, subependymal giant cell astrocytoma and skin changes as mentioned above. *(Sparagana and Roach, 115–119)*

10. **(B)** Neurofibromatoses type I gene occurs as a spontaneous mutation in 1/10,000 and can affect most organ systems. Initial signs and symptoms vary. In 1987, the National Institutes of Health issued a consensus statement enumerating the clinical diagnostic criteria for neurofibromatosis type I. They include 2 of the following: (1) 6 or more "cafe au lait" macules greater than 5 mm in prepubertal patients and greater than 15 mm in postpubertal patients; (2) 2 or more neurofibromas of any type or one plexiform neurofibroma; (3) axillary or inguinal freckling; (4) optic nerve glioma; (5) 2 or more Lisch nodules (iris hamartomas); (6) sphenoid wing dysplasia or cortical thinning of long bones, with or without pseudarthrosis; and (7) a first-degree relative (parent, sibling, or child) with NF-1 based on the preceding criteria. *(Karnes, 1071–1076)*

11. **(B)** Hereditary hemorrhagic telangiectasia (HHT), also known as Osler-Weber-Rendu disease, is a hereditary autosomal dominant syndrome characterized by easy bleeding vascular abnormalities. The classic picture is that of a familial pattern of telangiectases and epistaxis. The characteristic lesion is the telangiectasia: a 1- to 2-mm-diameter lesion consisting of a dilated vessel directly connecting an artery and a vein. Telangiectasias probably develop from dilated postcapillary venules. Telangiectasias usually appear on the skin and mucosal surfaces, especially on the nose.

Larger arteriovenous malformations (AVMs), consisting of thin-walled vascular spaces with single or multiple feeding arteries, occur mostly in the lungs, liver, and brain. These AVMs may reach a diameter of several centimeters. Vascular malformations may appear in any organ, however. Transforming growth factor beta is known to have a regulatory role in tissue repair and angiogenesis. Mutation on chromosome 9 seems to predispose to high prevalence of pulmonary AVMs. Pulmonary AVMs are found in 15% to 33% of patients with HHT and are usually fed by the pulmonary artery, draining through the pulmonary veins.

Seventy percent of pulmonary AVMs (PAVMs) occur in the lower lung fields and may enlarge with time or during pregnancy. They can result in a substantial right-to-left shunt, with significant hypoxemia. Serious complications may occur: bleeding can result in potentially life-threatening hemoptysis or hemothorax, and paradoxical emboli, bypassing the pulmonary capillary system via the PAVM, may give rise to ischemic cerebral events. This is the primary mechanism leading to cerebral infarction in patients with HHT (up to one-third of patients with PAVMs suffer from ischemic cerebral events). *(Haitjema et al., 714–719)*

12. **(A)** Sturge-Weber syndrome is a neurocutaneous syndrome characterized by port wine facial nevus-associated leptomeningeal and brain angiomas. The syndrome occurs sporadically but may result from a somatic mutation, disturbing the angiogenic process. *(Huq et al., 780–782)*

13. **(C)**

14. **(A)**

15. **(B)**

16. **(D)**

17. **(B)**

18. **(C)**

19. **(A)**

20. **(A)**

21. **(B)**

22. **(A)**

23. **(A)**

24. **(D)**

Explanations 13 through 24

Neurofibromatosis (NF) is a neurocutaneous condition, of which two types exist. NF type I (NF-I) occurs in about 1 in 3000 persons and accounts for 96% to 97% of all cases of NF. NF type II (NF-II) accounts for about 3% of cases. NF types I and II have autosomal dominant transmission. Almost every organ system can be involved in NF type I; thus, initial signs and symptoms vary. Lisch nodules and optic nerve glioma are among the diagnostic criteria of NF type I.

The most common benign tumors in patients with NF type I are neurofibromas. They are composed of schwann cells, fibroblasts, mast cells, and vascular elements. Plexiform neurofibromas are specific to NF-I. Schwannomas are

uncommon in patients with NF-I but when they occur, they exist on spinal nerve sheaths. It was suggested recently that when a single vestibular schwannoma is detected on an imaging study of the head, it is unlikely that the patient has NF-I.

Central nervous system manifestations of NF-I include aqueductal stenosis, hydrocephalus, and seizures. Of patients with NF-I, 25% to 40% may have learning disabilities, and 5% to 10% may have mental retardation. Essential hypertension may occur in patients with NF-I; hypertension may also be due to pheochromocytoma, renal artery stenosis, neurofibromas that compress the kidneys or renal arteries, renal artery dysplasia, Wilms' tumor, or coarctation of the abdominal or thoracic aorta. Dysplasia of the cerebral artery may occur, causing moyamoya syndrome.

The gene for NF-I is located on the long arm of chromosome 17 at 17q11.2. Neurofibromin is the protein encoded by the neurofibromatosis gene and may act as a tumor suppressor.

The diagnostic criteria for NF-II are either (1) bilateral eighth nerve masses or (2) a first-degree relative with NF-II and either a unilateral auditory nerve mass or two of the following: neurofibroma, meningioma, glioma, schwannoma, or juvenile posterior subcapsular lenticular opacity. Schwannoma is the most common tumor in NF type II. Such tumors may involve cranial as well as peripheral nerves. Schwannomas of spinal nerve sheath tumors are also common in patients with NF-II, and spinal cord ependymomas may occur. The gene for NF-II is located on chromosome 22 at 22q11. Merlin, the gene product of the chromosome of NF-II, is a tumor suppressor. *(Karnes, 1071–1076)*

25. **(A)**

26. **(D)**

27. **(B)**

28. **(E)**

29. **(C)**

30. (F)

31. (G)

Explanations 25 through 31

X-linked adrenoleukodystrophy (X-ALD) encompasses widely differing clinical phenotypes that reflect two distinct pathological mechanisms: an inflammatory demyelinating process that leads to a rapidly progressing fatal disorder; and a slowly progressing, distal axonopathy that leads primarily to adrenomyeloneuropathy in young adults. In all forms of X-ALD, very long-chain fatty acids (VLCFAs) accumulate in tissues and body fluids, due to impaired activation of these fatty acids.

Alexander's disease is a lethal leukodystrophy with a variable clinical course. The most common, infantile form is associated with megalencephaly, seizures, developmental retardation, and premature death. Juvenile and adult patients, on the other hand, experience ataxia, spasticity and bulbar signs, with relatively little loss of myelin. Neuroradiological and neuropathological studies show extensive white matter involvement with frontotemporal predominance. The pathological hallmark of Alexander's disease is the accumulation of intracellular inclusions (Rosenthal fibers) exclusively in astrocytes. These consist of aggregated glial fibrillary acidic proteins (GFAP) and small stress proteins.

Canavan's disease is an inherited infantile leukodystrophy that is associated with spongy degeneration of white matter, macrocephaly, severe psychomotor retardation, seizures, and premature death. It is characterized by aspartoacylase deficiency. The enzyme defect leads to the accumulation of N-*acetyl* aspartate (NAA) in brain and body fluids.

Cerebrotendinous xanthomatosis is a lipid storage disorder that is caused by deficiency of the mitochondrial enzyme sterol 27-hydroxylase, which leads to accumulation of cholesterol, and bile alcohols.

Globoid cell leukodystrophy (GLD), also called Krabbe disease, is an inherited neurological disease caused by mutations in the GALC gene, which encodes the lysosomal enzyme galactocerebrosidase that is responsible for the degradation of galactosylceramide and galactosylsphingosine.

The genetic deficiency of the lysosomal enzyme arylsulfatase A (ASA deficiency) causes the neurometabolic disease metachromatic leukodystrophy (MLD). Three major clinical variants have been characterized: late infantile, juvenile, and adult MLD. ASA-deficiency results in impaired degradation of the substrate galactosylsulfatide, which allows biochemical diagnosis of MLD on the basis of arylsulfatase A activity in leukocytes or fibroblasts and galactosylsulfatide excretion in urine. Pelizaeus-Merzbacher disease (PMD) is an X-linked dysmyelinating disorder caused by alterations in the proteolipid protein gene (PLP), which encodes two major proteins of CNS myelin: PLP and its spliced isoform DM20. *(Berger and Moser, 305–312)*

32. (B) Trinucleotide repeat expansion disorders may be arbitrarily divided into 2 types, based on the location of the mutation within their respective genes. This classification is useful because the location of the mutation may have implications regarding the mechanism of pathogenesis.

Type I disorders are those in which the expansion occurs in-frame (i.e., within the coding region) and results in an expanded stretch of amino acids generated by the abnormal gene. Huntington disease, kennedy disease, spinocerebellar ataxia types 1, 2, 3, 6, 7, and 17, dentatorubro-pallidoluysian atrophy, and oculopharyngeal muscular dystrophy are among type I expansion disorders.

Type II disorders are those in which the expansion occurs outside the coding region: either upstream of the coding sequence, downstream of the coding sequence, or within an intron. Spinocerebellar ataxia type 8, 10 and 12, fragile X syndrome, Jacobsen's syndrome, progressive myoclonic epilepsy type I, Friedreich ataxia, and myotonic dystrophy are type II diseases.

In type I disorders the mutant gene is transcribed and translated normally but leads to production of a protein harboring an expanded stretch of a particular amino acid. The trinucleotide expansions in type I disorders tend to be small, with a similar threshold for disease (36–40 trinucleotide repeats, with limited exceptions). To date, in each case of type I disease the mutant protein is endowed with a toxic "gain of function." In general, type I diseases are dominantly inherited (all except spinobulbar muscular atrophy), tend to be of late onset, and manifestations are limited to the nervous system.

Conversely, in type II disorders the coding sequence remains unchanged and the protein product is normal, yet mutations in untranslated regions of the gene lead to abnormal transcription or RNA processing, resulting in altered levels of gene expression. The trinucleotide expansions leading to type II disorders tend to be large, with hundreds to over one thousand trinucleotides. These mutations often result in "loss of function" of the relevant gene. Most of type II disorders are multisystem disorders and tend to have younger ages of onset than type I disorders. *(Taylor et al., 24–25)*

33. **(E)** Frontotemporal dementias occur either in familial forms or, more commonly, as sporadic cases. Neuropathologically, they are characterized by a remarkably circumscribed atrophy of the frontal and temporal lobes of the cerebral cortex, often with additional subcortical changes. An autosomal dominantly inherited familial form of frontotemporal dementia with parkinsonism was linked to chromosome 17q21.2. A major neuropathological characteristic of FTDP-17 is a filamentous pathology made of hyperphosphorylated tau protein. *(Goedert et al., 74–83)*

34. **(C)**

35. **(A)**

36. **(B)**

Explanations 34 through 36

Friedreich ataxia is the most common genetic ataxia and is of autosomal recessive inheritance, with progressive gait and limb ataxia as the cardinal features. It is associated with lower limb areflexia, dysarthria, pyramidal weakness, and sensory loss manifesting later in the course of the disease. The abnormal gene of Freidreich ataxia is located on chromosome 9. The abnormal gene contains an expansion of GAA trinucleotide that numbers between 200 and 900. (Normal chromosomes contain 10–21 GAA repeats). Secondary vitamin E deficiency (precipitated by a beta-lipoproteinaemia or other fat malabsorptive syndromes) is associated with ataxia.

The onset of symptoms occurs between 4 and 18 years of age, with progressive ataxia, areflexia, sensory loss, pyramidal signs, and sometimes cardiomyopathy. Ataxia with selective vitamin E deficiency was linked to chromosome 8q13 in 1993. Subsequently, the mutation was identified in the alpha-tocopherol transfer protein on chromosome 8. Ataxia telangiectasia is an autosomal recessive disease characterized by ataxia, diminished proprioception, areflexia, and dysarthria. The gene defect is located on chromosome 11q. The ataxia-telangiectasia mutated protein has sequence homologies to phosphatidylinositol-3 kinase and may be involved in a check-point response protein to DNA damage. *(Hammans, 327–332)*

37. **(D)** Spinocerebellar ataxia type 6 typically occurs at a later age than other spinocerebellar ataxias, which occur between the ages of 24 and 63 years. It accounts for 5.9% of autosomal dominant cerebellar ataxia in Japan and 13% of those in Germany. The disorder is characterized by gait and limb ataxia, dysarthria, nystagmus, slowing of saccades, signs of corticospinal tract disease, hypotonia, and proprioceptive sensory loss. Other less common features include ophthalmoparesis, spasticity, rigidity, sphincter disturbances, pes cavus or hammer toes, dystonia, and parkinsonism. The disease has a benign course and normal life span. *(Evidente et al., 475–490)*

38. **(A)** Spinocerebellar ataxias (SCAs) are a group of neurodegenerative diseases characterized by cerebellar dysfunction that may be associated with other neurological abnormalities. The expansions of coded CAG trinucleotide repeats was found to cause dominantly inherited SCAs such as SCAs 1, 2, 3, 6, 7, and dentatorubral-pallidoluysian atrophy (DRPLA). The abnormal

CAG triple repeat expansion gives rise to an elongated polyglutamine tract in the respective proteins, leading to a gain in function that is toxic to neurons. Spinocerebellar ataxia type 8 is associated with an expansion of a CTG repeat. *(Tan and Ashizawa, 191–195)*

39. (C)

40. (E)

41. (B)

42. (A)

43. (D)

Explanations 39 through 43

Huntington disease (HD) is an autosomal dominant disorder with high penetrance. The characteristic findings of progressive chorea and dementia are caused by severe neuronal loss, initially in the neostriatum and later in the cerebral cortex. HD was linked to chromosome 4p16.3. The abnormal gene was found to contain an unstable CAG repeat in the open reading frame of its first exon. Normal subjects have a median of 19 CAG repeats (range 11 to 34), whereas nearly all patients with HD have more than 40. The increased number of CAG repeats in the HD gene is expressed as an elongated Huntingtin protein with 40 to 150 glutamine residues.

Spinocerebellar ataxia 3 (SCA-3) or Machado-Joseph disease is characterized by ataxia and lack of coordination. The gene defect is located on chromosome 14 and the gene product is ataxin–3. Spinal bulbar muscular atrophy is an X-linked illness caused by expanded CAG repeats in the coding region of the androgen receptor gene. Dentatorubral-pallidoluysian atrophy (DRPLA) is caused by expanded polyglutamine tracts in the coding region of huntingtin. The gene defect is located on chromosome 12 and the gene product is atrophin. Myotonic dystrophy is CTG repeat triplets disease. The abnormal gene is located on chromosome 19 and the gene product is myotonin. *(Martin, 1970–1980; Price et al., 1079–1083)*

44. (D) Mitochondrial disorders can affect virtually every tissue. However, skeletal muscles and the brain are most often affected. Maternal transmission occurs since the maternal ovum is the source of most mitochondria in a person. The clinical findings depend upon the proportion of normal to abnormal mitochondria in a given patient. This phenomenon is called heteroplasmy. The rate of heteroplasmy differs, often drastically, among maternal family members, and proportion of abnormal mitochondria may vary from one organ to another organ in the same patient. Also, while one might assume that the more mutant DNA a cell has the more abnormalities it will exhibit, in practice the cell develops the disease when the proportion of mutant mitochondrial DNA reaches a threshold. Below this threshold, the cell is normal. This threshold varies among different tissues (some are more sensitive to energy deficiency than others) and different mutations. *(Conneally et al., 120)*

45. (A)

46. (B)

47. (B)

48. (A)

49. (C)

50. (A)

51. (C)

52. (D)

Explanations 45 through 52

In autosomal dominant disorders, a mutation occurring in a single gene on any of the 22 autosomes can produce clinical symptoms or signs. The carrier of a single mutation on one chromosome is called a heterozygote. Each child of an affected person has a 50% risk of inheriting the mutation and potentially developing the disease. Males and females are equally affected, the disease appears over multiple generations, and heterozygote mothers or fathers pass the gene on with equal risk to sons or daughters.

Examples of autosomal dominant neurologic disorders include: neurofibromatosis (NF-I and II), myotonic dystrophy (1 and 2), tuberous sclerosis, juvenile myoclonic epilepsy, Huntington disease, benign neonatal convulsions, and several forms of hereditary ataxias. With autosomal recessive inheritance, the heterozygote carriers of a single mutation are essentially always clinically normal. However, individuals who have inherited a mutation in the same gene from both parents (homozygotes) will show clinical manifestations of the disease. If both parents are carriers of a mutation in the same gene, then each of their children has a 25% risk for being homozygous and having the disease.

Autosomal recessive disorders are usually seen in only one generation, typically among siblings; both males and females can be affected. Examples of autosomal recessive neurologic disorders are phenylketonuria, infantile spinal muscular atrophy, Tay-Sachs disease, Wilson disease, metachromatic leukodystrophy, ataxia-telangiectasia, Lafora body myoclonic epilepsy, Canavan disease, ceroid lipofuscinoses, Friedreich's ataxia, and Niemann-Pick disease.

In X-linked disorders heterozygote female carriers are usually clinically normal, but occasionally have mild manifestations of the disease. In X-linked recessive disorders, each son of a carrier female is at 50% risk for the disease. Each daughter of a carrier female is at 50% risk for also being a carrier. If an affected male has children, his daughters are at 100% risk for being carriers (they must inherit his X chromosome) and his sons are at no risk to inherit the mutation (because they must inherit only the Y chromosome from their father). Thus, X-linked recessive disease shows almost exclusively affected males in multiple generations with transmission through normal carrier females and never shows male-to-male transmission.

Examples of X-linked recessive neurologic disorders include adrenoleukodystrophy, Pelizaeus-Merzbacher disease, Duchenne/Becker muscular dystrophy, Kennedy's spinobulbar muscular atrophy, fragile X mental retardation, Emery-Dreifuss muscular dystrophy, and Fabry lipid storage disease.

Mitochondrial DNA codes for 13 proteins involved in oxidative phosphorylation, ribosomal, and transfer RNAs. Mitochondrial DNA is inherited in the cytoplasm surrounding a mother's egg but not inherited from the sperm of the father. Therefore, mitochondrial disorders are transmitted only by mothers and never by fathers. Male and female children can both be affected. The disease has the potential to appear in all children of an affected mother. Each child of an affected mother may vary in the number of mitochondria they have inherited containing the DNA mutation. Furthermore, the proportion of mutant mitochondria may vary considerably from cell to cell in any given affected individual. Therefore, mitochondrial disorders often show extreme variability in clinical expression both within and between families. Point mutations in mitochondrial DNA tend to be inherited through females, whereas deletions of mitochondrial DNA tend to be sporadic events in isolated individuals. Mitochondrial disorders include the MERRF syndrome (myoclonus epilepsy and ragged-red fibers), the MELAS syndrome (mitochondrial encephalomyopathy, lactic acidosis, and stroke), Leber's hereditary optic atrophy, and Leigh's encephalopathy. *(Bird, 1–17)*

REFERENCES

Berger J, Moser HW, Forss-Petter S. Leukodystrophies: Recent developments in genetics, molecular biology, pathogenesis and treatment. *Curr Opin Neurol.* 2001;14: 305–312.

Bird TD. The language and basic concepts of medical genetics for neurologists. From *Genetics in Neurology.* AAN COURSES 2002.

Conneally M. Neurogenetics. *Continuum.* 2000;6.

Evidente VG, Gwinn-Hardy KA, Caviness JN, Gilman S. Hereditary ataxias. *Mayo Clin Proc.* 2000;75: 475–490.

Goedert M, Ghetti B, Spillantini MG. Tau gene mutations in frontotemporal dementia and parkinsonism linked to chromosome 17 (FTDP-17). Their relevance for understanding the neurogenerative process. *Ann N Y Acad Sci.* 2000;920:74–83.

Haitjema T, Westermann CJ, Overtoom TT, Timmer R, Disch F, Mauser H, Lammers JW. Hereditary hemorrhagic telangiectasia (Osler-Weber-Rendu disease): new insights in pathogenesis, complications, and treatment. *Arch Intern Med*. 1996;156:714–719.

Hammans SR. The inherited ataxias and the new genetics. *J Neurol Neurosurg Psychiatr*. 1996;61:327–332.

Huq AH, Chugani DC, Hukku B, Serajee FJ. Evidence of somatic mosaicism in Sturge-Weber syndrome. *Neurology*. 2000;59:780–782.

Karnes PS. Neurofibromatosis: a common neurocutaneous disorder. *Mayo Clin Proc*. 1998;73:1071–1076.

Martin JB. Molecular basis of the neurodegenerative disorders. *N Engl J Med*. 1999;340:1970–1980.

Price DL, Sisodia SS, Borchelt DR. Genetic neurodegenerative diseases: the human illness and transgenic models. *Science*. 1998;282:1079–1083.

Roach ES. Neurocutaneous syndromes. *Clin N Amer*. 1992;39:591–620.

Sparagana SP. Roach ES. Tuberous sclerosis complex. *Curr Opin Neurol*. 2000;13:115–119

Tan EK, Ashizawa T. Genetic testing in spinocerebellar ataxias: defining a clinical role. *Arch Neurol*. 2001;58: 191–195.

Taylor JP et al: Repeat expansion and neurological diseases. From *Genetics in Neurology*. AAN Courses 2002.

CHAPTER 12

Neuroophthalmology
Questions

1. Balint syndrome is characterized by all of the following EXCEPT

   (A) it results from bilateral extensive parietooccipital damage
   (B) difficulty initiating slow eye movement
   (C) simultagnosia
   (D) optic ataxia
   (E) ocular motor apraxia

Questions 2 through 6
Link each of the following types of nystagmus to the appropriate clinical syndrome.

   (A) Downbeat nystagmus
   (B) See-saw nystagmus
   (C) Spasmus nutans
   (D) Upbeat nystagmus
   (E) Vestibular nystagmus

2. Nystagmus frequently associated with vertigo and tinnitus

3. Nystagmus frequently associated with Arnold-Chiari malformation

4. Head turn, head nodding, and nystagmus

5. Nystagmus associated with posterior fossa tumor

6. Pendular nystagmus with one eye elevated and intorted, and the other eye depressed and extorted associated with suprasellar mass lesion

7. See-saw nystagmus is caused by all of the following EXCEPT

   (A) midbrain stroke
   (B) multiple sclerosis
   (C) Arnold-Chiari malformation
   (D) B12 Deficiency
   (E) head trauma

8. The most likely cause of convergence-retraction nystagmus in a 10-year-old boy is

   (A) congenital aqueductal stenosis
   (B) pinealoma
   (C) brain stem vascular malformation
   (D) multiple sclerosis
   (E) head trauma

9. Opsoclonus in an infant is most likely seen in a case of

   (A) hyperosmolar coma
   (B) brain stem encephalitis
   (C) neuroblastoma
   (D) lung cancer
   (E) toxic encephalopathy

10. Ocular myoclonus, caused by a lesion in the triangle of Guillain and Mollaret, involves all of the following anatomical sites EXCEPT

    (A) interstitial nucleus of Cajal
    (B) red nucleus
    (C) contralateral dentate nucleus
    (D) ipsilateral inferior olive
    (E) ipsilateral dentate nucleus

11. The most common cause of nontraumatic oculomotor nerve palsy with pupillary involvement is

   (A) diabetes
   (B) basilar artery aneurysm
   (C) schwannoma
   (D) aneurysm at the junction of the posterior communicating artery and the internal carotid artery
   (E) cavernous sinus thrombosis

12. Argyll-Robertson pupils may be caused by all of the following conditions EXCEPT

   (A) chronic ethanol abuse
   (B) multiple sclerosis
   (C) diabetes mellitus
   (D) HTN
   (E) sarcoidosis

13. All of the following vitamin deficiencies may cause optic atrophy EXCEPT

   (A) vitamin C
   (B) vitamin B$_{12}$
   (C) pyridoxine
   (D) riboflavin
   (E) folic acid

14. Which of the following is NOT true about ocular myasthenia?

   (A) Ocular involvement occurs in 90% of myasthenic patients in the course of the disease.
   (B) Ocular symptoms account for 75% of initial complaints.
   (C) Approximately 20% of patients with ocular onset of myasthenia progress to involve other muscle groups within 2 years.
   (D) Only one-third of patients with ocular myasthenia have positive acetylcholine receptors antibodies.
   (E) The major ophthalmologic complaints of ocular myasthenia are ptosis and diplopia.

15. Which of the following muscles is the most affected in Graves' disease?

   (A) Superior oblique
   (B) Inferior rectus
   (C) Medial rectus
   (D) Lateral rectus
   (E) Superior rectus

16. Which of the following is true about ophthalmoplegic migraine?

   (A) The onset is in the fourth decade of life.
   (B) The abducens nerve is more often affected than the oculomotor nerve.
   (C) The ophthalmoplegia resolves when the headache clears.
   (D) Pupils and accommodation are frequently involved.
   (E) The ophthalmoplegia is contralateral to the headache

Questions 17 through 22
Match each of the following types of retinal artery obstruction to its etiology.

   (A) Platelet fibrin emboli
   (B) Cholesterol emboli
   (C) Calcium emboli
   (D) Septic emboli
   (E) Myxomatous emboli
   (F) Fat emboli

17. Bacterial endocarditis

18. Bright orange-yellow refractile emboli

19. White intraarterial plug lodged at the bifurcation of the artery

20. Friable mass

21. Gray-white non refractible emboli

22. Long bone

Questions 23 through 29
Link each of the following neurocutaneous diseases to the appropriate visual manifestation.

(A) Neurofibromatosis type I
(B) Neurofibromatosis type II
(C) Tuberous sclerosis
(D) Von Hippel-Lindan
(E) Sturge-Weber syndrome
(F) Ataxia-telangiectasia
(G) Wyburn-Mason syndrome

23. Choroidal hemangioma

24. Bilateral bulbar and conjunctival telangiectasia

25. Posterior subcapsular cataract

26. Retinal hemangioblastoma

27. Retinal astrocytic hematoma

28. Racemose angioma

29. Lisch nodule

30. What is the most likely finding in the fundus examination of the early stage of Leber's disease?

(A) Optic nerve atrophy
(B) Papilledema
(C) Hyperemic optic nerve with telangiectasic capillaries
(D) Optic disc vasculitis
(E) Optic nerve drusen

31. A 25-year-old man with a 3 year history of diabetes underwent a routine ophthalmological examination. His visual acuity was normal. On funduscopic examination, the ophthalmologist noted the following in both eyes: glistening hyaline bodies, absence of disc hyperemia, exudates or hemorrhage. The disc borders are irregular, and the cup is absent. The retinal vessels have a central origin and are trifurcated. Spontaneous venous pulsations are present. This funduscopic report is consistent with

(A) papilledema from increased intracranial pressure
(B) drusen
(C) optic neuritis
(D) early diabetic neuropathy
(E) anterior ischemic optic neuropathy

Questions 32 through 34
Link each of the following eye movements to its most likely cause.

(A) Downbeat nystagmus
(B) Pendular seesaw nystagmus
(C) Square wave jerks

32. Episodic ataxia type II

33. Pituitary tumors

34. Progressive supranuclear palsy

35. Which of the following is TRUE about optic neuritis?

(A) Typically it occurs after the age of 60 years.
(B) Visual acuity is preserved until late in disease progression.
(C) It reduces color vision.
(D) Head MRI is usually normal.
(E) Oral corticosteroids are efficient in hastening recovery from the acute phase and in improving the long-term prognosis.

36. Which of the following is FALSE about anterior ischemic neuropathy?

(A) It is characterized by bilateral painful visual loss.
(B) Migraine is a risk factor in young patients.
(C) Spontaneous improvement of visual loss may occur.
(D) Fundoscopic examination may show flame-shaped hemorrhages near the optic disc margin.
(E) Small optic disc is a predisposing factor for developing nonarteritic form of ischemic optic neuropathy.

37. Disturbance of depth perception is produced by a lesion located in the

    (A) optic chiasm
    (B) optic tract
    (C) optic radiation
    (D) optic nerve
    (E) lateral geniculate body

38. Which of the following is inconsistent with the diagnosis of cortical blindness?

    (A) Loss of vision in both eyes
    (B) Preservation of extraocular movements
    (C) Retinal integrity
    (D) Absence of pupillary constriction to light
    (E) Preserved pupillary constriction to convergence

39. A 50-year-old man developed a subacute mild headache. Neurological examination demonstrated right lid ptosis, right miosis, and right anhydrosis. Cocaine and hydroxyamphetamine drops failed to dilate the affected pupil. The right pupil dilates on 2% epinephrine drops and becomes larger than the left. Among the following diseases, which one is consistent with the above findings?

    (A) Right hypothalamic infarction
    (B) Right lateral medullary infarction
    (C) Malignant mass in the apex of the right lung
    (D) Right brachial plexus trauma
    (E) Right internal carotid artery dissection

40. Which of the following supports the diagnosis of a dilated pupil from Adie's syndrome rather than pharmacologically induced mydriasis?

    (A) Oculomotor nerve palsy
    (B) Ptosis
    (C) Segmental contraction of the pupils on slit lamp examination
    (D) Ophthalmoplegia
    (E) Diplopia

Answers and Explanations

1. **(B)** Balint syndrome is an acquired ocular motor apraxia caused by an extensive bilateral parietooccipital lesion. There is a difficulty in initiating reflexive visually guided saccades and pursuit in all directions with intact vestibular eye movements. Other sign's of Balint syndrome include simultagnosia (inability to perceive more than one object at a time), optic ataxia (inaccurate visual guided pointing), and ocular motor apraxia (difficulty in initiating voluntary saccades). These symptoms are frequently associated with dementia and visual field defects. *(Kline and Bajandas, 68)*

2. **(E)**

3. **(A)**

4. **(C)**

5. **(D)**

6. **(B)**

Explanations 2 through 6

Vestibular nystagmus is characterized by a mixed direction, horizontal-torsional primary position nystagmus. It is of maximal amplitude when the gaze is directed toward the fast component. The nystagmus is suppressed by visual fixation and increased when fixation is removed. The fast phase usually beats away from the damaged end-organ. The nystagmus is usually associated with tinnitus, vertigo, and deafness. Downbeat nystagmus is usually associated with lesions at the craniocervical junction, such as Arnold-Chiari malformation, and is often accentuated during lateral down-gaze. The triad of head turning, head nodding, and nystagmus is highly suggestive of spasmus nutans. Symptoms begin in the first 18 months of life and resolve within the first decade of life. The nystagmus is horizontal or vertical, pendular, low in amplitude, and of high frequency. Upbeat nystagmus has an up phase while the eyes are in primary position of gaze. Reported causes include cerebellar degeneration, multiple sclerosis, brain stem stroke, posterior fossa tumor, and Wernicke's encephalopathy. See-saw nystagmus is a nystagmus with one eye elevated and intorted and the other depressed and extorted, frequently associated with suprasellar mass lesions. *(Kline and Bajandas, 82–85)*

7. **(D)** See-saw nystagmus has been associated with suprasellar mass lesions, midbrain stroke, multiple sclerosis, head trauma, Arnold-Chiari malformation, and congenital causes. *(Kline and Bajandas, 83–84)*

8. **(B)** Convergence-retraction nystagmus is a jerk convergence-retraction movement due to cocontraction of the extraocular muscles, especially on attempted convergence or upward gaze. Its etiology may depend on age. Congenital aqueductal stenosis is the most likely cause in a newborn. At the age of 10 years, pinealoma is the most likely cause. Head trauma and brain stem vascular malformations may cause convergence-retraction nystagmus in the 20- and 30-year-age groups, respectively. Multiple sclerosis (at the age of 40) and basilar artery stroke (at the age of 50) are the most likely causes of convergence-retraction nystagmus. *(Kline and Bajandas, 84)*

9. **(C)** Opsoclonus is a rapid, involuntary, multi-vectorial, and unpredictable conjugate fast eye movement that stops during sleep. Neuroblastoma is the most likely cause of opsoclonus in infant, as a paraneoplastic phenomenon. Autoim-mune brain stem encephalitis that is responsive to ACTH is also seen in infants. In adults, opsoclonus may occur as a paraneoplastic syndrome caused by lung, breast, or ovarian cancer. *(Kline and Bajandas, 87–88)*

10. **(A)** The triangle of Guillain and Mollaret is formed by the following anatomical sites: red nucleus, ipsilateral inferior olive, and contralateral dentate nucleus. *(Kline and Bajandas, 88)*

11. **(D)** In its course toward the cavernous sinus, the oculomotor nerve travels lateral to the posterior communicating artery. The pupillomotor fibers are situated in the periphery of the nerve and are affected early in case of compression of the nerve by an aneurysm at the junction of the posterior communicating and the internal carotid arteries. This is the most common cause of isolated third nerve palsy with pupillary involvement. In cases of ischemic lesions, such as in diabetes, the pathology is confined to the core of the nerve and spares the peripheral pupillomotor fibers. *(Brazis, 168; Kline and Bajandas, 108)*

12. **(D)** Argyll-Robertson pupils are characterized by miotic irregular pupils, absence of pupillary light response with brisk pupillary constriction to near stimuli, normal anterior visual pathway function, and poor dilatation in the dark. The lesion is most likely located in the region of the Sylvian aqueduct in the rostral midbrain, interfering with the light reflex fibers and supranuclear inhibitory fibers as they approach the Edinger-Westphal nuclei. More ventrally located fibers for near response are spared. The classic cause of Argyll-Robertson pupils is neurosyphilis. Other reported causes include diabetes mellitus, multiple sclerosis, sarcoidosis, and chronic alcoholism. *(Kline and Bajandas, 141–142)*

13. **(A)** Deficiency optic neuropathy is characterized by a progressive bilateral visual loss with central or centrocecal scotoma and optic atrophy. Vitamin deficiencies that may be responsible for optic atrophy include vitamin B_{12} or cobalamin, vitamin B_6 or pyridoxine, vitamin B_1 or thiamine, niacin, vitamin B_2 or riboflavin, and folic acid. *(Kline and Bajandas, 166)*

14. **(C)** Myasthenia involves skeletal but not visceral neuromuscular transmission. Therefore, the major ophthalmologic complaints are ptosis and diplopia. Ocular involvement occurs in 90% of myasthenics and accounts for the initial complaint in 75% of cases of myasthenia. Approximately 36% of patients with ocular onset progress to involve other muscle groups within 2 years. Acetylcholine receptor antibodies, if present, are diagnostic of myasthenia, but they are present in only one-third of patients with ocular myasthenia. *(Kline and Bajandas, 473; Kupersmith et al., 243–248)*

15. **(B)** A restrictive myopathy of ocular muscles may occur in Graves' disease, leading to ophthalmoparesis and diplopia. The inferior rectus is the most frequently involved muscle. Its fibrotic shortening leads to elevator palsy. Abduction weakness may occur in case of involvement of the medial rectus, mimicking an abducens nerve palsy. Superior and lateral rectus muscles and superior oblique are less frequently involved. *(Kline and Bajandas, 176; Kupersmith et al., 243–248)*

16. **(D)** The onset of ophthalmoplegic migraine is usually before the age of 10 years. There is always a history of typical migraine. The ophthalmoplegia is ipsilateral to the headache. The oculomotor nerve is affected 10 to 1 over the abducens nerve. The pupils and accommodation are frequently involved. The ophthalmoplegia occurs at the height of the headache, persisting after the headache clears. It may last days to weeks. *(Kline and Bajandas, 207)*

17. **(D)**

18. **(B)**

19. **(A)**

20. **(E)**

21. (C)

22. (F)

Explanations 17 through 22

Platelet fibrin emboli are white intraarterial plugs that lodge at bifurcations; they arise from ulcerative atheromas that may be located in the internal carotid artery. Cholesterol emboli are bright orange-yellow and refractile. The source may be carotid or aortic atheroma. Calcium emboli are gray-white and nonrefractile. They originate from the cardiac valves or the aortic wall, and are usually lodged in retinal arterioles near or on the optic disc. Septic emboli may originate from infected cardiac valves, especially aortic or mitral valves. The sources of fat emboli and myxomatous emboli are long bones and the heart, respectively. *(Kline and Bajandas, 212–214)*

23. (E)

24. (F)

25. (B)

26. (D)

27. (C)

28. (G)

29. (A)

Explanations 23 through 29

Neurofibromatosis type I occurs in approximately 1/3000 persons. It may be inherited as an autosomal dominant trait (the gene is located on chromosome 17q12-22) and produces neurofibromin, a protein that regulates a tumor suppressor gene named oncoprotein ras. The mutated gene leaves the ras unopposed to stimulate cell growth. Clinical manifestations are of cutaneous, ocular, neurological, and visceral organs. Lisch nodules are ocular melanocytic hamartomas, brown or yellow in color. Dome-shaped lesions protrude from the iris surface. They are uncommon prior to age 6, but increase in number with age. Other ocular lesions include eyelid, orbital neurofibromas, and optic nerve gliomas.

Neurofibromatosis type II is characterized by bilateral acoustic neurons. It occurs in 1/50,000 persons. It is inherited as an autosomal dominant trait. The gene is located on chromosome 22 (22q12), a tumor suppressor gene that suppresses a protein called schawannomin. Cutaneous lesions and peripheral neurofibromas are rare. Ocular lesions include posterior subcapsular cataracts, epiretinal membranes, and retinal hamartomas.

Tuberous sclerosis is an autosomal dominant disease with an incidence from 1/6000 to 1/10,000 persons. Spontaneous mutations may occur in up to 66% of cases. The condition is caused by defects, or mutations, on two genes, TSC1 and TSC2; both are believed to be tumor suppressor genes. Only one of the genes needs to be affected for TSC to be present. The TSC1 gene is on chromosome 9 and produces a protein called hamartin. The TSC2 gene is on chromosome 16 and produces the protein tuberin. Seventy-five percent of TSC patients have ocular lesions including retinal astrocytic hamartomas. Multiple lesions are found in one eye; 25% of patients have bilateral lesions.

Von Hippel-Lindau disease occurs in 1/36,000 persons. It is inherited as an autosomal dominant disease with incomplete penetrance. The gene is located on chromosome 3 (3q26) and has a tumor-suppressing function. Ocular manifestations include retinal hemangioblastoma, which is found in both eyes in 50% of patients and 60% of patients have multiple lesions in one eye.

Ocular manifestations of Sturge-Weber syndrome include glaucoma, which is found in 60% of patients before the age of 2 and choroidal hemangioma, which is seen in 40% of patients with Sturge-Weber syndrome. It is located ipsilaterally to the facial angioma (also referred to as port-wine stain), which is one of the criteria for the diagnosis of the disease.

Wyburn-Mason syndrome is also known as retinocephalic vascular malformation. Ocular manifestations include arteriovenous malformation of the retinal, orbital, and optic nerves. Arteriovenous malformation of the retina, also known as racemose angioma, is usually unilateral and most often located in the posterior pole. Arteriovenous malformations are also found in the central nervous system and are symptomatic in 50% of patients.

Ataxia-telangiectasia is inherited as an autosomal recessive trait. Its gene is located on chromosome 11 (11q22-23). The gene encodes a protein called ATM, which is important for cell cycle control and DNA repair. Ocular manifestations of the disease include bilateral bulbar conjunctiva, telangiectasia, and ocular motility disturbances. These include, at the beginning, ocular apraxia that may progress to impairment of smooth pursuit and eventually to complete supranuclear ophthalmoplegia. *(Kline and Bajandas, 249–255)*

30. **(C)** Leber's hereditary optic neuropathy is a maternally inherited disease linked to abnormalities in mitochondrial DNA. In the early stage of the disease, funduscopic examination may show hyperemia of the optic disc, dilatation, and tortuosity of vessels. A classic triad is seen in many cases of Leber's hereditary optic neuropathy, including circumpapillary telangiectatic microangiopathy, swelling of the nerve fiber layer around the disc (pseudoedema), and absence of leakage from the disc or papillary region on fluorescein angiography, distinguishing Leber's hereditary optic neuropathy from a truly swollen disc. *(Walsh and Hoyt, 304–308)*

31. **(B)** This vignette raises the differential diagnosis of an abnormal funduscopic examination in a 25-year-old diabetic male. Although papilledema from increased intracranial pressure is a medical emergency that should not be missed, other less ominous causes of abnormal disc appearance should be considered, such as congenital anomalies, inflammatory processes, ischemia, and diabetic retinopathy. Increased intracranial pressure is characterized clinically by nausea, morning headache, transitory visual obscuration, and ataxia. Visual examination may show an enlarged blind spot and visual field constriction. Color vision and visual acuity are preserved early in the disease. Funduscopy may show the absence of retinal venous pulsations, disc hyperemia, preserved cup, cotton-wool spots, exudates and blurring of vessels in peripapillary area. In this patient the absence of any physical sign suggesting increased intracranial pressure, the preservation of the retinal venous pulsations, and the absence of hyperemia argue against the diagnosis of papilledema.

Optic neuritis may complicate the course of multiple sclerosis rather than diabetes. The patient may report retro-orbital pain on eye movement. Visual examination may demonstrate loss of central acuity and color discrimination, while funduscopic examination may show unilateral disc swelling. The disc appearance may be normal with retrobulbar involvement. The patient in this vignette is asymptomatic and has normal visual acuity. Optic neuritis is unlikely to be the diagnosis.

Ischemic optic neuropathy is the most common cause of acute painless monocular visual loss in the elderly population. It may be seen in patients after the age of 50 years. Diabetes and hypertension are predisposing factors. Funduscopic examination may demonstrate segmental disc edema. Ischemic optic neuropathy is unlikely to be the diagnosis in this patient as he has normal visual acuity. In diabetic retinopathy, funduscopic examination may show microaneurysms, hemorrhages that may occur within the compact middle layers of the retina, hard exudates and retinal edema. Diabetic retinopathy is due to microangiopathy affecting the retinal precapillary arterioles, capillaries, and venules. The funduscopic findings in this patient are not suggestive of diabetic retinopathy. The patient in this vignette is asymptomatic, has normal visual acuity and bilateral irregular disc border with absent cup on funduscopic examination. These findings are highly suggestive of drusen. This is a congenital elevation of the optic disc not associated with cotton-wool spots, peripapillary swelling or hemorrhage. Retinal venous pulsations are preserved. Retinal vessels may appear to originate from the center of the disc. There are no exudates, neovascularization or hyperemia. *(Laskowitz et al., 323–353)*

32. (A)

33. (B)

34. (C)

Explanations 32 through 34

Downbeat nystagmus is a vertical jerk nystagmus. It is exacerbated by looking down and laterally. It is poorly suppressed by visual fixation. Downbeat nystagmus is encountered when lesions affect the vestibular pathways, or in drug intoxication. Downbeat nystagmus is also a feature of episodic ataxia type II, a calcium channelopathy. Pendular see saw nystagmus consists of elevation and intorsion of one eye and synchronous depression and extorsion of the other eye in the first half cycle, followed by change in direction during the next half cycle. It is encountered in diseases affecting the crossing axons of the optic chiasm such as pituitary tumors. Square wave jerks are small conjugate saccades that briefly take the eye away from the fixation position and then return it there. It is a prominent finding in progressive supranuclear palsy. It occurs also in healthy subjects. *(Serra and Leigh, pp. 615–618)*

35. (C) Optic neuritis is an inflammatory disorder of the optic nerve. Its incidence is higher among adults younger than 46 years, where it is the most common cause of acute optic neuropathy. Most cases are idiopathic or associated with MS. Its clinical features may include periocular pain, particularly with eye movement, and progressive visual loss over several days. Visual acuity, color vision, and visual fields are reduced early in disease onset. Funduscopy may show normal optic nerve, or optic disc edema. Head MRI may show white-matter abnormalities identical to those seen in multiple sclerosis in 50% to 70% of cases. Low doses of oral prednisone have no demonstrable efficacy in the recovery of visual function in acute monosymptomatic optic neuritis. Although high dose oral or parenteral methylprednisolone has been shown to have an effect in hastening the recovery of the acute phase of optic neuritis; it does not confer long term benefit on the visual function. *(Kaufman et al., pp. 2039–2044)*

36. (A) Anterior ischemic optic neuropathy (AION) results from an ischemic lesion of the laminar and prelaminar portions of the optic nerve. The disease occurs in patients over 50 years. Diabetes mellitus, hypertension, and giant-cell arteritis are predisposing factors. Migraine and systemic vasculitis particularly increase the risk of AION in young patients. Congenital small optic disc with absent or small central cup is thought to be the major predisposing factor for developing non arteritic AION.

Clinically, AION is characterized by a sudden monocular and painless loss of vision. In about 40% of cases of the nonarteritic form the loss of vision may improve spontaneously over weeks or months. Funduscopic examination may show either hyperemic or pallid disc swelling, with flame-shaped hemorrhages near the margins of the disc. *(Walsh and Hoyt, 138–140)*

37. (A) In addition to the bitemporal field defects, patients with optic chiasmus lesions may develop a disturbance of depth perception. Clinically, the patient complains of difficulties with near tasks such as using precise tools. In such tasks the required convergence causes crossing of the two blind temporal hemifields. This produces a completely blind triangular area of field with its apex at fixation. The image of an object beyond fixation falls on blind nasal retinas and thus disappears; binocular vision, however, is preserved. *(Walsh and Hoyt, 323–327)*

38. (D) Pupillary constriction to light and to convergence is preserved in cortical blindness. Retinal structures are preserved, except if the blindness is caused by prenatal or perinatal injury. *(Walsh and Hoyt, 358–362)*

39. (E) The patient described in this vignette has Horner syndrome. This syndrome can be confirmed and further characterized by pharmacologic tests. The cocaine test is the most commonly used test to confirm the diagnosis. Cocaine blocks the reuptake of norepinephrine into the sympathetic nerve endings. In the normal eye, it causes dilatation of the pupil. This dilatation only occurs if there is continuous release of norepinephrine from the sympathetic nerves.

In case of sympathetic denervation, cocaine fails to dilate the affected pupil.

Hydroxyamphetamine can be used to differentiate between postganglionic and preganglionic Horner syndrome. Hydroxyamphetamine acts by releasing norepinephrine from adrenergic stores in nerve endings. In case of damage to the postsganglionic neuron (third order neuron), norepinephrine stores are depleted, thus hydroxyamphetamine fails to dilate the denervated pupil.

In this vignette, the affected pupil failed to dilate after exposure to cocaine and hydroxyamphetamine. Postganglionic sympathetic neuron dysfunction is the most likely cause. Evidence of denervation supersensitivity to adrenergic substances of the postganglionic neuron is supported by the full dilation of the right pupil after exposure to a 2% solution of epinephrine, a weak direct-acting topical adrenergic drug. Postganglionic Horner syndrome may occur in diseases of the internal carotid artery, such as internal carotid artery dissection or atherosclerosis, and in cavernous sinus infection or tumors.

Lesions of the hypothalamus and lateral medulla cause damage to the first order neuron of the sympathetic pathway. Tumors of lung apex and brachial plexus damage may cause a preganglionic (second order) neuron lesion. *(Walsh and Hoyt, 434–774)*

40. **(C)** Holmes-Adie tonic pupil syndrome is caused by a generalized peripheral or autonomic neuropathy that also affects the ciliary ganglion or the short ciliary nerves. Clinically, the patient has a unilateral or bilaterally dilated pupil(s) that may be confused with pharmacologically induced mydriasis.

The distinction between these two entities can be made by slit lamp examination. Patients with Holmes-Adie tonic pupils have segmental contraction of the iris sphincter. In pharmacological anticholinergic blockade, the sphincter is entirely paralyzed and there is no segmental contraction with light stimulation. *(Walsh and Hoyt, 450–455)*

REFERENCES

Brazis PW. *Localization in Clinical Neurology*. 3rd ed. Boston, MA: Little, Brown;1996.

Kaufman DI. Trobe JD. Eggenberger ER. Whitaker JN. Practice parameter: the role of corticosteroids in the management of acute monosymptomatic optic neuritis. Report of the Quality Standards Subcommittee of the American Academy of Neurology. *Neurolog*. 2000;54: 2039–2044.

Kline & Bajandas: *Neuroophtalmology Review Manual*. 5th ed. New York, NY: Slack;2001.

Laskowitz D, Liu GT, Galetta SL. Acute visual loss and other disorders of the eyes. *Neurolog Clin*. 1998;16: 323–353.

Serra A, Leigh RJ. Diagnostic value of nystagmus: spontaneous and induced ocular oscillations. *J Neurol, Neurosurg Psychiatr*. 2003;73:615–618.

Miller NR, Newman NJ (eds.). *Walsh & Hoyt's Clinical Neuro-Ophthalmology: The Essentials*. 5th ed. New York, NY: Lippincott, Williams & Wilkins;1999.

CHAPTER 13

Neurooncology
Questions

1. What is the most likely diagnosis of a well-circumscribed lobulated mass displacing the brain that, on microscopic examination, exhibits perivascular pseudorosettes?

    (A) Oligodendroglioma
    (B) Pilocytic astrocytoma
    (C) Fibrillary astrocytoma
    (D) Germ cell tumor
    (E) Ependymoma

2. Ependymomas have

    (A) a predominant male to female incidence
    (B) a predominant supratentorial location in the adult population
    (C) thoracic predominance when located in the spinal cord
    (D) an association with neurofibromatosis type II when there is multifocal spinal cord involvement
    (E) a peak incidence at the age of 23 years

3. Myxopapillary ependymomas occur most frequently in the

    (A) fourth ventricle
    (B) third ventricle
    (C) cervical spinal cord
    (D) conus-cauda-filum terminal
    (E) lumbar spinal cord

4. The most frequent location of choroid plexus papillomas in children is

    (A) lateral ventricle
    (B) third ventricle
    (C) suprasellar region

    (D) cerebellopontine angle
    (E) multifocal ventricular involvement

5. The most common location of germ cell tumors in the central nervous system is the

    (A) basal ganglia
    (B) thalamus
    (C) pineal region
    (D) cerebellum
    (E) brain stem

6. Hormonal assays indicate that most meningiomas express receptors to

    (A) androgen
    (B) glucocorticoid
    (C) estrogen
    (D) progesterone
    (E) somatostatin

7. The most frequent location of intracranial meningiomas is

    (A) olfactory groove
    (B) parasagittal/falcine
    (C) sphenoidal ridge
    (D) optic sheath
    (E) choroid plexus

8. Psammoma bodies are seen in

    (A) glioblastoma
    (B) pituitary adenoma
    (C) ependymoma
    (D) medulloblastoma
    (E) meningioma

9. What is the most common location of intracranial schwannomas?

(A) Facial nerve
(B) Abducens nerve
(C) Trigeminal nerve
(D) Oculomotor nerve
(E) Optic nerve

10. The presence of a biphasic architectural pattern composed of Antoni A and Antoni B areas is a hallmark of

(A) meningiomas
(B) gliomas
(C) ependymomas
(D) oligodendrogliomas
(E) schwannomas

11. Neurofibromas are composed of

(A) Schwann cells
(B) astrocytes
(C) oligodendrocytes
(D) melanocytes
(E) neuronal cells

12. The most frequent pituitary secreting adenomas is the

(A) prolactinoma
(B) growth hormone adenoma
(C) TSH secreting adenoma
(D) ACTH secreting adenoma
(E) FSH/LH secreting adenoma

13. What is the dominant type of hormone secreting cell seen in the normal anterior lobe of the pituitary gland?

(A) Prolactin-secreting cells
(B) Adrenocorticotrophin-secreting cells
(C) Thyrotrophin-secreting cells
(D) Growth hormone-secreting cells
(E) Luteinizing stimulating hormone-secreting cells

14. An astrocytoma of intermediate differentiation with the presence of nuclear atypia and mitotic activity, but without necrosis or endothelial proliferation, is best classified as

(A) pilocytic astrocytoma (WHO Grade I)
(B) fibrillary astrocytoma (WHO Grade II)
(C) anaplastic astrocytoma (WHO Grade III)
(D) glioblastoma multiforme (WHO Grade IV)
(E) pleomorphic xanthoastrocytoma (WHO Grade II)

15. Which of the following immunohistochemical reactions helps to differentiate glioblastoma from metastatic melanoma?

(A) Glial fibrillary acidic protein
(B) S-100 protein
(C) HMB 45
(D) Vimentin
(E) Keratin

16. All of the following tumors often appear as a cystic lesion with an enhancing mural nodule on gadolinium-enhanced MRI imaging EXCEPT

(A) oligodendroglioma
(B) ependymoma
(C) pilocytic astrocytoma
(D) hemangioblastoma
(E) ganglion cell tumor

17. Which of the following neoplasms is typically located near the foramen of Monro as an intraventricular mass?

(A) Lymphoma
(B) Medulloblastoma
(C) Oligodendroglioma
(D) Dysembrioplastic neuroepithelial tumor
(E) Central neurocytoma

Questions 18 through 22
Link each of the following molecular abnormalities to the most likely nervous system neoplasm.

(A) p 53 suppressor on 17p 13.1
(B) CDKN2 suppressor
(C) N-myc oncogene

(D) Neurofibromin

(E) Tubulin

18. Tuberous sclerosis

19. Anaplastic astrocytoma

20. Neuroblastoma

21. WHO Grade II astrocytoma

22. von Recklinghausen neurofibromatosis

23. The presence of cellular pleomorphism, nuclear atypia, and marked mitotic activity with the absence of necrosis and endovascular proliferation is highly suggestive of

(A) WHO Grade I astrocytoma

(B) WHO Grade II astrocytoma

(C) WHO Grade III astrocytoma

(D) glioblastoma multiforme

(E) gemistocytic astrocytoma

24. The most consistent chromosomal abnormality in glioblastoma multiforme is

(A) gain of chromosome 7

(B) gain of chromosome 17p

(C) loss of chromosome 1p

(D) loss of chromosome 11p

(E) loss of chromosome 9q

25. PTEN gene (Phosphatase and tensin homologue gene located on chromosome 10) mutations occur most commonly in cases of

(A) oligodendroglioma

(B) medulloblastoma

(C) pilocytic astrocytoma

(D) anaplastic astrocytoma

(E) de novo glioblastoma

26. Which of the following molecular features is shared between well-differentiated oligodendrogliomas and anaplastic oligodendrogliomas?

(A) Loss of heterozygosity on chromosome 15

(B) Deletion of CDKN2A gene

(C) Loss of heterozygosity on chromosome 4

(D) Loss of heterozygosity on chromosome 1p

(E) Mutation of the PTEN gene

27. What is the most common endocrine abnormality seen in suprasellar germ cell tumors?

(A) Precocious puberty

(B) Diabetes insipidus

(C) Impotence

(D) Acromegaly

(E) Amenorrhea

28. The most efficacious single agent in the chemotherapeutic treatment of malignant gliomas is

(A) nitrosourea derivatives (BCNU, CCNU)

(B) procarbazine

(C) temozolomide

(D) vincristine

(E) carboplatine

29. Which of the following statements is true about primary central nervous system lymphoma in immunocompetent patients?

(A) It is more common before the age of 40.

(B) Glucocorticoids should be administrated before stereotactic biopsy.

(C) The survival rate significantly improves with tumor resection.

(D) B lymphocyte phenotype is found in more than 80% of cases.

(E) It is resistant to radiation therapy.

30. The most frequent brain tumor in the pediatric population is

(A) craniopharyngioma

(B) brain stem glioma

(C) medulloblastoma

(D) germ cell tumor

(E) ependymoma

31. Which of the following statements is true about medulloblastoma?

    (A) It typically arises from the vermis and the roof of the fourth ventricle.
    (B) Its peak incidence is at the age of 20 years.
    (C) Hydrocephalus is usually seen late in the course of the disease.
    (D) High tyrosine protein kinase C receptors expression may be an indicator of poor prognosis.
    (E) Radiotherapy has a modest benefit in the management of medulloblastoma.

32. Which of the following criteria suggests a higher risk for disease recurrence in the case of medulloblastoma?

    (A) Posterior fossa location of the tumor
    (B) Age of the patient over 4 and under 21 years at the time of the diagnosis
    (C) Decreased tyrosine kinase C receptor activity
    (D) Total resection of nondisseminated tumor
    (E) None of the above

33. Cerebrospinal fluid alphafetoprotein may be elevated in

    (A) choroid plexus tumors
    (B) ependymomas
    (C) medulloblastomas
    (D) germ cell tumors
    (E) craniopharyngiomas

34. The most frequent origin of brain metastasis is

    (A) breast cancer
    (B) lung cancer
    (C) skin cancer
    (D) kidney cancer
    (E) unknown primary site

35. The most frequent origin of metastasis causing epidural spinal cord compression is

    (A) prostate
    (B) lung
    (C) lymphoma
    (D) GI tract
    (E) breast

Answers and Explanations

1. **(E)** Ependymomas arise throughout the neuraxis, often in an intraventricular location. In the adult population, 60% of ependymomas are supratentorial and 40% are infratentorial. Among the pediatric population, ependymomas are the third most common intracranial tumor after pilocytic astrocytomas and primitive neurectodermal tumors. About 30% of them appear before the age of 3 years and about 50% before the age of 5 years. Nearly 90% of pediatric ependymomas are intracranial and only 10% are intraspinal. Approximately, two-thirds of intracranial ependymomas in children occur in the infratentorial compartment. Classic ependymomas grow as demarcated soft, gray masses that arise in the ventricular system. In the posterior fossa, they may fill the fourth ventricle and pass through its exit foramina. On microscopic examination, ependymomas are generally composed of uniform cells with indistinct cytoplasmic borders and round or oval nuclei. The nuclear/cytoplasmic ratio varies; it is usually high, but infrequent nodules of densely packed cells may be scattered throughout paucicellular areas. The pseudorosette is a perivascular anuclear zone of radial fibrillary processes that taper toward a vessel and is a hallmark of ependymomas. Less commonly, ependymomas show the characteristic epithelial features of true ependymal pseudorosettes. *(Parisi, 6–8)*

2. **(D)** Most ependymomas occur in childhood, with a peak incidence between 1 and 5 years. Males and females are nearly equally affected. In the adult population, infratentorial ependymomas are more common. Ependymomas represent 60% of intramedullary gliomas of the spinal cord, most arising in the filum terminale (as myxopapillary variants) and occurring primarily in adults. Multifocal spinal cord ependymomas are associated with neurofibromatosis type II. *(Parisi, 6–8)*

3. **(D)** Myxopapillary ependymomas appear as well-defined, sausage-shaped lesion located in the cauda equina and tend to distend it. Hemorrhagic rupture of these tumors may result in seeding of the subarachnoid space. *(Parisi, 6–8)*

4. **(A)** The site of predilection for the development of choroid plexus papillomas is the lateral ventricle in children, and the fourth ventricle in adults. *(Parisi, 9–10)*

5. **(C)** Central nervous system germ cell tumors are most common in children and adolescents, with a peak incidence between the ages of 10 and 12 years. They are more common in males than females, with an overall male to female ratio of 2.5/1. The most common locations of germ cell tumors are the pineal and the suprasellar regions. Occasionally, these tumors may occur in the basal ganglia, thalamus, and other sites in the central nervous system. *(Jones, 2)*

6. **(D)** Meningiomas may become clinically evident during pregnancy or during the luteal phase of the menstrual cycle, suggesting that growth of meningiomas may be hormonally related. Hormone assays indicate that most meningiomas express receptors to progesterone, rather than estrogen or both hormones. *(Parisi, 1)*

7. **(B)** Approximately 90% of meningiomas are intracranial, while 9% are intraspinal. The most frequent intracranial location is the skull base (planum spheroidale, sphenoid wing, the petrous ridge, etc.), and at sites of dural reflection (falx, tentorium, etc.). Other less frequent locations include the tuberculum sella, olfactory groove, foramen magnum, optic nerve sheath, and choroid plexus. *(Parisi, 11; Whittle et al., 1535–1543)*

8. **(E)** Psammoma bodies are concentrically laminated calcifications seen in meningiomas. *(Parisi, 2)*

9. **(C)** Schwannomas account for approximately 8% of all primary intracranial neoplasms. The most common intracranial schwannomas develop from the vestibular nerve and occupy the posterior cranial fossa. The second most common intracranial schwannomas develop from the trigeminal nerve and account for less than 8% of intracranial schwannomas. Trigeminal schwannomas are encapsulated masses that are predominantly solitary. They are more common in females with an age range of 35 to 60 years. Facial nerve schwannomas are less frequent than trigeminal schwannomas, followed by glossopharyngeal, vagus, and spinal accessory nerve schwannomas. Schwannomas involving the oculomotor, trochlear, abducens, and hypoglossal nerves are rare. Intraparenchymal schwannomas are very rare. Since the olfactory and optic nerves do not have a Schwann cell layer, they do not develop schwanommas. *(Parisi, 6–7)*

10. **(E)** The microscopic hallmark of schwannomas is a biphasic histological pattern composed of distinct compact (Antoni A) areas intermixed with loose microcytic (Antoni B) areas. The Antoni A regions are cellular but lack the mitotic figures of a malignant nerve-sheath tumor. The identification of an encapsulated schwann cell tumor implies a benign nature. The Antoni B areas are hypocellular and lack a patterned arrangement. Cells are loosely arranged in a myxoid matrix accompanied by thin strands of collagen. Occasional mast cells may be identified in the Antoni B area. *(Parisi, 7)*

11. **(A)** Schwann cells, perineural cells, and fibroblasts are all present in neurofibromas. *(Parisi, 9)*

12. **(C)** Pituitary adenomas represent the third most common primary intracranial neoplasm encountered in neurosurgical practice, with a reported annual incidence ranging from 1 to 14.7 per 100,000 persons. It may account for approximately 10% to 15% of primary brain tumors. Prolactinomas have the highest incidence among pituitary-secreting tumors. They account for 40% to 60% of functioning adenomas and are the most common subtype of pituitary tumor diagnosed in adolescents. Men are generally diagnosed in their fourth and fifth decades, whereas women are generally diagnosed earlier. GH-secreting adenomas represent nearly 30% of all functioning tumors, followed by ACTH adenomas, which account for 15% to 25% of all functioning adenomas. TSH- and LH/FSH-secreting tumors are the least frequent functioning pituitary adenomas. An immunocytochemical study of 100 subclinical pituitary adenomas discovered at autopsy found that 50% of them were null cell adenomas (nonhormone-secreting adenoma) and 45% were prolactinomas. *(Freda and Wardlaw, 3859–3866; Lafferty and Chrousos, 4317–4323; McComb et al., 488)*

13. **(D)** The normal adenohypophysis pituitary gland comprises growth hormone-secreting cells (somatotroph cells), prolactin-secreting cells (lactotroph cells), ACTH-secreting cells (corticotroph cells), LH/FSH-secreting cells (gonadotroph cells), and TSH-secreting cells. The total composition of secreting cells in the pituitary gland is as follows:

- 50% growth hormone-secreting cells
- 10% to 30% prolactin-secreting cells
- 10% to 20% ACTH-secreting cells
- 10% LH/FSH-secreting cells
- 5% TSH-secreting cells *(Scheithauer, 2)*

14. **(C)** The World Health Organization has assigned four grades to the spectrum of astrocytic tumors: grade I (pilocytic astrocytoma), grade II (diffuse astrocytoma), grade III (anaplastic astrocytoma), and grade IV (glioblastoma multiforme). The pilocytic astrocytoma is one of the most benign forms of astrocytic tumors. The 10-year survival in supratentorial cases is generally over 90% in most studies, after gross total resection, and 74% after subtotal resection. Most, but not all,

pilocytic astrocytomas occur in children or young adults. They are most abundant in the cerebellum, where they represent the majority of childhood astrocytomas. They are also found in the region of the third ventricle, thalamus, hypothalamus, and neurohypophysis, where they can be difficult to treat due to their location near clinically sensitive brain structures.

"Pilocytic" means "hair cell," referring to one of the major microscopic features of this tumor, namely parallel bundles of elongated, fibrillar cytoplasmic processes resembling mats of hair. These hair-like processes contain large amounts of glial fibrils that stain well with either PTAH (Mallory phosphotungstic acid and hematoxylin stain) or immunoperoxidase for GFAP (glial fibrillary acidic protein).

Diffuse (low-grade) Grade II astrocytomas are well-differentiated, diffusely infiltrative neoplasms, composed of fibrillary astrocytes with nuclear atypia but no mitoses. Anaplastic astrocytomas are Grade III astrocytomas. They are characterized by an intermediate differentiation, increased cellular density, increased nuclear pleomorphism, and moderately increased nuclear hyperchromatism plus mitoses. The lack of endothelial proliferation and foci of coagulation necrosis in anaplastic astrocytic gliomas distinguishes them from glioblastomas, but individual cells with pyknotic nuclei may be interspersed in anaplastic astrocytomas.

Glioblastoma multiforme (Glioblastoma) is classified as a Grade IV astrocytoma. It is a glioma that may be uniformly undifferentiated, but may contain focal areas of differentiation, including oligodendroglioma, and rarely ependymoma-like elements. Endothelial proliferation (increased density of cells in vascular walls), necrosis, nuclear atypia, and mitotic activity are the most important characteristic of grade IV astrocytoma. The pleomorphic xanthoastrocytoma is a bizarre supratentorial astrocytoma of young individuals that often involves both leptomeninges and cerebral cortex. It is occasionally hemorrhagic. Its fibrillary, pleomorphic, hyaline, and lipid-laden multinucleated giant cells are clues to its diagnosis. Protein granular degeneration may be prominent, similar to that seen in pilocytic astrocytomas. Intracellular lipid content varies from abun-

dant to absent between individual tumors. Astrocytomas are characterized by strong GFAP-positive cells, often with histiocytic features. *(Scheithauer, 1–2)*

15. **(C)** HMB 45 staining is useful because it is specific for melanoma. Both melanoma and glioblastoma can react with S-100 proteins and vimentin. Glioblastomas may or may not react with GFAP (Glial fibrillary acidic protein) and keratin. Glioblastomas lack reactivity to HMB 45, whereas metastatic melanoma reacts specifically with this immunohistochemical stain, which is helpful in differentiating between these two tumors. *(Scheithauer, 15)*

16. **(A)** The following tumors may appear cystic with an enhancing mural nodule: Pleomorphic xanthoastrocytoma, pilocytic astrocytoma, ganglion cell tumors, hemangioblastoma, and ependymoma. *(Burger, 295)*

17. **(E)** Central neurocytomas are rare large intraventricular globular masses, commonly straddling the midline in the region of the septum pellucidum. They can obstruct the flow of cerebrospinal fluid, resulting in increased intracranial pressure and hydrocephalus. Other intraventricular masses arising near the foramen of Monro include colloid cysts, subependymomas, and subependymal giant cell astrocytomas. *(Burger, 296)*

18. **(E)**

19. **(B)**

20. **(C)**

21. **(A)**

22. **(D)**

Explanations 18 through 22

Mutations of two different genes (TSC1 at 9q34 and TSC2 at 16p13.3) result in the tuberous sclerosis complex (TSC). It is inherited as an autosomal dominant trait with a high rate of spontaneous mutations in the TSC genes (65% to 75% of patients arise from new mutations).

Tubulin is the gene product of TSC2. Although the phenotypic expression of TSC is highly variable, it is not determined by the specific gene mutation. In fact, even affected members of the same family often develop very different manifestations. Neurofibromin belongs to the family of GTPase-activating proteins (GAPs), which turn off the growth-promoting function of the Ras family of proteins by stimulating the hydrolysis of GTP bound to Ras. Without enough neurofibromin, Ras remains unchecked, resulting in cellular overgrowth and tumors. Mutation of neurofibromin gene causes Neurofibromatosis 1 (NF1), also known as von Recklinghausen disease. It is an autosomal dominant condition caused by mutations of the NF1 gene, which is located on chromosome 17q11.2.

Mutation in the p53 tumor-suppressor gene may be seen in WHO Grade II astrocytoma. The gene is located on chromosome 17p13.1. It encodes nuclear phosphoprotein, a transcription factor which enables passage through cell cycle. The most common genetic abnormality observed in anaplastic astrocytomas and glioblastomas is cell cycle regulatory pathway defects, such as inactivation of the CDKN2A and B genes. The N-myc gene plays an essential role in organogenesis. Gene overexpression due to genomic amplification has been observed in many human tumors such as the common childhood tumor neuroblastoma. *(Davis, 846–847; Rasheed et al., 162–167; Sparagana and Roach, 115–119; Tai et al., 255–262)*

23. **(C)** WHO Grade III astrocytomas (also called anaplastic astrocytomas) diffusely infiltrate the surrounding brain parenchyma and have an intrinsic tendency for malignant progression to glioblastoma. Histological examination shows greater cellular and nuclear atypia than seen in grade II astrocytoma, but there is absence of necrosis and microvascular glomeruli or festoons seen in glioblastoma. Glioblastoma multiforme is the most common primary malignant tumor in adults and is characterized by the presence of endothelial proliferation (increased density of cells in vascular walls), necrosis, nuclear atypia, and mitotic activity. Grade II astrocytomas are slow-growing, diffusely infiltrating, well-differentiated astrocytomas. Histologically, they are composed of well-differentiated astrocytes exhibiting moderate cellular density and nuclear atypia. Gemistocytic astrocytoma is a variant of astrocytoma with a tendency towards rapid progression to glioblastoma. Pilocytic astrocytomas (WHO Grade I) are typically circumscribed, slow-growing, cystic neoplasms. Histologically, they are characterized by a biphasic pattern of compact bipolar cells and loose textured, multipolar cells, the presence of Rosenthal fibers, microcysts, and eosinophilic granular bodies. *(Hildebrand, 11)*

24. **(A)** The most consistent chromosomal changes in glioblastoma multiforme are gains of chromosome 7, losses of chromosomes 9p, 10 and 17p, and genetic amplification represented by the presence of double-minute chromosomes (Small extrachromosomal segments of amplified DNA sequences containing oncogenic alleles). *(Hildebrand, 12)*

25. **(E)** The PTEN gene (phosphatase and tensin homologue deleted from chromosome 10) encodes a protein that dephosphorylates phospatidylinositol-3,4,5-triphosphate (PIP3), thus inactivating a cellular growth pathway. Growth factor receptors activate phospatidylinositide-3-kinase (PI3K), which phosphorylates phospatidylinositol-4,5-diphosphate (PIP2) to PIP3, thus activating protein kinase B (PKB). Activated PKB stimulates cell growth, and blocks apoptosis. PTEN shuts off this pathway, suppressing oncogenesis. Analyses of LOH (loss of heterozygosity) have consistently shown losses of all or part of chromosome 10 in more than 80% of glioblastoma cases and have showed a common deletion region in distal 10q. PTEN mutations and overexpression of EGFR (epidermal growth factor receptors) are more common in primary de novo tumors rather than secondary progressing glioblastoma multiformes. *(Rasheed et al., 162–167; Weiss, 543–548)*

26. **(D)** Anaplastic oligodendrogliomas share many molecular features with well-differentiated oligodendrogliomas, including loss of heterozygosity for 19q, 1p, or both. In contrast to well-differentiated oligodendrogliomas, anaplastic oligodendrogliomas can exhibit allelic loss of 9p,

homozygous deletion of the CDKN2A gene, and losses involving chromosomes 4, 14, 15, and 18. Anaplastic oligodendrogliomas with 1p deletions, especially if coupled with 19q loss, have a better response to chemotherapy and improved prognosis. *(Hildebrand, 15)*

27. **(B)** Diabetes insipidus is the most likely endocrine manifestation of germ cell tumors in the suprasellar areas. Precocious puberty is the most frequent endocrine disorder seen in hamartoma and hypothalamic glioma. Impotence, amenorrhea, galactorrhea, and acromegaly are seen in pituitary tumors. *(Hildebrand, 31)*

28. **(A)** Nitrosourea derivatives (BCNU, CCNU) remain for many neurooncologists the most effective single agents with a 20% to 30% partial or complete response rate and 20% to 30% rate of stabilization. *(Hildebrand, 48)*

29. **(D)** The incidence of primary central nervous system lymphoma (PCNSL) in immunocompetent patients increased fivefold during the last decades for unknown reasons. Most central nervous system lymphomas occur in patients over the age of 50 years, with a median onset of 58 years. There is a slight preponderance of men among immunocompetent patients. PCNSL has a poor prognosis if untreated, with a median survival of 3 to 4 months. The predominant locations of PCNSL are the corpus callosum, frontal lobes, and deep periventricular structures of the brain. Most PCNSLs are non-Hodgkin lymphomas, with approximately 80% of them are non-Hodgkin B cell lymphoma. The clinical features of the disease may include deterioration of cognitive function, headache, and seizures. When lymphoma is suspected, a biopsy should be performed before starting treatment, particularly with glucocorticosteroids. In about 50% of patients, the tumor responds to steroid administration and occasionally may transiently disappear completely, compromising the pathologic diagnosis and delaying treatment. PCNSL can be initially highly sensitive to the combination of radiation therapy and glucocorticosteroids, which increases the median of survival from a few to 12 to 18 months. High doses of methotrex-

ate can extend 5-year survival rates to about 20%, but when combined with radiation therapy, it is associated with significantly delayed neurotoxicity, especially in individuals over the age of 60. However, tumor resection does not significantly improve survival. *(DeAngelis, pp. 687–691; Hildebrand, 54–56)*

30. **(C)** Medulloblastoma is the most common malignant brain tumor of childhood with a peak incidence around the first decade of life and a male-to-female preponderance of about 2 to 1. It is a member of the primitive neuroectodermal tumor family of central nervous system neoplasms and is considered a Grade IV lesion by the World Health Organization. *(Reddy and Packer, 681–685)*

31. **(A)** Medulloblastomas are invasive embryonal tumors of the cerebellum with a tendency to metastasize in the central nervous system (CNS). They represent 10% to 20 % of brain tumors and 30% of tumors localized in posterior fossa. The peak incidence of medulloblastoma is in the first decade of life, with an annual incidence of 0.5 per 100,000 children. In the brain, medulloblastoma typically arises in the vermis of the cerebellum or roof of the fourth ventricle, causing ataxia and signs of hydrocephalus early on. At the time of the diagnosis, over 80% of children have hydrocephalus. Tyrosine protein kinase C receptor (TrkC) is expressed on mature granular cells. It is also the receptor for neurotropin-3, which is one of the regulators of cerebellar granular cell development. TrkC expression in medulloblastoma correlates with a favorable clinical outcome. The management of patients with medulloblastoma includes surgical resection followed by craniospinal radiation. With this treatment, patients with average-risk disease (patients who have localized tumor totally or nearly totally resected by surgery) have approximately a 60% 5-year progression-free survival. The addition of chemotherapy to the management of high-risk patients with medulloblastoma (patients with disseminated disease or partially resected tumor) may improve the outcome. *(Reddy and Packer, 681–685; Hildebrand, 61)*

32. (C) Factors associated with poor outcome in medulloblastoma include nonposterior fossa location, disseminated tumor, nondisseminated incompletely resected tumor with residual tumor greater than 1.5 cm in its greatest dimension, decreased tyrosine protein kinase C receptor activity, and age less than 3 years at the time of diagnosis. *(Hildebrand, 61)*

33. (D) Alpha fetoprotein and β-HcG are elevated in the cerebrospinal fluid of the majority of patients with mixed germ cell tumors, while only β-HcG is elevated in patients with choriocarcinomas. *(Hildebrand, 72)*

34. (B) Brain metastases are seen in approximately 15% to 20% of cancers. The most frequent primary tumor associated with brain metastasis is nonsmall cell lung cancer, which represents about 50% of brain metastases. Breast cancer is the second most frequent cause of brain metastases and represents about 19% of all brain metastases. Skin/melanoma brain metastases represent about 10.5% of total brain metastasis, whereas GI metastases account for about 10% of all brain metastases. Unknown primary site metastases represent 11% of brain metastases. *(Kleihues et al., 252; Hildebrand, 76)*

35. (E) The most frequent origin of metastasis, causing epidural spinal cord compression, is the breast (it represents 22% of epidural metastasis). Other origins include lung, prostate, and malignant lymphoma with about 15%, 10%, and 10% of epidural spinal cord compression cases, respectively. *(Kleihues et al., 252)*

REFERENCES

Burger PC. Pathologic analysis of central nervous system surgical specimens. *Neuropathology review.* AFIP Course 2002.

Davis RL. Neurofibromin progress on the fly. *Nature.* 2000;403:846–847, 2000.

DeAngelis LM. Primary central nervous system lymphoma. *Curr Opin Neurol.* 1999;12:687–691.

Freda PU, Wardlaw SL. Diagnosis and treatment of pituitary tumors. *J Clin Endocrinol Metab.* 1999;84:3859–3866.

Hildebrand J, ed. Clinical relevance of advances in molecular biology. From Tumors of the brain and spinal cord. *Continuum.* 2001:7.

Jones RV. Germ cell tumors of the central nervous system. *Neuropathology review.* AFIP Course 2002.

Kleihues P et al. *Pathology & Genetics of Tumors of the Nervous System. World Health Organization Classification of Tumors.* Lyons, France: IARC Press; 2000.

Lafferty AR, Chrousos GP. Pituitary tumors in children and adolescents. *J Clin Endocrinol Metab.* 1999;84:4317–4323.

McComb DJ, Ryan N, Horvath E, Kovacs K. Subclinical adenomas of the human pituitary. *Arch Path Lab Med.* 1983;107:488–491.

Parisi JE. Other glial tumors. *Neuropathology review.* AFIP Course 2002.

Rasheed BK. Wiltshire RN. Bigner SH. Bigner DD. Molecular pathogenesis of malignant gliomas. *Curr Opin Oncol.* 1999;11:162–167.

Reddy AT. Packer RJ. Medulloblastoma. *Curr Opin Neurol.* 1999;12:681–685.

Scheithauer BW. *Pituitary tumors.* Neuropathology review. AFIP Course 2002.

Sparagana SP, Roach ES. Tuberous sclerosis complex. *Curr Opin Neurol.* 2000;13:115–119.

Tai KF, Rogers SW, Pont-Kingdon G, Carroll WL. Definition of the human N-myc promoter region during development in a transgenic mouse model. *Pediatr Res.* 1999;46:255–262.

Weiss WA. Genetics of brain tumors. *Curr Opin Pediatr.* 2000;12:54354–8.

Whittle IR, Smith C, Navoo P, Collie D. Meningiomas. *Lancet.* 2004;363:1535–1543.

CHAPTER 14

Movement Disorders
Questions

1. The combination of generalized seizures with ataxia and dementia is seen in all of the following conditions EXCEPT

   (A) Huntington disease
   (B) neuronal ceroid lipofuscinosis
   (C) Lafora disease
   (D) GM2 gangliosidosis
   (E) mitochondrial encephalomyelopathy

2. Alien limb occurs significantly in case of

   (A) Huntington disease
   (B) corticobasal degeneration
   (C) Parkinson disease
   (D) Wilson disease
   (E) carbon monoxide intoxication

3. Which of the following is true about the dorsal prefrontal circuit?

   (A) It originates in the frontal convexity and projects to the nucleus accumbens.
   (B) The circuit involves the ventral posterolateral nucleus of the thalamus.
   (C) Lesion of the circuit results in deficits in executive function and motor programming.
   (D) The mini mental test is typically impaired in cases of prefrontal cortex lesion.
   (E) The prefrontal circuit is particularly spared in Huntington disease.

4. Lesion of the lateral orbitofrontal circuit results in

   (A) contralateral hemiplegia
   (B) depression
   (C) reduced executive function
   (D) apathy
   (E) disinhibition

5. Lesion of the anterior cingulate circuit results in

   (A) apathy
   (B) euphoria
   (C) agitation
   (D) hallucination
   (E) loss of executive function

6. Which of the following movement disorders carries the highest risk of depression with suicide?

   (A) Huntington disease
   (B) Parkinson disease
   (C) Progressive supranuclear palsy
   (D) Wilson disease
   (E) Gille de la Tourette syndrome

7. The main movement disorder associated with apraxia is

   (A) Parkinson disease
   (B) Huntington disease
   (C) Creutzfeldt-Jacob disease
   (D) corticobasal degeneration
   (E) Wilson disease

8. Which of the following is characteristic of dementia in Parkinson disease?

   (A) Aphasia
   (B) Agnosia
   (C) Psychomotor slowing
   (D) Amnesia
   (E) Apraxia

9. Cerebral blood flow studies showed that when untreated Parkinson disease patients are asked to perform a paced movement with a joystick, there is a decrease of the blood flow in the

   (A) sensorimotor cortex
   (B) lateral premotor cortex
   (C) lateral parietal cortex
   (D) contralateral anterior cingulate
   (E) ipsilateral lentiform nucleus

10. Age-related mitochondrial deletion is most frequently seen in the

    (A) putamen
    (B) globus pallidus
    (C) hippocampus
    (D) cerebellum
    (E) cerebral cortex

11. Inherited dystonia is caused by a defect of the oxidative phosphorylation complex involving

    (A) complex I (NADH)
    (B) complex II (Succinate)
    (C) complex III (Ubiquinone)
    (D) complex IV (Cytochrome oxidase)
    (E) complex V (Adenosine triphosphate)

12. The neurotoxin 1 methyl-4-phenyl-1,2,3,6 tetrahydropyridine (MPTP) may cause Parkinson disease. It acts by

    (A) inhibiting monoamine oxidase B in basal ganglia neurons
    (B) increasing ATP generation
    (C) blocking complex I of the oxidative phosphorylation complex

    (D) blocking complex II of the oxidative phosphorylation complex
    (E) blocking complex V of the oxidative phosphorylation complex

13. Proximal limb kinetic apraxia is caused by a lesion in the

    (A) primary motor cortex
    (B) supplementary motor cortex
    (C) lateral premotor cortex
    (D) cingulate motor area
    (E) parietal cortex

14. The motor component of the basal ganglia-thalamocortical circuits is processed by the

    (A) caudate
    (B) globus pallidus internal segment
    (C) nucleus accumbens
    (D) globus pallidus external segment
    (E) putamen

Questions 15 through 22
Link each of the following neurotransmitters or neuroanatomical structures to the appropriate basal ganglia pathway (direct and indirect).

    (A) Direct pathway of the basal ganglia
    (B) Indirect pathway of the basal ganglia
    (C) Both
    (D) Neither

15. GABA

16. Enkephalin

17. Substance P

18. Globus pallidus internal segment

19. Globus pallidus external segment

20. Subthalamic nucleus

21. Glutamine

22. Glycine

23. A 65-year-old man died from a progressive dementia complicating a parkinsonian syndrome poorly responsive to levodopa. Pathological examination showed a shrinking globus pallidus associated with atrophy of the subthalamic nucleus and pallor of the substantia nigra with enlargement of the aqueduct of sylvius. The most likely diagnosis is

   (A) Huntington disease
   (B) progressive supranuclear palsy
   (C) multisystem atrophy
   (D) Parkinson disease
   (E) corticobasal degeneration

24. Which of the following is associated with an increased risk of Parkinson disease?

   (A) Vitamin E
   (B) Manganese
   (C) Caffeine
   (D) Cigarette smoking
   (E) Alcohol

25. Which of the following is true about 1-methyl-4-phenyl-1,2,3,6 tetrahydropyridine (MPTP)?

   (A) MPTP induced parkinsonism has more resting tremor than idiopathic Parkinson disease.
   (B) MPTP is oxidized inside the neuron into MPP+.
   (C) MPTP inhibits mitochondrial respiration in astrocytes.
   (D) MPP+ inhibits mitochondrial complex I, which results in failure of ATP synthesis.
   (E) MPTP has a cocaine-like mechanism of action.

26. Which of the following is the most disabling in Parkinson disease?

   (A) Tremor
   (B) Akinesia
   (C) Rigidity
   (D) Postural instability
   (E) Depression

Questions 27 through 34
Link the following.

   (A) D1 receptors
   (B) D2 receptors
   (C) Both
   (D) Neither

27. Olfactory tubercle

28. It stimulates adenylate cyclase

29. Clozapine

30. Bromocriptine

31. 5q31-q34

32. 3q13.3

33. Medulla

34. Haloperidol

35. The administration of L dopa, three times per day, to a 73-year-old man diagnosed with early stage Parkinson disease may show a sustained motor response because of

   (A) hypersensitivity to L dopa
   (B) presynaptic storage of exogenous dopamine
   (C) half-life of L dopa (8 hours)
   (D) post synaptic storage of L dopa
   (E) none of the above

Questions 36 through 43
Link the following.

   (A) Anticholinergic drug
   (B) MAOB inhibitor drug
   (C) Anti-NMDA receptor effect
   (D) Dopamine agonist drug
   (E) COMT drug
   (F) Glutamic acid releases inhibition

36. Entacapone

37. Pergolide

38. Tolcapone

39. Selegiline

40. Benztropine

41. Pramipexole

42. Remacemide

43. Riluzole

44. The most common neurobehavioral abnormality observed in Parkinson disease is

(A) depression
(B) personality change
(C) panic attacks
(D) illusion
(E) hallucination

45. Which of the following differentiate supranuclear palsy from Parkinson disease?

(A) Staring gaze
(B) Absence of tremor
(C) Flexed posture
(D) Hypersensitivity to dopamine
(E) Gait disturbance late in the progression of the disease

46. The earliest sign of progressive supranuclear palsy is

(A) dysarthria
(B) visual symptoms
(C) gait difficulties
(D) dysphagia
(E) dementia

47. Which of the following is NOT in favor of the diagnosis of supranuclear palsy?

(A) Absence of tremor
(B) Vertical gaze palsy
(C) Preserved horizontal oculocephalic reflex
(D) Early cerebellar sign
(E) Neck rigidity greater than limb rigidity

Questions 48 through 53
Link the following.

(A) Parkinson disease
(B) Progressive supranuclear palsy
(C) Both
(D) Neither

48. Cerebral cortical and midbrain atrophy on MRI of the head

49. Neurofibrillary tangles

50. Symmetric axial rigidity with postural instability

51. Positive L dopa response in early stage of the disease

52. Cerebellar atrophy

53. Down-gaze palsy

54. Which of the following cerebral cortical layers are the most affected in case of progressive supranuclear palsy?

(A) Layers I and II
(B) Layers III and V
(C) Layers IV and VI
(D) Layers III and IV
(E) Layers V and VI

Questions 55 through 59
Link each of the following toxic causes of Parkinson disease to the corresponding anatomical damage in the basal ganglia.

(A) Caudate
(B) Putamen
(C) Globus pallidus
(D) Substantia nigra

55. MPTP

56. Manganese

57. Cyanide

58. Methanol

59. Carbon monoxide

60. A bilateral decrease of signal intensity on head MRI T-2 weighted images in the globus pallidus of a 20-year-old man with a history of Parkinson syndrome is highly suggestive of

(A) Hallervorden–Spatz disease
(B) neuroacanthocytosis
(C) Rett syndrome
(D) MPTP intoxication
(E) diffuse Lewy body disease

61. Tremor is most commonly caused by which of the following drugs?

(A) Phenytoin
(B) Phenobarbital
(C) Valproic acid
(D) Carbamazepine
(E) Lamotrigine

62. Which of the following is true about the huntingtin protein?

(A) It is formed by consecutive proline residues encoded by a CCG repeat.
(B) Its gene is located on the long arm of chromosome 4.
(C) It is expressed in neuronal and non neuronal cells.
(D) The pattern of huntingtin expression is parallel to areas of huntington pathology.
(E) Huntingtin is a nuclear protein; its location is altered in case of Huntington disease.

63. Which of the following is true about the clinical features of Huntington disease?

(A) The severity of chorea correlates with the disease progress.
(B) Chorea is the most disabling symptom.
(C) Excecutive function is selectively lost.
(D) Apraxia is the earliest sign of cognitive impairment.
(E) Opticokinetic nystagmus is typically conserved.

64. The unpleasant sensation of internal restlessness that is partially relieved by volitional movement in a patient on chronic neuroleptic treatment is called

(A) dystonia
(B) akathisia
(C) choreic movement
(D) tics
(E) myoclonus

65. What is the initial treatment of choice for a 15-year-old teenager who is complaining of motor tics related to Tourette syndrome?

(A) Clonidine
(B) Haloperidol
(C) Fluoxetine
(D) Botulinum toxin
(E) Clonazepam

66. Which of the following is true about the disturbance of eye movements in cases of cerebellar lesion?

(A) Saccadic dysmetria results from a lesion of the dorsal vermis.
(B) Gaze-evoked nystagmus is seen in case of a lesion of the fastigial nucleus.
(C) Lesion of the nodulus results in impaired smooth tracking.
(D) Lesion of the floculus results in impairment of the duration of the vestibular response.
(E) Parafloculus lesion causes saccadic dysmetria.

67. Which of the following molecular abnormalities is related to stiff-man syndrome?

(A) Abnormal CAG repeat
(B) Abnormal CCG repeat
(C) Glutamic acid decarboxylase antibodies
(D) Abnormal cooper metabolism
(E) Alpha synuclein abnormality

68. Which of the following gene mutations is seen in Parkinson disease?

(A) Huntingtin gene
(B) Alpha synuclein
(C) Adhalin gene
(D) Dystrophin gene
(E) Synaptophysin gene

Answers and Explanations

1. **(A)** Progressive myoclonic epilepsy (PME) is a slowly progressive autosomal recessive disorder occurring in late childhood or early adulthood. Generalized seizures, ataxia, and dementia are prominent features. Linkage analysis has shown that the gene responsible is located on the long arm of chromosome 21q22.3. The common causes of PME are neuronal ceroid lipofuscinosis, mitochondrial encephalomyelopathy, sialidosis, Lafora disease, Baltic myoclonus, GM2 ganglisidosis, and dentatorubropallidoluysian atrophy. *(Evidente et al., 475–490)*

2. **(B)** Alien limb is defined as the lack of recognition of movement in the affected limb, or a feeling that one limb is foreign associated to observable involuntary motor activity. The upper extremity is the most frequently affected limb. Signs include the failure to perceive ownership of one's limb in the absence of visual cues, an impression that the visual limb is foreign, personification of the affected limb, and autonomous motor activity deemed by the patient as beyond voluntary control. Alien limb syndrome is a well-established part of the corticobasal degeneration. It is reported to complicate the course of the disease in nearly 50% of cases. Vascular etiology is most commonly reported in ischemic or hemorrhagic lesions of the anterior cerebral artery. Surgical lesions such as corpus callosotomy and thalamotomy have been associated with alien limb. Other causes of alien limb include Alzheimer's disease and Creutzfeldt-Jacob disease. *(Hanna and Doody, 135–145)*

3. **(C)** The dorsal lateral prefrontal circuit originates in the frontal lobe convexity and projects to the dorsolateral head of the caudate and subsequently to the dorsomedial globus pallidus and rostral substantia nigra. These structures project to ventral anterior and medial dorsal thalamic nuclei, which connect back to the dorsolateral prefrontal cortex. Lesion of this circuit results in deficit in executive function and motor programming. The patient exhibits difficulties in maintaining or shifting set, generating organizational strategies, and retrieving memory. The dorsolateral prefrontal circuit is assessed by the Wisconsin Card sort test. The circuit is disturbed in Huntington disease, as the degenerative process involves the caudate nucleus. *(Watts and Koller, 15)*

4. **(E)** The lateral orbitofrontal circuit of the frontal subcortical pathways originates in the inferolateral prefrontal cortex and projects to the ventromedial caudate nucleus, which then projects to the dorsomedial globus pallidus and substantia nigra. The return pathway is via the ventral anterior and dorsothalamic nuclei, which project back to the orbitofrontal cortex.

   Lesion of the orbitofrontal circuit causes personality changes with irritability and disinhibition (similar to personality changes seen in idiopathic calcification of the basal ganglia and neuroacanthocytosis). *(Watts and Koller, 16)*

5. **(A)** The anterior cingulate circuit of the subcortical frontal lobe pathway originates in the anterior cingulate gyrus and projects to the ventral striatum, which include the nucleus accumbens, olfactory tubercles, and parts of the caudate and putamen. The ventral striatum then sends afferents to the globus pallidus and substantia nigra, which in turn project to the paramedian part of

the medial dorsal thalamus. The thalamus projects back to the cingulate gyrus. Lesion of the anterior cingulate circuit causes apathy, reduced drive and initiative, and decreased motivation. Akinetic mutism and profound apathy may result from bilateral lesions of the anterior cingulate circuit. *(Watts and Koller, 16)*

6. **(A)** Depression may complicate the course of a number of movement disorders. Among all movement disorders, Huntington disease carries the highest risk of depression with suicide. Depression may affect half of the patients, with 30% meeting the criteria of major depression. Suicide is four to six times more common in Huntington disease patients than in other depressed patients. In one study including Huntington disease patients and their relatives, the rate of death caused by suicide reached 7.3%. Depression may complicate the course of Parkinson disease patients in approximately 40%. Depression is seen in 20% to 30% of patients with the diagnosis of Wilson disease. Depression is less frequently seen in progressive supranuclear palsy, and Gilles de la Tourettes' disorders. *(Di Maio et al., 293–295; Poewe and Luginger, S2–6; Watts and Koller, 17)*

7. **(D)** Apraxia is the inability to perform motor acts despite intact comprehension, cooperation, and motor and sensory skills. Corticobasal degeneration is the main movement disorder associated with apraxia (reported in 71% of cases in one series). The disorder is attributed to neuronal loss and achromasia in the frontoparietal cortex. *(Watts and Koller, 23)*

8. **(C)** Studies of the frequency of dementia in patients with Parkinson disease (PD) have found rates ranging from 8% to 81%. The addition of mental impairment to the motor symptoms of PD increases the functional impairment and the need for health care in patients with PD. The dementia in PD is of the subcortical type. It is characterized by a psychomotor slowing (also called bradyphrenia), memory retrieval deficits, abnormal cognition with impaired ability to manipulate knowledge, and disturbed executive function. Aphasia, apraxia, agnosia, and amnesia are absent. *(Watts and Koller, 23)*

9. **(D)** When normal subjects perform paced movements with a joystick in freely selected directions with their right hand, there is an increase of the cerebral blood flow in the contralateral lentiform nucleus and sensorimotor cortex, and bilateral increase of the blood flow of the anterior cingulate, supplementary motor cortex, lateral premotor cortex, and dorsolateral prefrontal cortex. When an untreated Parkinson disease patient performs the same task, there is normal activation of sensorimotor cortex, lateral premotor cortex, and lateral parietal association areas. There is, however, decreased activation of the contralateral lentiform nucleus, anterior cingulate, supplementary motor area, and dorsolateral prefrontal area. *(Watts and Koller, 33)*

10. **(A)** The susceptibility of the central nervous system to somatic mitochondrial mutations is high and occurs with age in specific brain regions. The caudate and putamen are the locations of the highest accumulation of mitochondrial DNA mutations, whereas the cerebellum and myelinated axons have the lowest level of mitochondrial DNA mutations. *(Watts and Koller, 54)*

11. **(A)** Complex I specific activity as determined by the nicotinamide adenine dinucleotide ubiquinone assay is reduced in brains of patients with inherited dystonia compared to controls. *(Watts and Koller, 58)*

12. **(C)** 1-methyl-4-phenyl-1,2,3,6-tetrahydropyridine (MPTP) induces parkinsonism by causing selective degeneration of nigral neurons. 1-Methyl-4-phenylpyridinium ion (MPP+), the oxidative metabolite of MPTP, is actively taken up into dopaminergic neurons through the dopamine transporters and concentrated within dopaminergic neurons. In nigral neurons, MPP+ inhibits complex I of the mitochondrial electron transport chain and the A-ketoglutarate dehydrogenase complex (KGDHC) of the Krebs cycle. This has been considered as the major mechanism of neuronal death in MPTP-induced PD, although other mechanisms such as apoptosis have also been postulated. *(Mizuno et al., 893–902)*

13. **(C)** The control of proximal limb musculature and interlimb coordination is related to the lateral

premotor area of the cortex. This is suggested by the heavy projections from this region to the medial pontomedullary reticular formation, which spinal projections constitute the bulk of the ventromedial descending brain stem system that is associated with control of the proximal musculature. Lesion of the lateral premotor cortex causes a proximal limb kinetic apraxia that contrasts sharply with the bimanual distal apraxia of the supplementary motor cortex. Such patients may have difficulties making coordinate rotatory movements of both shoulders whereas independent movement of either shoulder is performed with ease, within the limits of any associated weakness. *(Watts and Koller, 76)*

14. **(E)** Motor circuitry is initiated in cortical regions that transmit parallel glutaminergic projections to the striatum. The motor component of the basal ganglio-thalamocortical circuits is processed by the putamen; whereas the caudate and nucleus accumbens mediate cognitive, emotive, and limbic processes. *(Hallett, 177–183; Watts and Koller, 100)*

15. **(C)**

16. **(B)**

17. **(A)**

18. **(C)**

19. **(B)**

20. **(B)**

21. **(B)**

22. **(D)**

Explanations 15 through 22

The spiny neurons of the putamen are the principal input/output cells of the striatum. These cells project to the internal segment of the globus pallidus via two separate pathways: direct and indirect pathways. The direct pathway involves a subpopulation of spiny cells using GABA and substance P as neurotransmitters, and projecting directly to the internal segment of the globus pallidus and the substantia nigra pars reticulata, which are the output nuclei of the basal ganglia. The indirect pathway involves another subpopulation of spiny cells that use GABA and enkephalin as neurotransmitters and project to the external segment of the globus pallidus, which sends GABAergic projections to the subthalamus. The subthalamic nucleus projects to the internal part of the globus pallidus and substantia nigra, using glutamate as a neurotransmitter. This model of neurotransmission suggests that there is an equilibrium between the direct pathway, tending to reduce the basal ganglia output, and the indirect pathway, tending to increase the output from the internal segment of the globus pallidus and substantia nigra. *(Watts and Koller, 99–100)*

23. **(B)** The pathologic features mentioned in this question are highly suggestive of progressive supranuclear palsy (PSP). Typical PSP patients present with early postural instability, supranuclear vertical gaze palsy, parkinsonism (bradykinesia and axial more than limb rigidity) resistance to levodopa therapy, pseudobulbar palsy, and subcortical dementia. Subsequent to the onset of postural instability, dysarthria and bradykinesia are the most common problems. An absent, poor, or waning response to levodopa is a characteristic feature defining the atypical parkinsonian disorders. Often, although not always, patients with these disorders may exhibit axial more than limb muscle involvement.

Several features should make us suspect that a patient may suffer from PSP. Early instability and falls, particularly during the first year of symptom onset, should suggest the diagnosis of PSP. However, early instability and falls may also rarely develop in patients with corticobasal degeneration (CBD), when asymmetric symptoms develop in the lower extremities. Instability and falls may also develop early in multiple system atrophy (MSA), although these symptoms are usually present when patients already exhibit autonomic disturbances.

Marked slowing of vertical saccades usually precedes the development of vertical supranuclear gaze palsy and should readily point toward the diagnosis of PSP. The saccades in

CBD may have increased latency but normal speed, and are similarly affected in the vertical and horizontal planes, whereas in MSA the saccades have normal speed and latency. Patients with PSP may present prominent early or severe speech and swallowing difficulties and may exhibit oversized mouthfuls or over-stuffing the mouth when eating, but these features may also be present in CBD.

Neuropathologically, PSP is characterized by abundant neurofibrillary tangles and/or neuropil threads in particular areas of the basal ganglia and brain stem; neuronal loss and gliosis are variable. Neurofibrillary tangles, neuronal loss, and gliosis in PSP affect the striatum, pallidum, subthalamic nucleus, substantia nigra, oculomotor complex, periaqueductal gray, superior colliculi, basis pontis, dentate nucleus, and prefrontal cortex. *(Litvan, 41–48)*

24. **(B)** The only definite risk factor for Parkinson disease is age. However, epidemiological studies have suggested an increased risk of Parkinson in males, those with a family history of the disease, exposure to iron, farming, rural residence, steel alloy industries, and herbicide and pesticide exposure. Manganese was found to increase the incidence. Smoking cigarettes is consistently associated with a decreased risk for Parkinson disease. However, whether this association is truly caused by cigarette smoking, or instead reflects a personality characteristic or another behavior associated with smoking is not known. Caffeine was recently reported to decrease the risk of Parkinson disease. Other factors associated with decreased risk of Parkinson disease include vitamin E, tocopherol, and alcohol consumption. *(Ross et al., 2674–2679; Tanner and Aston, 427–430)*

25. **(D)** MPTP-induced parkinsonism is very much like idiopathic Parkinson disease, except for the resting tremor, which is less frequent with MPTP intoxication. In the brain, MPTP is taken up into astrocytes, where it is oxidized to MPP+ by monoamine oxidase B. MPP+ is then actively taken up into nigrostriatal neurons through dopamine transporters and concentrated in dopaminergic neurons. MPP+ inhibits mitochondrial respiration in the dopaminergic neurons,

which causes the selective death of that type of cell. MPP+ inhibits mitochondrial complex I and NADH-linked state 3 respiration causing a loss of oxidative phosphorylation mechanism and fall in the ATP level. *(Watts and Koller, 162)*

26. **(D)** Among the cardinal signs of Parkinson disease, postural instability is usually the last sign to appear, the most disabling and the least treatable. Postural instability results from the combination of changes in postural adjustment, loss of postural reflexes, rigidity, and akinesia. *(Watts and Koller, 187)*

27. **(C)**

28. **(A)**

29. **(D)**

30. **(B)**

31. **(A)**

32. **(D)**

33. **(D)**

34. **(B)**

Explanations 27 through 34

Dopamine receptors are divided into five subtypes based on their action on adenylate cyclase: D1-like receptors include D1 and D5 and are able to stimulate adenylate cyclase. D2-like receptors include D2, D3, and D4 and are able to inhibit adenylate cyclase. D1 receptors are encoded by a gene located on chromosome 5, D2 and D4 receptor genes are located on chromosome 11, D3 receptors are coded by a gene located on chromosome 3, and D5 receptors are encoded by a gene located on chromosome 4. D1 and D2 receptors are located mainly in the striatum and substantia nigra in the postsynaptic areas, although D2 and D3 receptors also have presynaptic locations. The olfactory tubercle contains both D1 and D2 receptors; the medulla contains D4 receptors. D2 receptors have bromocriptine as an agonist and haloperidol as an antagonist. Clozapine is a selective D4 receptor antagonist. *(Watts and Koller, 202)*

35. **(B)** Despite the short half-life of L dopa (60 minutes), patients in early stages of the disease may experience a sustained motor response with the administration of L dopa three or four times per day. This sustained response is speculated to be caused by storage of exogenous dopamine in presynaptic terminals in survival dopaminergic striatal cells. *(Watts and Koller, 204)*

36. **(E)**

37. **(D)**

38. **(E)**

39. **(B)**

40. **(A)**

41. **(D)**

42. **(C)**

43. **(F)**

Explanations 36 through 43

Neuroprotective therapies can be defined as medical or surgical interventions that favorably alter the underlying etiology or pathogenesis and thus delay the onset, slow, or even halt the progression of the neurodegenerative process such as Parkinson disease (PD). Selegiline was found to prevent parkinsonism induced by the oxidated form of 1-methyl-4-phenyl-1,2,3,6-tetrahydropyridine (MPTP), which has stimulated interest in an antioxidative therapy to retard the progression of PD. Selegiline acts as a "suicide substrate" for monoamine oxidase (MAO) type B, irreversibly inhibiting this enzyme. Selegiline has a levodopa-sparing effect, and it smoothes out levodopa-related motor fluctuations, possibly by prolonging dopamine-induced responses in midbrain dopaminergic neurons.

Remacemide, an anticonvulsant with anti-NMDA effects, has been shown to enhance the effects of levodopa in parkinsonian rats and monkeys. It may have a neuroprotective effect in PD and Huntington disease. The rationale behind using remacemide as a neuroprotective agent is that in Parkinson disease, there is an increased activity in the subthalamic nucleus and internal segment of the globus pallidus. The subthalamic nucleus provides an excitatory glutaminergic input to the internal part of the globus pallidus. Glutamate inhibition would be expected to improve parkinsonism.

Riluzole, a drug approved for the treatment of amyotrophic lateral sclerosis, acts primarily by inhibiting glutamic acid release and noncompetitively blocking NMDA receptors, and as such it may exert antiexcitotoxic effects similar to those of NMDA antagonists.

Tolcapone and entacapone are catechol-O-methyl transferase (COMT) inhibitors that may be used as an adjuvant therapy to dopamine for the management of PD.

Dopamine agonists exert their pharmacological effect by directly activating dopamine receptors, bypassing the presynaptic synthesis of dopamine. Several new dopamine agonists, cabergoline, pramipexole and ropinirole, have been added to the previously known potent antiparkinsonian drugs bromocriptine and pergolide. Pramipexole differs from the ergot dopamine agonists such as bromocriptine and pergolide in its preferential affinity for the D3 receptor subtype. The drug has been shown to be safe and effective when used as monotherapy in the early stages of PD. Benztropine has an anticholenergic action. *(Jankovic, 785–790)*

44. **(A)** Depression is the most frequent neurobehavioral abnormality seen in Parkinson disease, with a prevalence of 25% to 40%. Depression may appear before the emergence of the first motor signs and does not correlate with the severity of the disease. Psychotic signs such as illusion or hallucination are among the most disabling complications of L dopa treatment in Parkinson disease. They are seen in 8% to 15% of patients with Parkinson disease, especially elderly patients who show signs of impaired cognition and have longer duration on L dopa treatment. Other neurobehavioral abnormalities seen in Parkinson disease include sleep

alterations, personality change, anxiety, and panic attacks. *(Watts and Koller, 257–259)*

45. (B) Progressive supranuclear palsy is characterized by gait disturbance with multiple falls, erect posture with retrocollis, contracted facial muscles, bradykinesia, predominantly proximal rigidity, vertical supranuclear gaze abnormalities, and spastic dysarthria. Progressive supranuclear palsy can be differentiated from Parkinson disease by the presence of contracted rather than flaccid face, undirected rather than staring gaze, erect rather than flexed posture, spastic dysarthria, and absence of rest tremor. *(Watts and Koller, 279)*

46. (C) Early instability and falls, supranuclear vertical gaze palsy and poor response to levodopa are features highly suggestive of the diagnosis of progressive supranuclear palsy (PSP). Other features of PSP include subcortical dementia and pseudobulbar palsy. Marked slowing of vertical saccades is seen earlier than the development of vertical supranuclear palsy in PSP. Instability and falls may also develop in corticobasal degeneration as well as in early multiple system atrophy (MSA), although these symptoms are usually present when patients already exhibit autonomic disturbances. The saccades in CBD may have increased latency but normal speed, and are similarly affected in the vertical and horizontal planes, whereas in MSA the saccades have normal speed and latency. *(Litvan, 41–48)*

47. (D) The presence of early or prominent cerebellar signs, unexplained polyneuropathy, and prominent noniatrogenic dysautonomia other than isolated postural instability contradict the diagnosis of progressive supranuclear palsy. *(Watts and Koller, 280)*

48. (B)

49. (B)

50. (B)

51. (A)

52. (D)

53. (B)

Explanations 48 through 53

MRI of the head does not show specific abnormalities in most patients with the diagnosis of progressive supranuclear palsy. However, it may show more prominent cerebral cortical atrophy than in Parkinson disease. In moderate to advanced stages, there may be a thinning of the anteroposterior diameter of the midbrain tectum and tegmentum with atrophy of the colliculi and disproportionate enlargement of the sylvian fissures and posterior third ventricle. Cerebellar atrophy is seen in multisystem atrophy. The presence of neurofibrillary tangles is necessary for the neuropathological diagnosis of progressive supranuclear palsy. Most of these neurofibrillary tangles are rounded in shape, whereas in Alzheimer's disease most of them have a flame-shaped form. Clinically, patients with progressive supranuclear palsy have a symmetric neurological deficit, prominent axial rigidity, postural instability, and severe vertical gaze restriction. In Parkinson disease, the neurological symptoms are not symmetric, axial rigidity and postural instability are less prominent than in progressive supranuclear palsy, and there is a good response to L dopa early in the course of the disease. *(Watts and Koller, 281–283)*

54. (E) The cerebral cortex is one of the major areas of primary involvement in progressive supranuclear palsy. Motor strip 4 and the ocular motor association areas are the most important sites of pathology. Area 17, the primary visual cortex, is the least affected. The large pyramidal and small neurons of layers V and VI are the most affected layers of the cerebral cortex in progressive supranuclear palsy; layers III and V are the most affected in Alzheimer's disease. *(Watts and Koller, 283)*

55. (D)

56. (C)

57. (C)

58. (B)

59. (C)

Explanations 55 through 59

MPTP induces parkinsonism by selective damage to the substantia nigra. MPTP is converted by glial cells to MPDP+, which is then converted to MPP+ and enters dopaminergic neurons through a dopamine uptake system. MPP+ induces mitochondrial damage, causing cell death. Overexposure to manganese may cause Parkinson syndrome by inducing selective neuronal loss in the globus pallidus, probably by increasing auto-oxidation of dopamine by a higher valence ion, causing an increase in the generation of free radicals. Carbon monoxide intoxication may cause Parkinson syndrome, with more damage in the white matter and globus pallidus. Carbon monoxide causes tissue anoxia. The globus pallidus is vulnerable to anoxic injury, probably from intrinsic metabolic susceptibility. Pathological changes after acute cyanide intoxication have demonstrated selective destruction of the basal ganglia, especially the globus pallidus. Cyanide radicals inactivate cytochrome oxidase and other oxidative systems, leading to cell death. Methanol intoxication causes a bilateral necrosis of the putamen, optic atrophy, and widespread lesions of the cerebral cortex. Methanol is metabolized to formic acid, which achieves high concentration in the putamen and causes selective damage there. *(Watts and Koller, 315–332)*

60. (A) Hallervorden–Spatz syndrome (HSS) is a rare autosomal recessive disease that has been mapped to chromosome 20p12.3–p13. The symptoms usually start in childhood and involve the cognitive, speech, and motor domains. Children demonstrate signs of cognitive and motor regression, the speech becomes dysarthric, and extrapyramidal symptoms appear.

Typical symptoms at onset involve difficulty walking or postural abnormalities. Personality changes and cognitive changes infrequently are the presenting symptoms. Rigidity gradually progresses. Spasticity associated with hyperreflexia is seen in over half of the cases. Dysarthria becomes evident in all cases. Dystonia, chorea, and tremor are also seen. Ophthalmic abnormalities are seen in HSS patients including pigmentary retinopathy and optic atrophy. Movement disorders associated with HSS include rigidity, which can involve half of the body, axial structures, arms, legs or be generalized. Dystonia is also seen, typically involving the facial musculature and the feet.

Parkinsonism as an initial manifestation is rare, and usually occurs only in adult-onset cases. In rare adult-onset cases presenting symptoms can be indistinguishable from PD. The cognitive abnormalities are common in HSS. They may precede the motor symptoms of the disease. Seizures can also be seen in this disorder. The disease usually starts between the ages of 7 and 12 years. The disorder typically progresses and leads to death within 20 years.

Definitive diagnosis of HSS can only be made histologically. Presumptive clinical diagnosis is based on the constellation of the clinical signs, supported by the neuroimaging data. CT scanning may reveal cerebral atrophy with increased ventricular size. Mineralization of the globus pallidus is also seen. Hyperlucency of the putamen and globus pallidus is seen on CT scanning. MR imaging is more sensitive. There is decreased T–2 weighted and proton density signal in the globus pallidus, which is caused by iron deposition. In some patients there is a hyperintense area within the area of hypointensity, the "eye of the tiger" sign. Pathologically, the hallmark of the disease, is rust-brown discoloration of the pars reticulata of the substantia nigra and the internal segment of the globus pallidus. The pigmentation is caused not only by the abnormal iron deposition, but also by high concentration of the organic pigments lipofuscin and neuromelanin. *(Colcher and Simuni, 629–649)*

61. (C) Valproic acid is the most common cause of tremor among antiepileptic medications. Chronic treatment with valproic acid may cause a tremor in up to 25% of patients. Occasionally, phenytoin and carbamazepine have been reported to cause tremor. *(Watts and Koller, 350)*

62. **(C)** An aberrant expansion of glutamines in the protein huntingtin causes Huntington disease (HD), a neurodegenerative disorder that strikes in middle age. The HD gene is located on the short arm of chromosome 4. It is a CAG repeat located in exon1 of a 67 exon gene, which is transcribed into huntingtin. Huntingtin is expressed in neuronal and non-neuronal tissues, suggesting that its normal function is not confined to cells in the areas of HD. Huntingtin is a cytoplasmic protein that conserves its location in HD.

The pattern of huntingtin expression does not parallel the region of HD neuropathology. Only a small subset of neurons that express huntingtin in neuronal popuplation succumb to the effect of HD. It has been presumed that mutant huntingtin with its extra glutamines is toxic to neurons, possibly because it has a tendency to form aggregates. In HD, there is selective destruction of the medium-sized spiny neurons in the striatum of the brain, which has been attributed either to the accumulation of mutant huntingtin aggregates or to the continued expansion of glutamine repeats. Mutant huntingtin affects cortical neurons, producing brain-derived neurotrophic factor (BDNF), which is necessary for the survival of striatal neurons.

One proposal suggests that partial loss of the beneficial effects of wild-type huntingtin combined with the toxicity of the mutant huntingtin conspire to selectively destroy the striatum of the brain. Huntingtin is a widely expressed protein that resides in the cell cytoplasm and may be important for transport of vesicles in the endosomal and secretory pathways, and for preventing cells from undergoing apoptosis. Mutant huntingtin is proteolytically processed, and the resulting amino-terminal fragments containing the glutamine expansions form aggregates that are deposited in nuclear and cytoplasmic inclusions in the brains of HD patients. *(Trottier and Mandel, 445–446; Watts and Koller, 484–485)*

63. **(C)** Chorea, although of cosmetic concern, is not disabling per se and does not correlate with the severity of the disease. Patients may be able to ambulate and accomplish activities of daily living despite suffering from severe chorea. Bradykinesia, rigidity, dystonia, and postural instability are more disabling. Dementia in Huntington disease is of the subcortical type. There is prominence of slowed thinking, impairment of sequencing, with the absence of cortical deficit, such as aphasia, agnosia and apraxia. Diminished executive function includes loss of the ability to plan, sequence, and carry out complex tasks. Eye movement abnormalities occur early in the course of Parkinson disease. Optokinetic nystagmus is impaired in both vertical and horizontal directions as well as voluntary initiation of ocular saccades. *(Watts and Koller, 492–493)*

64. **(B)** Akathisia is an unpleasant sensation of internal restlessness that is partially relieved by volitional movements occurring in a patient who has received chronic neuroleptics. *(Watts and Koller, 319)*

65. **(A)** Clonidine, an alpha-adrenergic agonist originally approved for treatment of hypertension, is actually the treatment of choice for children with mild or moderate tics. Clonidine has the potential for decreasing impulsiveness and improving attention span along with decreasing tics. The most common side effects are sedation and orthostatic hypotension. Dizziness can occur at higher doses. Guanfacine is similar to clonidine and is also marketed as an antihypertensive agent. It has shown some promise as a medication capable of both decreasing tics and improving behavior. Clonidine is often the drug of first choice for children with tics or Tourette syndrome who require symptomatic help. This is because the tic problem is often accompanied by attentional or other behavioral difficulties.

The dopamine-blocking agent haloperidol was found to be effective in treating tics. Although newer neuroleptic agents are available, haloperidol has always been the gold standard by which all new medications have been judged. Experience indicates that haloperidol can reduce tics in approximately 70% of treated persons, but over 50% of treated patients will complain of side effects. Only 25% of patients report significant improvement without side effects. The potential side effects of all neuroleptics are similar to those seen with haloperidol, most commonly fatigue and increased appetite. Others include depression and school or work phobia. A third type of medication used for the control of tics has been clonazepam. Traditionally used as a medication either for control of seizures or anxiety, this has helped individual patients. The dosage is titrated in a weekly basis until a clinical effect is observed or until there are side effects. Other medications that have been reported to improve tics include tetrabenzamine, local injection of botulinum toxin, and calcium channel antagonists. *(Watts and Koller, 573)*

66. **(A)** Cerebellar control of extraocular movements is performed mainly by the following structures: the dorsal vermis and underlying fastigial nucleus, the floculus and parafloculus, and the nodulus. Lesions of the dorsal vermis and fastigial nucleus result in saccadic dysmetria, typically with hypermetric movements and at time with macrosaccadic oscillations. Lesions of the flocculus and paraflocculus cause gaze-evoked nystagmus, rebound nystagmus, downbeat nystagmus, impaired smooth tracking, glissadic post saccadic drift, and disturbance in adjusting the gain of the vestibulo-ocular reflex. Lesions of the nodulus lead to an increase in the duration of the vestibular response. *(Watts and Koller, 580)*

67. **(C)** Stiff-man syndrome is a rare disorder of the CNS, which is characterized clinically by fluctuation and progressive muscle rigidity and spasms. The diagnosis relies also on the presence of continuous motor unit activity, without evidence of neuromyotonia, extrapyramidal or pyramidal dysfunction, or focal lesions of the spinal cord. Rigidity and spasms may dominate in the axial muscles, or in one or more distal limbs. Fifty percent to 60% of these patients have autoantibodies in the serum and CSF directed against glutamic acid decarboxylase (GAD), an enzyme present in GABA-ergic neurons and pancreatic beta-cells, and a high proportion of them have other autoimmune diseases including diabetes mellitus. *(Folli, 618)*

68. **(B)** Two distinctive mutation have been identified in the (alpha)-synuclein gene (SNCA) located on chromosome 4q have been linked to a familial form of Parkinson disease. A-Synuclein is a highly conserved, abundant 140-amino-acid protein of unknown function that is expressed mainly in presynaptic nerve terminals in the brain. *(Lang and Lozano, 1044–1053)*

REFERENCES

Colcher A, Simuni T. Other Parkinson syndromes. *Neurol Clin.* 2001;19:629–649.

Di Maio L, Squitieri F, Napolitano G, Campanella G, Trofatter JA. Conneally PM. Suicide risk in Huntington disease. *J Med Genet.* 1993;30:293–295.

Erenberg, Gerald, Tics, Tourette Syndrome, and Associated Conditions. Cleveland Clinic Foundation Cleveland, OH

Evidente VG, Gwinn-Hardy KA, Caviness JN, Gilman S. Hereditary ataxias. *Mayo Clin Proc.* 2000;75:475–490.

Folli F. Stiff man syndrome, 40 years later. *J Neurol, Neurosurg & Psychiatry.* 1998;65:618.

Hallett M. Physiology of basal ganglia disorders: an overview. *Can J Neurol Sci.* 1993;20:177–183.

Hanna PA. Doody RS. Alien limb sign. *Adv Neurol.* 2000; 82:135–145.

Jankovic J. New and emerging therapies for Parkinson disease. *Arch Neurol.* 1999;56:785–790.

Lang AE. Lozano AM. Parkinson disease. First of two parts. *N Engl J Med.* 1998;339:1044–1053.

Litvan I. Diagnosis and management of progressive supranuclear palsy. *Sem Neurol.* 2001;21:41–48.

Mizuno Y, Hattori N, Matsumine H. Neurochemical and neurogenetic correlates of Parkinson disease. *J Neurochem.* 1998;71:893–902.

Poewe W. Luginger E. Depression in Parkinson disease: impediments to recognition and treatment options. *Neurology.* 52(Suppl 3):S2–6,

Ross GW, Abbott RD, Petrovitch H, et al. Association of coffee and caffeine intake with the risk of Parkinson disease. *JAMA.* 2000;283:2674–2679.

Tanner CM, Aston DA. Epidemiology of Parkinson disease and akinetic syndromes. *Curr Opin Neurol.* 2000;13:427–430.

Trottier Y, Mandel JL. Biomedicine. Huntingtin–profit and loss] *Science.* 2001;293:445–446.

Watts RL, Koller WC. Movement disorders. Neurological principle and practice. 1997;New York: McGraw-Hill.

CHAPTER 15

Neuropathology
Questions

1. Which of the following is a pathological nuclear inclusion?

   (A) Marinesco body
   (B) Lipofuscin
   (C) Lewy bodies
   (D) Cowdry type A
   (E) Hirano body

2. Neurofibrillary tangles are NOT found in

   (A) normal aging
   (B) Alzheimer's disease
   (C) Huntington disease
   (D) progressive supranuclear palsy
   (E) postencephalitic Parkinson disease

3. Bunina bodies are found in

   (A) Pick disease
   (B) amyotrophic lateral sclerosis
   (C) multiple system atrophy
   (D) Alzheimer's disease
   (E) normal aging

4. Alzheimer type II glia are seen in

   (A) Canavan disease
   (B) Alzheimer's disease
   (C) Parkinson disease
   (D) Huntington disease
   (E) supranuclear palsy

5. Brain herniation through a skull defect is called

   (A) fungating herniation
   (B) subfalcine herniation
   (C) tonsillar herniation
   (D) central herniation
   (E) unclear herniation

Questions 6 through 10
Link the following histological structures to the appropriate central nervous system infection.

   (A) Cowdry A
   (B) Owl's eye cells
   (C) Negri bodies
   (D) Oligodendrocytes with inclusion
   (E) Spongiform changes in the cortex

6. Creutzfeldt-Jacob disease

7. rabies encephalitis

8. herpes encephalitis

9. progressive multifocal leukodystrophy

10. CMV encephalitis

11. Mumps virus has an affinity for which of the following central nervous system cells?

   (A) Neurons
   (B) Astrocytes
   (C) Ependymal cells
   (D) Oligodendrocytes
   (E) Microglia

12. HIV encephalitis is characterized by

   (A) microglial nodules with perivascular or parenchymal multinucleated cells
   (B) periventricular mixed large and small B cells
   (C) hemorrhagic necrotizing lesions in the cortex, basal ganglia, and brain stem with Cowdry type A nuclear inclusions and small cytoplasmic basophilic inclusions
   (D) Cowdry type B nuclear inclusions
   (E) meningoencephalitis with ventriculitis

13. The most common histological characteristic of lacunar strokes is

   (A) atherosclerosis
   (B) mycotic aneurysm
   (C) amyloid deposition
   (D) lipohyalinosis
   (E) coagulation necrosis

14. Cytokeratine is useful for the diagnosis of

   (A) pituitary adenoma
   (B) meningioma
   (C) melanoma
   (D) glioma
   (E) craniopharyngioma

Questions 15 through 22
Link each of the following immunohistochemical stains to the appropriate type of brain tumors.

   (A) Alpha fetoprotein
   (B) Desmin
   (C) Cytokeratin
   (D) Epithelial membrane antigen
   (E) L26
   (F) Transthyretin
   (G) HMB-45
   (H) Neurofilament

15. Meningioma

16. Choroid-plexus tumor

17. Neurofibroma

18. Endodermal sinus tumor

19. Medullomyoblastoma

20. Chordoma

21. Melanoma

22. B-cell lymphoma

23. Deletion of chromosome 19q occurs in

   (A) ependymoma
   (B) glioblastoma
   (C) oligodendroglioma
   (D) schwannoma
   (E) meningioma

24. The presence of cellular monotony, uniform cell density, and nuclei surrounded by a rim of clear cytoplasm giving a "fried egg" appearance is most suggestive of

   (A) oligodendroglioma
   (B) ependymoma
   (C) meningioma
   (D) dysembryoplastic neuro-epithelial tumor
   (E) pilocytic astrocytoma

25. This coronal section of the brain shows

   (A) nocardia abscess
   (B) mucormycosis
   (C) plasmodium falciparum malaria
   (D) brain metastasis
   (E) cysticercosis

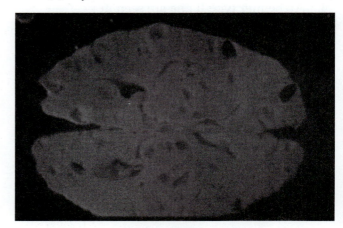

See color plate 1

26. The following shows

 (A) tachyzoites of toxoplasma gondii
 (B) CMV inclusion cells
 (C) Hirano body
 (D) Lewy body
 (E) Cowdry type A inclusion

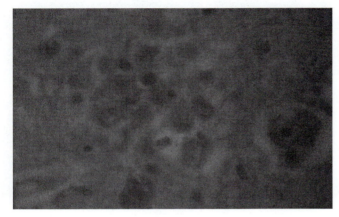

See color plate 2

27. This slide shows

 (A) cavernous hemangioma
 (B) temporal arteritis
 (C) arteriovenous malformation
 (D) polymyositis
 (E) cerebral amyloid angiopathy

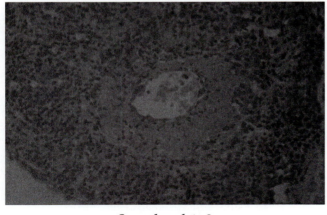

See color plate 3

28. This slide shows

 (A) acute inflammatory demyelinating neuropathy
 (B) vasculitic neuropathy
 (C) Charcot-Marie-Tooth neuropathy
 (D) leprosy neuropathy
 (E) diabetic neuropathy

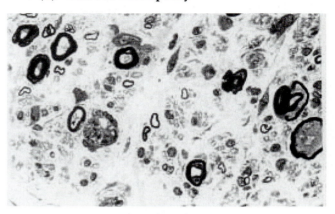

See color plate 4

29. This slide shows

 (A) acute inflammatory demyelinating neuropathy
 (B) vasculitic neuropathy
 (C) Charcot-Marie-Tooth neuropathy
 (D) leprosy neuropathy
 (E) diabetic neuropathy

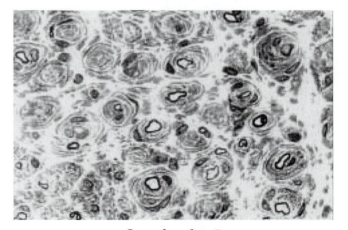

See color plate 5

30. This lesion is an illustration of

 (A) polimyelitis
 (B) Brown-Sequard syndrome
 (C) Krabbe's disease
 (D) vacuolar myelopathy
 (E) multiple sclerosis

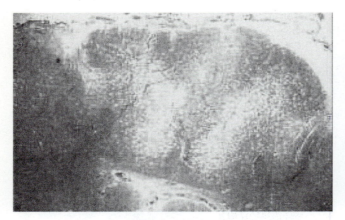

See color plate 6

31. This lesion corresponds to

(A) central pontine myelinolysis
(B) multiple sclerosis
(C) progressive multifocal leukoencephalopathy
(D) ischemic stroke
(E) Krabbe's disease

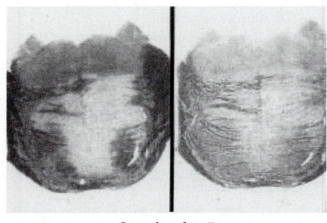

See color plate 7

32. This is a

(A) neurofibrillary tangle
(B) neuritic plaque
(C) Lewy body
(D) Bunina body
(E) Hirano body

See color plate 8

33. This slide shows

(A) Lewy bodies
(B) Bunina bodies
(C) neurofibrillary tangles
(D) Lafora bodies
(E) Cowdry A inclusions

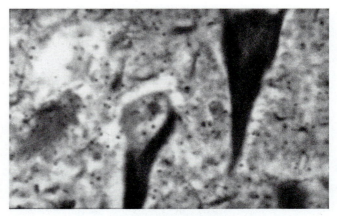

See color plate 9

34. This slide shows

(A) Cowdry A inclusions
(B) Marinesco bodies
(C) Bunina bodies
(D) Lafora bodies
(E) Lewy bodies

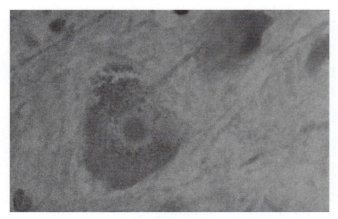

See color plate 10

35. This section of the brain shows a lesion that corresponds to

   (A) Wernicke encephalopathy
   (B) carbon monoxide intoxication
   (C) central pontine myelinolysis
   (D) Parkinson disease
   (E) Huntington disease

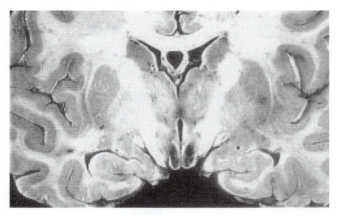

See color plate 11

36. The lesion in this brain section corresponds to

   (A) chronic ethanol intoxication
   (B) carbon monoxide intoxication
   (C) chronic phenytoin toxicity
   (D) methanol intoxication
   (E) lead intoxication

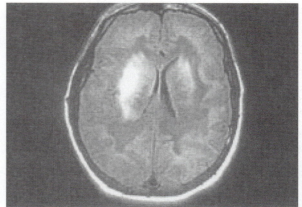

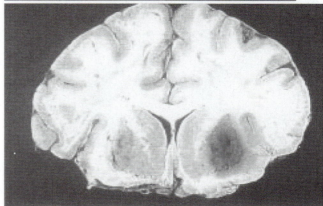

See color plate 12

37. This picture illustrates

   (A) heterotopia
   (B) agyria
   (C) polymicrogyria
   (D) porencephaly
   (E) holoprosencephaly

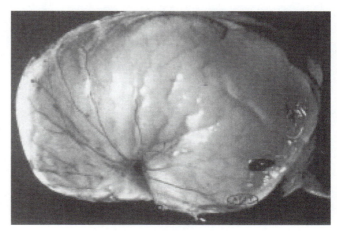

See color plate 13

38. This picture shows

(A) polymicrogyria
(B) pachygyria
(C) heterotopia
(D) porencephaly
(E) agenesis of the corpus callosum

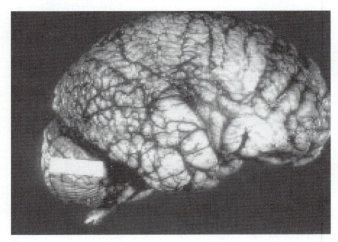

See color plate 14

39. This slide shows

(A) porencephaly
(B) holoprosencephaly
(C) agenesis of the corpus callosum
(D) heterotopia
(E) cortical dysplasia

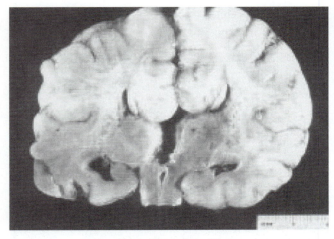

See color plate 15

40. This is a CT scan of the head and biopsy slide of a 40-year-old man who developed a new onset of seizure. What is the most likely diagnosis?

(A) Glioblastoma multiform
(B) Clear cell ependymoma
(C) Fibrillary astrocytoma
(D) Oligodendroglioma
(E) Dysembrylastic neuroepithelial tumor

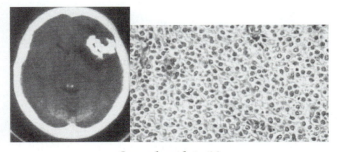

See color plate 16

41. This slide shows

(A) ependymoma
(B) medulloblastoma
(C) fibrillary astrocytoma
(D) subependymoma
(E) colloid cyst of the third ventricle

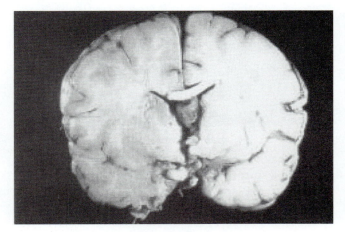

See color plate 17

42. This slide illustrates

(A) psammoma bodies
(B) Lewy bodies
(C) neuritis plaques
(D) Cowdry type A inclusions
(E) Hirano bodies

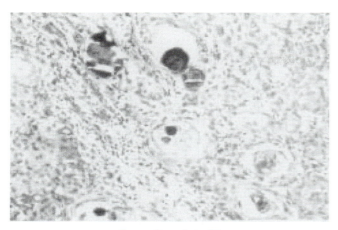

See color plate 18

43. This slide illustrates a metastatic brain disease. The most likely primary tumor is

(A) renal cell carcinoma

(B) melanoma

(C) GI adenocarcinoma

(D) squamous cell carcinoma

(E) breast cancer

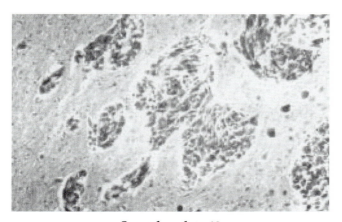

See color plate 19

Questions 44 through 51
Link the following.

(A) Normal muscle

(B) Central core disease

(C) Nemaline myopathy

(D) Ragged-red fibers

(E) Dermatomyositis

(F) Target fibers

(G) Infantile spinal muscular atrophy

(H) Polymyositis

44.

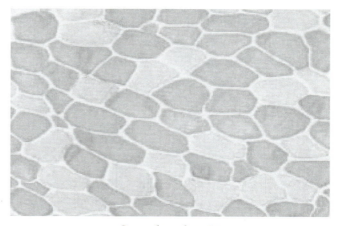

See color plate 20

45.

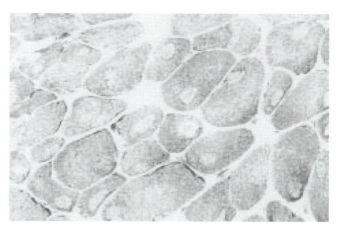

See color plate 21

46.

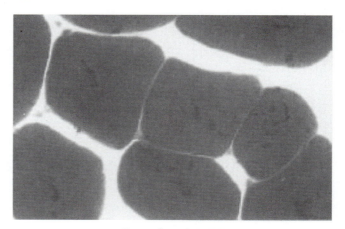

See color plate 22

47.

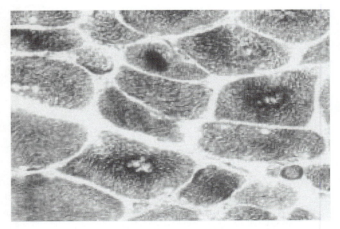

See color plate 23

48.

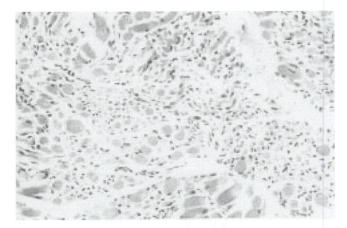

See color plate 24

49.

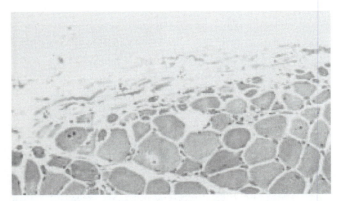

See color plate 25

50.

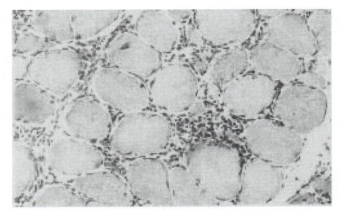

See color plate 26

51.

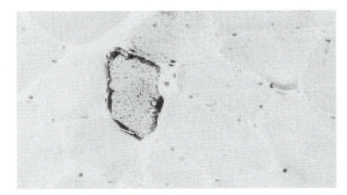

See color plate 27

Answers and Explanations

1. **(D)** Nuclear inclusions are divided into pathological and nonpathological types. Nonpathological nuclear inclusions include:

   - Nucleolus: it is the site of processing and partial assembly of ribosomes, which are required for cytoplasmic protein synthesis. It is prominent in large neurons, including motor neurons and Purkinje cells.
   - Marinesco body: a small round eosinophilic paranucleolar inclusion seen in normal aging. It stains with ubiquitin. Its ultrastructure is composed of intermediate filaments. It is commonly located in pigmented neurons of the substantia nigra, pyramidal cells of the hippocampus, and tegmentum of the brain stem.

   Pathological nuclear inclusions include viral inclusions:

   - Cowdry type A is an amorphous, large spherical eosinophilic inclusion that displaces the nucleus and chromatin to the periphery, and may be surrounded by a halo. It is usually indicative of viral infection
   - Cowdry type B is a small eosinophilic inclusion that does not displace the nucleus. Its origin may be viral or nonviral.

   Lipofuscin is a normal cytoplasmic inclusion. It is composed of lipid, protein, and carbohydrate. It is produced by lysosomes by oxidation of lipid and lipoproteins. Hippocampal pyramidal neurons, thalamus, and motor neurons of the brain stem and spinal cord are among the common locations of lipofuscin cytoplasmic inclusions.

   Hirano bodies are cytoplasmic inclusions. They are eosinophilic refractile inclusions found within the cytoplasm and adjacent to neurons. They stain positively for actin, tau protein, and vinculin. They are seen most frequently in Pick and Alzheimer's disease, and are most commonly located in the hippocampus. *(Davis and Robertson, 3–5; Sandberg, 7–8)*

2. **(C)** Neurofibrillary tangles are abnormal cytoplasmic inclusions. They are coarse fibrillary inclusions, some of which are composed of hyperphosphorylated tau proteins that may be ubiquitinated or glycated. They are flame shaped in pyramidal neurons and take on a globose appearance in neurons of the locus ceruleus. They are commonly located in the hippocampus and the temporal lobe. They are seen in normal aging, progressive supranuclear palsy, postencephalitic Parkinson disease, Alzheimer's disease, and amyotrophic lateral sclerosis-parkinsonism-dementia complex of Gum. *(Davis and Robertson, 28–30; Sandberg, 9)*

3. **(B)** Bunina bodies are abnormal cytoplasmic inclusions. They are small bead-like eosinophilic inclusions, most commonly found in motor neurons of patients with ALS. *(Davis and Robertson, 42–44; Sandberg, 9–10)*

4. **(A)** Alzheimer type II cells are astrocytic cells with enlarged nuclei and marginated chromatin. They are commonly located in the globus pallidus, cerebellar dentate nucleus, and cerebral cortex. They are seen in hepatic encephalopathy, Wilson disease, and Canavan disease. *(Davis and Robertson, 470–471; Sandberg, 13)*

5. **(A)** Fungating herniation is a herniation of the brain through a defect in the skull secondary to

trauma or surgery. It is caused by increased intracranial pressure and is often associated with fatal outcome. *(Sandberg, 5)*

6. (E)

7. (C)

8. (A)

9. (D)

10. (B)

Explanations 6 through 10

The neuropathological characteristics of Creutzfeldt-Jacob disease are spongiform changes in the cortex, subcortical astrogliosis, and deposition of prion proteins. The normal prion protein is encoded by a gene located on chromosome 20 and is converted into an abnormal one. Partial breakdown of prion protein may produce protein products that spontaneously polymerize into amyloid fibers.

Rabies encephalitis is transmitted to humans, in most cases, through the infected saliva that is injected in soft tissue at the site of a bite from an animal such as a fox or a dog. The etiologic agent of rabies is a rhabdovirus that contains a single-stranded RNA. Histopathological features of rabies encephalitis are cytoplasmic negri bodies, best seen in large neurons of the hippocampus, brain stem, and Purkinje cells.

The pathological hallmarks of herpes encephalitis are necrotizing lesions of the limbic areas and Cowdry type A intranuclear inclusion bodies, which are amorphous large, spherical eosinophilic inclusion that displace the nucleolus and chromatin to the periphery.

Microglial nodules and necrotizing lesions in the region of the conus medullaris, cauda equina, and the periventricular areas are characteristic of central nervous cytomegalic virus infection. They are associated with the presence of cytomegalic cells, also known as Owl's cells.

Progressive multifocal leukoencephalopathy (PML) is caused by infection from JC virus, a papova (papilloma-polyoma-vacuolating) virus. The hallmark pathological features of PML are oligodendrocytes with inclusion bodies and multiple frequently coalescing large and small foci of demyelination. JC virus causes lytic infection of oligodendrocytes that leads to demyelination and to the development of corresponding signs. The cut surface of the fixed brain affected by PML appears asymmetrically pitted by small foci of gray discoloration mixed with larger confluent areas of abnormal parenchyma, which may be centrally necrotic. The lesions tend to be most numerous in the cerebral white matter, but also involve the cerebral cortex and deep gray matter. On microscopic examination, there are multiple foci of demyelination. Some are small and rounded, others confluent and irregular and occasionally centrally necrotic. The homogeneous amphophilic inclusions, seen in oligodendrocytes, largely fill the nuclei and consist of closely packed polyomavirus particles that can be identified on electron microscopy. *(Davis and Robertson 977–981, 1002–1010, 1018–1022, 1032–1034)*

11. (C) Mumps virus infects ependymal cells. Herpes and polio viruses infect neuronal cells, whereas JC virus attacks both astrocytes and oligodendrocytes. Microglial cells are preferentially infected by herpes virus. *(Takano et al., 2215–2221)*

12. (A) The combination of multinucleated giant cells, microglial nodules, and perivenular inflammation has been termed HIV encephalitis and has been identified in 30% to 90% of patients dying with AIDS. There is frequently a diffuse pallor of the myelin, particularly in deep areas of the centrum semiovale, with microscopic evidence of macrophage activation, astrocytosis, and productive HIV infection. Cerebral atrophy is common in patients with HIV-Dementia (HIV-D), often occurring in a frontotemporal distribution. The pathology of HIV-D is that of a chronic encephalitis with marked macrophage activation. Multiple small nodules containing macrophages, lymphocytes, and microglia are scattered throughout gray and white matter of the brain, appearing more commonly in white matter and subcortical gray matter of the thalamus, basal ganglia, and brain stem. These inflammatory nodules are not specific to HIV-1 infection and occur in other infections, including toxoplasmosis and CMV encephalitis.

Multinucleated giant cells are also characteristically seen, and their presence correlates with the degree of dementia and the detection of HIV-1 DNA. These giant cells are thought to reflect HIV-1 replication because giant multinucleated cells form in HIV-infected macrophage cultures.

Gross pathologic examination of primary central nervous system lymphoma (PCNSL) reveals a bulky tumor with indistinct borders, often contiguous with meningeal or ventricular surfaces. Most lesions are supratentorial. Whereas solitary lesions occur in one-third of cases, multiple lesions are evident in most cases. These lesions are histologically diffuse, with perivascular involvement, high mitotic rates, and variable degrees of necrosis and microglial reaction. Immunohistochemical studies of PCNSL identify these tumors as B cells in origin.

Cytomegalovirus has been identified in astrocytes, neurons, oligodendroglia, and capillary endothelia. Four pathologic lesions are associated with cytomegalovirus encephalitis in patients with AIDS:

1. Isolated cytomegalic cells: cytomegalic cells without associated microglial nodules or inflammation.
2. Microglial nodules: dense cellular aggregates of macrophages, rod cells, or both; typically well demarcated from the adjacent parenchyma and more common in gray matter than in white matter. Few microglial nodules (only 7% to 12%) contain cytomegalic inclusions.
3. Focal parenchymal necrosis: discrete foci of parenchymal necrosis with cytomegalic cells and macrophages.
4. Cytomegalovirus ventriculoencephalitis: focal or diffuse destruction of the ependymal lining and necrosis of periventricular parenchymal tissue associated with dense accumulation of cytomegalic cells in the ependymal and periependymal areas. Ventriculomegaly, necrosis, and hemorrhage or fibrinous exudates covering the ventricular system may be evident on gross inspection.

Varicella zoster virus causes meningoencephalitis with ventriculitis. CNS toxoplasmosis is the most common cause of focal brain lesions in patients with AIDS. The pathology of CNS toxoplasmosis may include necrosis and hemorrhage of choroid plexus. *(Arribas et al., 577–587; Ciacci et al., 213–221; McArthur et al., 129–150)*

13. **(D)** Lipohyalinosis, a destructive vasculopathy linked to severe hypertension, affects arteries 40 to 200 μm in diameter. The arterial lumen is compromised not by an intimal process but by thickening of the vessel wall itself. Subintimal lipid-laden foam cells and pink-staining fibrinoid material thicken the arterial walls, sometimes compressing the lumen. In places, the arteries are replaced by tangles and wisps of connective tissue that obliterate the usual vascular layers. The small, deep infarcts that result from occlusion of these arteries are usually called lacunes. Small, deep infarcts can also result from miniature atheromas (microatheromas) that form at the origin of penetrating arteries, as well as by plaques within the parent arteries that obstruct or extend into the branches (junctional plaques). Rarely, they are occluded by microemboli. *(Goetz, 913–914)*

14. **(E)** Cytokeratin immunohistochemical stains are useful in the diagnosis of craniopharyngioma, carcinoma, chordoma, and epithelial cyst. *(Kubo et al., 131–134)*

15. **(B)**

16. **(F)**

17. **(H)**

18. **(A)**

19. **(B)**

20. **(C)**

21. **(G)**

22. **(E)**

Explanations 15 through 22

Immunohistochemistry is the most common method used to identify cell types, tumor phenotypes, and to classify tumors. Endodermal sinus tumor stains positively for alpha fetoprotein. Desmin is used to identify rhabdosarcoma and medullomyoblastoma. Cytokeratin is used to identify craniopharyngioma as well as chordoma and epithelial cysts. Meningioma, carcinoma, and epithelial cysts stain positively for epithelial membrane antigen. L 26 identifies B-cell lymphoma, whereas HMB 45 identifies melanoma. Transthyretin stains choroid plexus tumors, whereas neurofilament stains neurofibroma, ganglion cell tumors, and pineocytoma. (McKeeveer, 19–21)

23. **(C)** Several genetic alterations are known to exist in human gliomas. In brief, these include alterations of chromosomes 9p, 10p, 10q, 11p, 13q, 17p, 19q, and 22p in diffuse fibrillary astrocytomas, and the loss of 1p and 19q combined or in isolation in both pure and mixed oligodendrogliomas. The loss of heterozygosity (LOH) of 1p and 19q appears to be specific to tumors of oligodendroglial origin, and this change is shared in both the astrocytic and the oligodendroglial portion of mixed oligo-astrocytomas, suggesting that these are clonal. The high frequency of 1p and 19q loss in oligodendrogliomas suggests that these regions also harbor tumor suppressor genes. (Perry, 705–710)

24. **(A)** Cellular monotony is the main microscopic feature of oligodendroglioma. This is formed by monomorphous cells characterized by uniformly round, more often than oval, nuclei with open chromatin. Nuclei are surrounded by either a rim of clear cytoplasm, resulting in the classic fried egg appearance, or a scant slightly eccentric rim of pink cytoplasm and few processes. (Parisi, 1–2)

25. **(E)** This slide illustrates a brain with disseminated cysticercosis. It is the commonest parasitic infection of the CNS in Mexico, as well as in other parts of the world, such as South America, India, and certain European countries. The number of cysts within the CNS varies from one to several hundred. They occur in the parenchyma (especially the gray matter), meninges, or ventricles. The viable intraparenchymal cysticerci are usually 1 to 2 cm in diameter and contain a single invaginated scolex. After degeneration, they become fibrotic and are represented by a firm white nodule. (Davis and Robertson, 896–898)

26. **(A)** Central nervous system toxoplasmosis is the most common cause of focal brain lesions in patients with AIDS. On macroscopic examination, the brain typically contains multifocal necrotic lesions of variable size. The basal ganglia are often involved, but any part of the brain may be affected. On microscopic examination, necrotizing abscesses or foci of coagulative necrosis are surrounded by mononuclear and polymorphonuclear inflammatory cells, newly formed capillaries, reactive astrocytes, and microglia. Intracellular and extracellular toxoplasma tachyzoites (also known as endozoites or trophozoites), as well as pseudocysts as illustrated in this slide, are usually abundant. (Davis and Robertson, 887–890)

27. **(B)** This slide illustrates temporal arteritis (giant cell arteritis). Giant cell arteritis is an autoimmune disease that involves large- and medium-sized arteries including the carotid and vertebral arteries and their major branches. It is characterized, on pathological examination, by a widespread granulomatous inflammation of the arterial walls and can cause cerebral infarction. Multinucleated giant cells are usually evident, and their cytoplasm may contain fragments of elastic lamina. (Davis and Robertson, 800–801)

28. **(A)** This slide shows various stages of demyelination and remyelination with myelin loss that may result in naked axons. This is highly suggestive of acute demyelinating inflammatory polyneuropathy. The pathological examination is characterized also by macrophages, which penetrate the Schwann cell basal lamina, displace a rim of Schwann cell cytoplasm, and strip away otherwise normal-appearing myelin. (Schmidt, 5–6)

29. **(C)** This slide shows axonal demyelination and remyelination with the development of concentric periaxonal Schwann cell processes in the form of an onion bulb. This is highly suggestive of hypertrophic neuropathy such as Charcot-Marie-Tooth neuropathy. *(Schmidt, 9–10)*

30. **(D)** Vacuolar myelopathy is the most common disease of the spinal cord in AIDS patients. It is characterized by a spongy vacuolation of myelin sheets in the posterior and lateral columns, as illustrated in this slide. There is vacuolation of the spinal white matter in the posterior columns and lateral corticospinal tracts. Breakdown of myelin, and later axons, is accompanied by an accumulation of macrophages containing debris. *(Davis and Robertson, 996–997)*

31. **(A)** The two slides illustrate pontine sections; the left image uses a LF(B)PAS stain that demonstrates myelin loss, while the image on the right uses a Bielschowsky stain that shows relative preservation of axons. These slides are highly suggestive of central pontine myelinolysis. Central pontine myelinolysis (CPM) is a monophasic demyelinating disease that predominantly involves the basis pontis. It usually occurs as a complication of rapid correction of hyponatremia. The mechanism of the demyelination is poorly understood. On macroscopic examination, the basis pontis typically includes a fusiform region of gray discoloration, which is abnormally soft and appears granular. On sectioning, the extent of the lesion is variable. Its cross-sectional area is usually greatest in the upper part of the pons, where only a narrow rim of subpial tissue may be spared. It may involve the middle cerebral peduncles, but rarely extends rostrocaudally beyond the confines of the pons and lower midbrain. The lesion may be asymmetric, being largely or completely confined to one side of the pons. On microscopic examination, CPM appears as an active demyelination. The lesions contain reactive astrocytes and large numbers of foamy lipid-laden macrophages, but only very scanty lymphocytes. *(Davis and Robertson, 518–520)*

32. **(B)** This slide shows a neuritic plaque seen in Alzheimer's disease (AD). Amyloid plaques are one of the pathological characteristics of AD. They are formed by extracellular proteinaceous deposits, either as amyloid filaments or in non-filamentous form, with variable associated abnormalities involving neuronal processes that traverse the abnormal region. The abnormal neuronal processes are termed dystrophic neurites. Plaques associated with abnormal neurites are termed neuritic plaques. Plaques are widely distributed in the brain of patients with AD. The neocortex and hippocampus are always involved. Plaques may also be present in the basal ganglia, the hypothalamus, the tegmentum of the midbrain and pons, and the subcortical white matter. *(Davis and Robertson, 1071–1073; Hart, 1–3)*

33. **(C)** This slide illustrates neurofibrillary tangles, intraneuronal abnormalities seen in Alzheimer's disease. Neurofibrillary tangles (NFTs) are neuronal inclusions composed largely of filamentous aggregates of hyperphosphorylated tau proteins that are variably ubiquitinated and glycated. In silver preparation, several morphologic forms of NFT can be identified. The shape of the NFT is probably determined by that of the neuron containing it. Ultrastructural investigation reveals that NFTs are composed of paired helical neurofilaments with a maximum diameter of 20 nm and a periodic narrowing to 10 nm every 80 nm. *(Davis and Robertson, 1073–1076; Hart, 1–3)*

34. **(E)** This slide shows eosinophilic cytoplasmic neuronal inclusions corresponding to a Lewy body. Lewy bodies are seen in idiopathic Parkinson disease as well as in diffuse Lewy body disease. *(Davis and Robertson, 38–41; Hart, 5)*

35. **(A)** This is a coronal brain section showing confluent petechial hemorrhages in the mammillary bodies consistent with Wernicke encephalopathy. It is caused by deficiency of thiamine. Lesions are usually discernible in the mammillary bodies, but may also involve parts of the hypothalamus, the medial thalamic nuclei, the floor of the third ventricle, the periaqueductal gray, the colliculi, the nuclei in the pontomedullary tegmentum (particularly the dorsal motor nuclei of the vagus), the inferior olives, and the cerebral

cortex. Typically, the involved regions are slightly shrunken and show brown discoloration due to hemosiderin deposition, and there may be petechial hemorrhages. The periventricular and periaqueductal lesions often spare a slender strip of subependymal tissue. In some patients, particularly those with previously treated disease, the mammillary bodies may be only mildly discolored and other lesions may be inconspicuous. On microscopic examination, acute lesions are edematous with relative preservation of neurons, variable necrosis of intervening tissue, and loss of myelinated fibers. Capillaries may appear strikingly prominent due to endothelial hyperplasia and cuffing by macrophages. *(Davis and Robertson, 536–538; Rushing, 9)*

36. **(D)** This patient's FLAIR MRI of the head shows a bright signal in the putamen area that correlates with the ischemic necrosis seen in the brain coronal section, which also shows a left putamen hemorrhagic lesion. Selective bilateral lesions of the putamen are highly suggestive of methanol intoxication. Acute methanol intoxication causes generalized edema of the brain, which usually shows features of global hypoxic injury. There may be scattered petechial hemorrhages and larger, symmetric foci of hemorrhagic infarction in the putamen and claustrum. Some patients develop extensive white matter necrosis. Degeneration of retinal ganglion cells results in optic nerve atrophy and gliosis. *(Davis and Robertson, 520–521; Rushing, 9)*

37. **(B)** This picture illustrates agyria. It results from injury of the germinal cells as they reach the cortex and results in abnormalities of gyral development. The thick cortical ribbon is disproportionately represented when compared to the relative paucity of the centrum semiovale. The characteristic histological appearance is a four-layer cortex instead of six layers of normal neocortical pattern:

- Molecular layer
- Thin, external neuronal layer
- Sparsely cellular layer with a tangential myelin fiber plexus

- Thick, inner neuronal layer, which splits in its deeper zone into columns of cells *(Davis and Robertson, 294–296; Henry, 13–14)*

38. **(A)** This picture illustrates polymicrogyria. Polymicrogyria is characterized by a hyperconvoluted cortical ribbon of miniature, individually thin gyri, which are often fused together or piled on top of one another. The macrogyric cerebral surface is irregular, and has been likened to cobblestones. Sections of the cerebrum reveal heaped up or submerged gyri that widen the cortical ribbon. Polymicrogyria may be:

- Widespread in one or both hemispheres
- Bilateral and symmetric in a particular arterial territory (usually the middle cerebral artery)
- Confined to the opercular region or depths of the insula
- Around porencephalic or hydranencephalic defects
- Focal in almost any neocortical area, except the cingulate or striate cortex.

    On microscopic examination, the cortical gray matter is abnormally thin and excessively folded, and there is fusion of adjacent gyri and abnormal cortical lamination. *(Davis and Robertson, 294–296; Henry, 14)*

39. **(C)** This picture illustrates an agenesis of the corpus callosum. *(Henry, 16)*

40. **(D)** The head CT of the patient shows a tumor with a gyriform pattern of calcification involving the left frontal lobe. The microscopic features of the tumor include cellular monotony, cells with round nuclei and perinuclear halos, resulting in the classic fried egg appearance. These findings are highly suggestive of oligodendrioglioma. *(Parisi, 1–3)*

41. **(E)** This slide shows a colloid cyst. Its location in the third ventricle, usually near the choroid plexus and foramen of Monro, helps distinguish the colloid cyst from other cysts that superficially resemble it (enterogenous cysts, ependymal cysts, and Rathke's cleft cysts) but occur in different locations. The simple columnar and

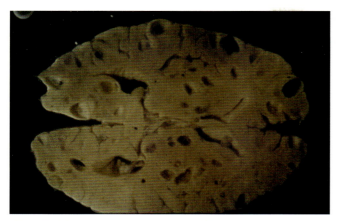

Plate 1: Corresponds to question 25.
Horizontal section of a human brain containing numerous lesions.

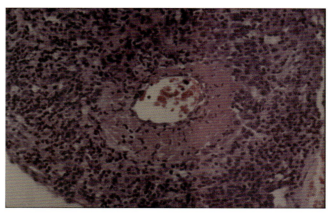

Plate 3: Corresponds to question 27.
Arterial wall infiltration of inflammatory cells.

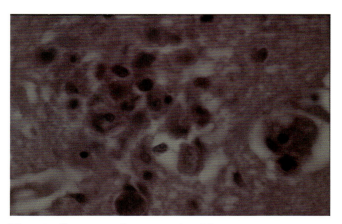

Plate 2: Corresponds to question 26.
High-power microscopic examination of an inflammatory brain lesion.

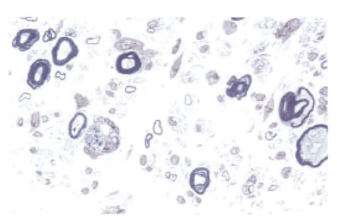

Plate 4: Corresponds to question 28.
Microscopic section of a peripheral nerve.

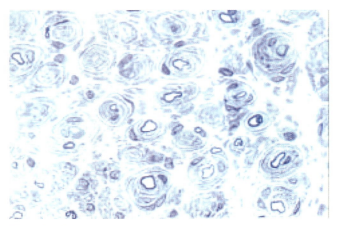

Plate 5: Corresponds to question 29.
Toluidine blue stains of a peripheral nerve section.

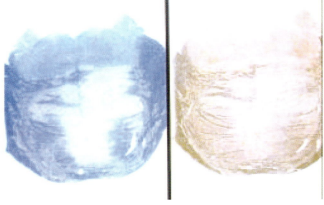

Plate 7: Corresponds to question 31.
The two slides illustrate central nervous system sections; using (*left*) a LF(B)PAS stain, and (*right*) a Bielschowsky stain.

Plate 6: Corresponds to question 30.
A 27-year-old died after he developed a progressive, painless, weakness in the leg, sensory loss, imbalance, and sphincter dysfunction. The pathological examination of his spinal cord is illustrated in this plate.

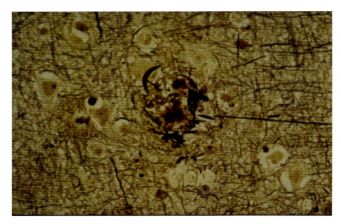

Plate 8: Corresponds to question 32.

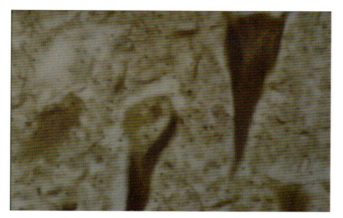

Plate 9: Corresponds to question 33.

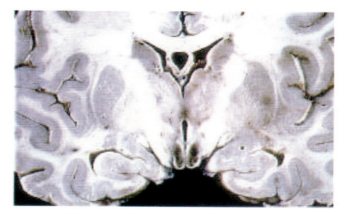

Plate 11: Corresponds to question 35.
Coronal section of the brain.

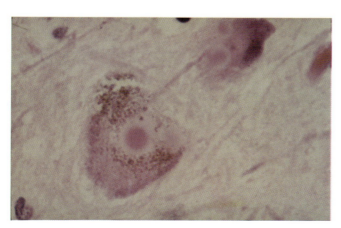

Plate 10: Corresponds to question 34.
Microscopic section of the substantia nigra.

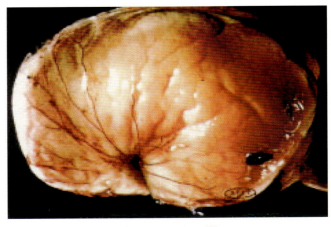

Plate 13: Corresponds to question 37. Brain of a term infant (lateral view).

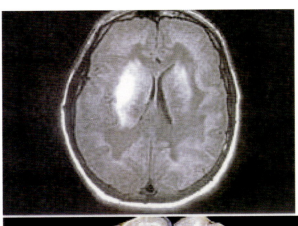

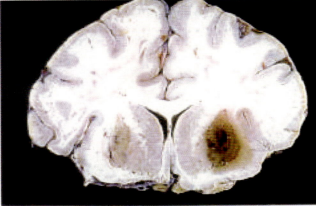

Plate 12: Corresponds to question 36. FLAIR head MRI (*top*) and the corresponding coronal section of the brain (*bottom*).

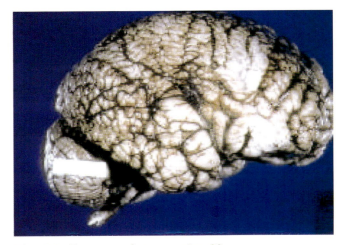

Plate 14: Corresponds to question 38. Brain of a term infant (lateral view).

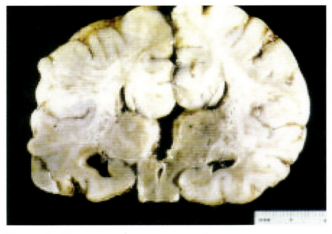

Plate 15: Corresponds to question 39.
Brain section (coronal view).

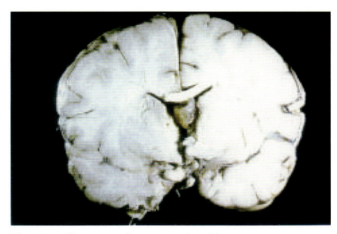

Plate 17: Corresponds to question 41.
Brain section (coronal view).

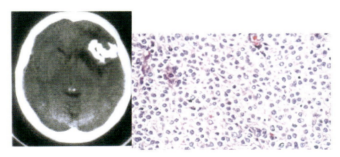

Plate 16: Corresponds to question 40.
A 40-year-old man developed a new onset of seizure. His head CT showed a left frontal lesion. The pathological examination of his lesion is illustrated in this plate.

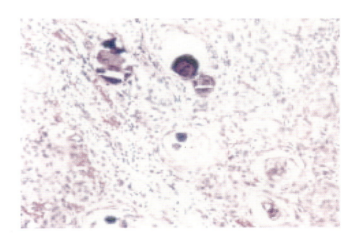

Plate 18: Corresponds to question 42.

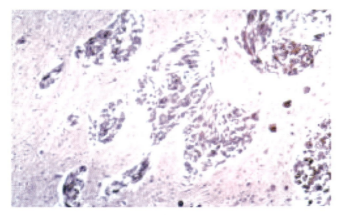

Plate 19: Corresponds to question 43.
Metastatic brain disease.

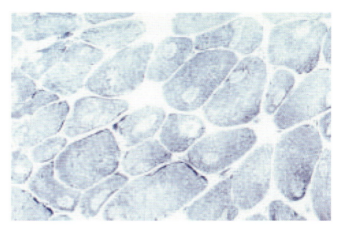

Plate 21: Corresponds to question 45.
Frozen muscle section stained with the oxidative stain NADH.

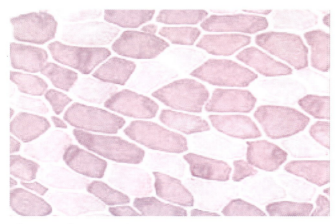

Plate 20: Corresponds to question 44.
Frozen muscle section stained with ATPase.

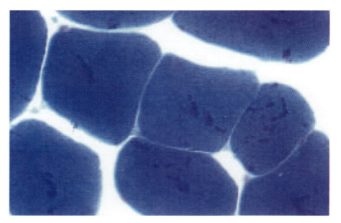

Plate 22: Corresponds to question 46.
Frozen muscle section stained with Gomori trichrome stain.

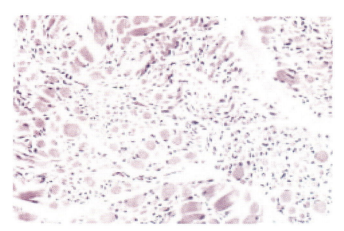

Plate 24: Corresponds to question 48.
Frozen muscle section stained with routine H&E stain.

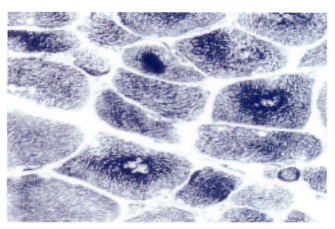

Plate 23: Corresponds to question 47.
Frozen muscle section stained with the oxidative stain NADH.

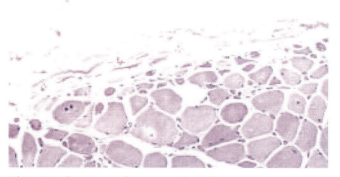

Plate 25: Corresponds to question 49.
Frozen muscle section.

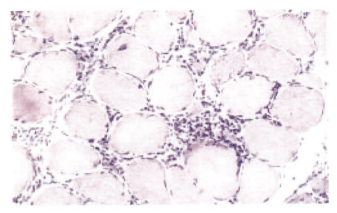

Plate 26: Corresponds to question 50.
Muscle section stained with routine H&E stain.

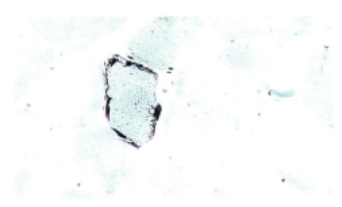

Plate 27: Corresponds to question 51.
Muscle section stained with modified Gomori trichrome stain.

cuboidal epithelium, which may be flattened to simple squamous epithelium, often contains a mixture of ciliated and nonciliated cells. *(Parisi, 10–11)*

42. **(A)** The slide shows psammoma bodies from a psammomatous meningioma. Meningothelial whorls and psammoma bodies typify meningiomas. Psammoma bodies are concentrically laminated calcifications, and are crowded with psammoma bodies. They are often spinal in location. This benign variant is recognized as meningioma by finding syncytial cells between the conspicuous, concentrically laminated psammoma bodies. *(Davis and Robertson, 212)*

43. **(B)** This picture shows a metastatic melanoma with cells containing abundant melanin. *(Davis and Robertson, 307)*

44. **(A)**

45. **(B)**

46. **(C)**

47. **(F)**

48. **(G)**

49. **(E)**

50. **(H)**

51. **(D)**

Explanations 44 through 51

The slide in question 44 demonstrates a normal muscle. Normal frozen muscle stains for ATPase at pH 9.4, and this differentiates Type I from type II fibers. At the alkaline pH, the type II fibers are dark and the type I fibers are light. There is a normal mosaic pattern of both types of fibers with approximately two-thirds being type II and one third type I.

The slide in question 45 illustrates central core disease. This is an autosomal dominant disorder and the gene defect is located on chromosome 19. Mutation on the ryanodine receptor contains a Ca release channel. Type I fibers have a central pale area fiber representing the lack of oxidative enzymes. The core tends to be single and central within the affected fiber. Structured cores have preserved cross banding, whereas unstructured cores have lost their cross binding.

The slide in question 46 shows nemaline rod myopathy, a congenital myopathy of autosomal or recessive inheritance. The diagnosis is suggested by the variable number of rods in the trichome stains.

The slide in question 47 shows target fibers in a denervating disease. Target fibers are seen in atrophic fibers and consist of central non staining areas surrounded by a darkened rim of oxidative enzymes.

The slide in question 48 shows panfascicular atrophy, suggestive of infantile muscular atrophy.

The slide in question 49 shows the perifascicular atrophy of dermatomyositis.

The slide in question 50 shows lymphocytes infiltrating the endomysium between fibers, suggesting the diagnosis of polymyositis.

The slide in question 51 shows a modified Gomori trichome stain of mitochondrial myopathy, which stains the mitochondria red, hence the term ragged red fibers. *(Heffner, 1–13)*

REFERENCES

Arribas JR, Storch GA, Clifford DB, Tselis AC. Cytomegalovirus encephalitis. *Ann Intern Med.* 1996; 125:577–587.

Ciacci JD, Tellez C, VonRoenn J, Levy RM. Lymphoma of the central nervous system in AIDS. *Sem Neurol.* 1999;19:213–21,1999.

Davis RL, Robertson DM, eds. *Textbook of Neuropathology.* 3rd ed. Baltimore, MD: Williams & Wilkins; 1997.

Goetz CG, Pappert EJ, eds. *Textbook of Clinical Neurology.* Philadelphia, PA: WB Saunders;1999.

Hart MN. Degenerative disease of the CNS. From *Neuropathology review.* AFIP Course 2002.

Heffner RR. Neuromuscular diseases. From *Neuropathology review.* AFIP Course 2002.

Henry JM. Pediatric neuropathology. From *Neuropathology review.* AFIP Course 2002.

Kubo O, Tajika Y, Uchimuno H, Muragaki Y, Shimoda M, Hiyama H, Morishita K, Takakura K. Immunohistochemical study of craniopharyngiomas. *Noshuyo Byori*. 1993;10:131–134.

McArthur JC, Sacktor N, Selnes O. Human immunodeficiency virus-associated dementia. *Sem Neurol*. 1999;19:129–150.

McKeeveer PE. New methods of brain tumor analysis. From *Neuropathology review*. AFIP Course 2002.

Parisi JE. Other glial tumors. From *Neuropathology review*. AFIP Course 2002.

Perry JR. Oligodendrogliomas: clinical and genetic correlations. *Curr Opin Neurol*. 2001;14:705–710.

Rushing EJ. Toxic metabolic disorders and nutritional deficiencies. From *Neuropathology review*. AFIP Course 2002.

Sandberg. GD. Introduction to neuropathology. From *Neuropathology Review*. AFIP Course. 2002.

Schmidt RE. Disease of the peripheral nervous system. From *Neuropathology review*. AFIP Course 2002.

Takano T, Takikita S, Shimada M. Experimental mumps virus-induced hydrocephalus: viral neurotropism and neuronal maturity. *NeuroReport*. 1999;10:2215–2221.

CHAPTER 16

Neuroradiology
Questions

1. These studies show

    (A) right middle cerebral artery infarction
    (B) bilateral anterior cerebral artery infarction
    (C) right anterior cerebral artery infarction
    (D) bilateral middle cerebral artery infarction
    (E) subdural hematoma

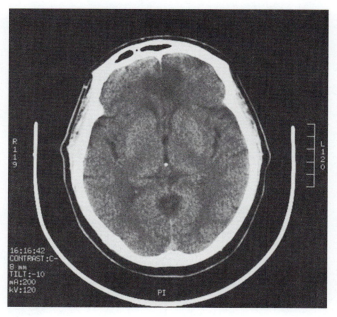

FIG. 1a

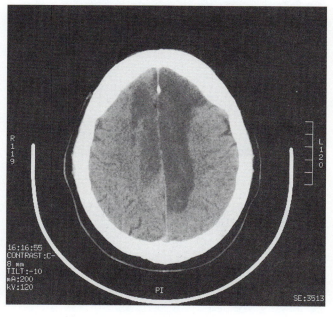

FIG. 1b

2. These images show the head MRI of a 43-year-old man with a history of progressive ataxia. The most likely diagnosis is

(A) pilocytic astrocytoma

(B) hemangioblastoma

(C) medulloblastoma

(D) metastatic tumor

(E) meningioma

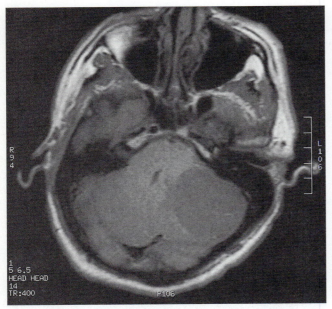

FIG. 2a

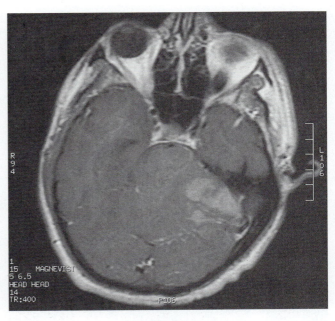

FIG. 2c

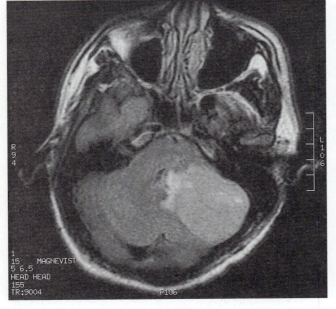

FIG. 2b

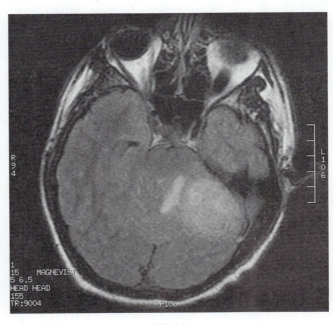

FIG. 2d

3. These images show the head MRI of a 65-year-old man who became acutely confused. The most likely diagnosis is

(A) amyloid angiopathy
(B) metastatic lung cancer
(C) metastatic melanoma
(D) glioblastoma multiforme
(E) hemorrhagic stroke

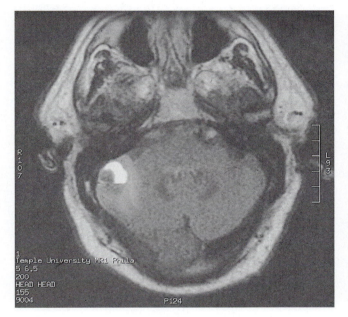

FIG. 3a

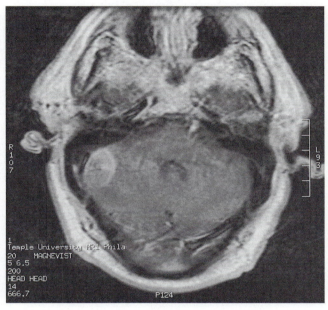

FIG. 3c

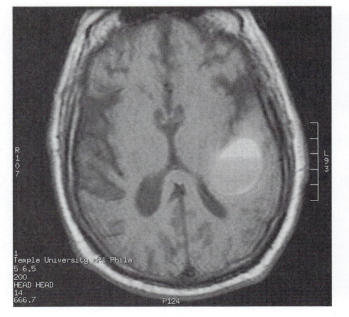

FIG. 3b

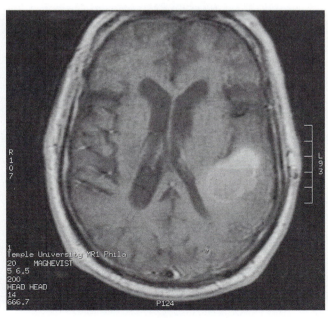

FIG. 3d

4. These are T1-weighted images of a gadolinium-enhanced head MRI of a 50-year-old asymptomatic man. The most likely diagnosis is

   (A) anterior cerebral artery aneurysm

   (B) arachnoid cyst

   (C) ependymoma

   (D) metastasis

   (E) meningioma

5. Which of the following clinical manifestations would one expect to see in a 56-year-old man with the following head MRI?

   (A) Left side weakness

   (B) Left oculomotor palsy

   (C) Anosmia

   (D) Left facial palsy

   (E) Vertical gaze palsy

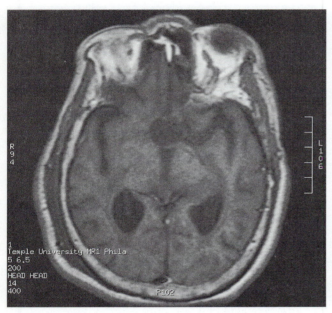

FIG. 4a

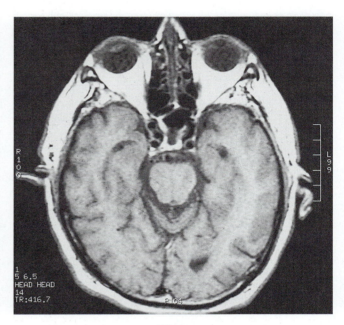

FIG. 5a

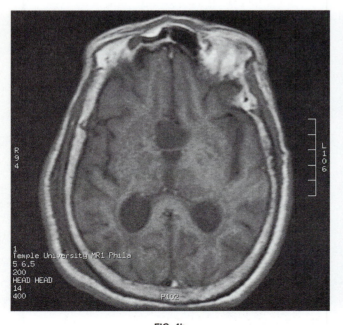

FIG. 4b

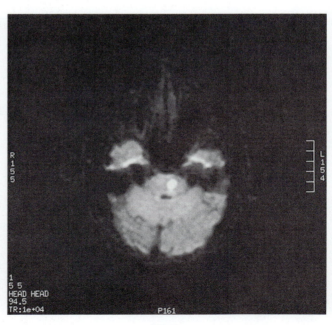

FIG. 5b

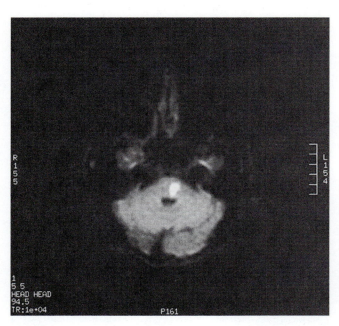

FIG. 5c

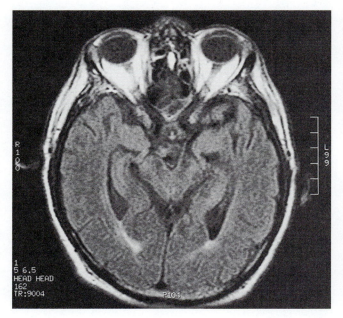

FIG. 5d

6. The most likely diagnosis suggested by this head MRI is

(A) craniopharyngioma

(B) pituitary adenoma

(C) thrombosed aneurysm

(D) brain metastasis

(E) primary central nervous system lymphoma

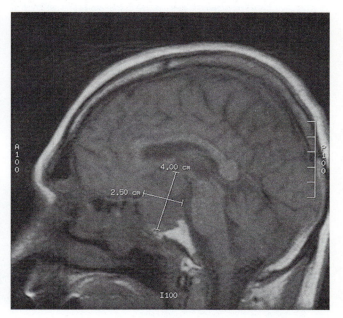

FIG. 6a

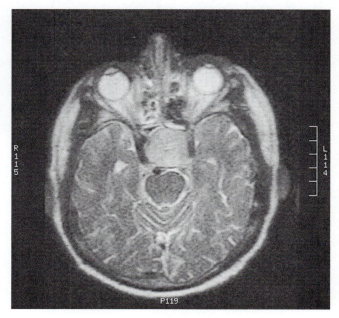

FIG. 6b

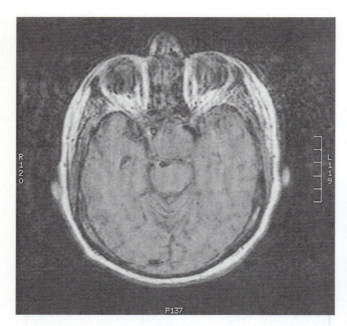

FIG. 6c

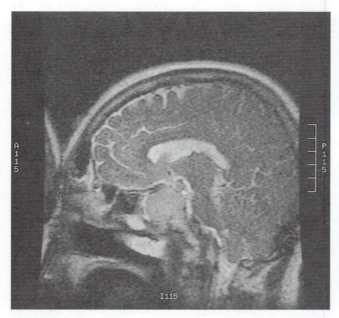

FIG. 6d

7. This head MRI of a newborn baby girl at 38 weeks gestation shows

   (A) cystic encephalomalacia
   (B) lissencephaly
   (C) polymicrogyria
   (D) schizencephaly
   (E) focal cortical dysplasia

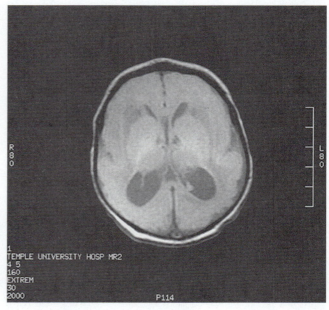

FIG. 7a

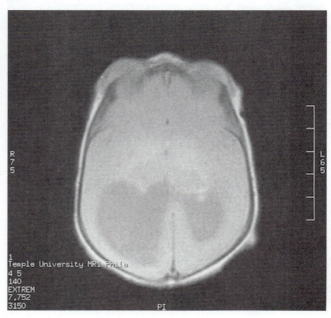

FIG. 7b

8. These are the imaging studies of an 80-year-old man with acute onset of left side weakness and slurred speech. The most likely diagnosis is

(A) metastatic melanoma
(B) metastatic choriocarcinoma
(C) cavernous hemangiomas
(D) arteriovenous malformation
(E) aneurysm

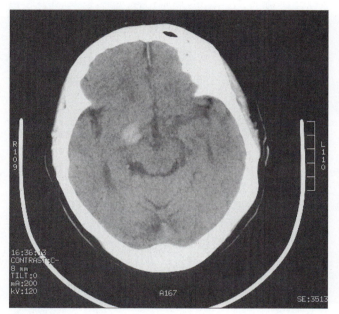

FIG. 8a

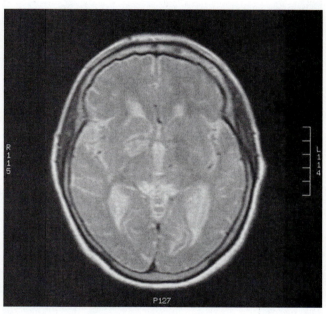

FIG. 8c

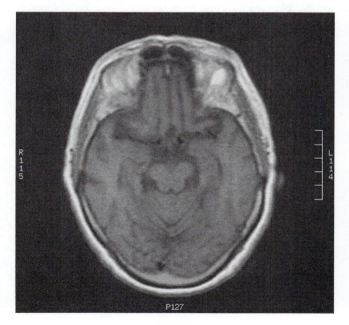

FIG. 8b

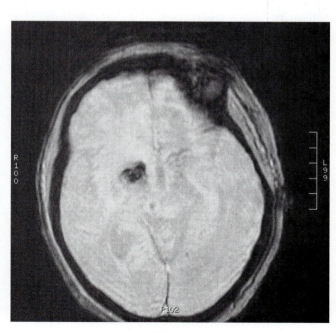

FIG. 8d

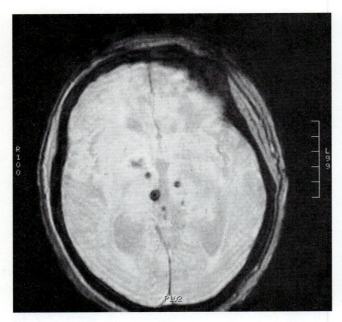

FIG. 8e

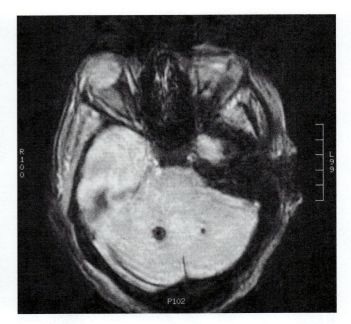

FIG. 8g

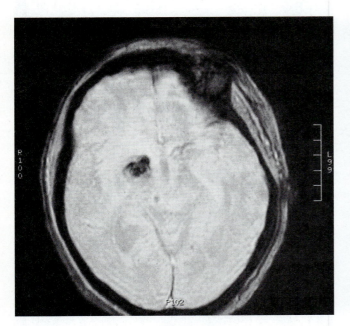

FIG. 8f

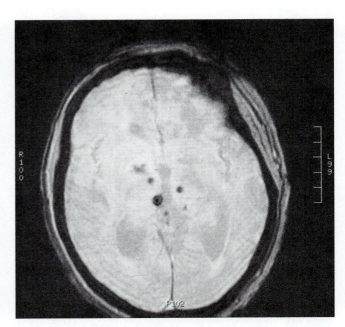

FIG. 8h

9. This is the head CT and MRI of a 39-year-old woman with a history of AIDS who developed progressive left side weakness. The most likely diagnosis is

   (A) progressive multifocal leukodystrophy
   (B) central nervous system lymphoma
   (C) brain metastasis
   (D) glioblastoma multiforme
   (E) bacterial abscess

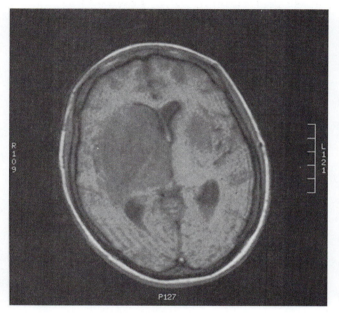

FIG. 9a

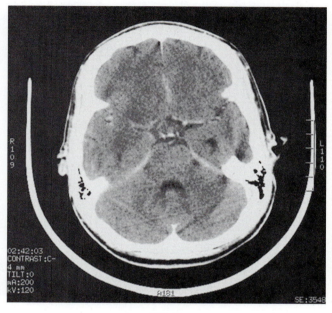

FIG. 9c

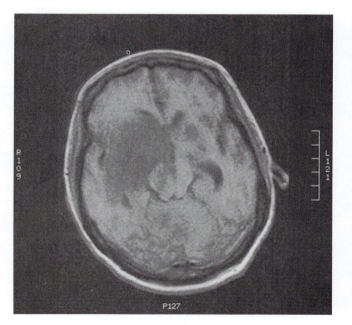

FIG. 9b

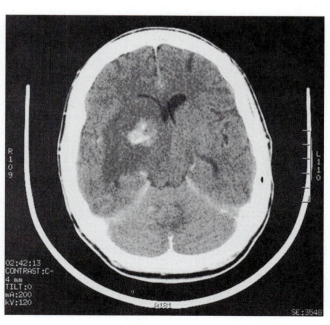

FIG. 9d

10. This is a head CT scan and MRI of a 62-year-old woman with no past medical history, who was hospitalized with a chief complaint of change in her mental status. The most likely diagnosis is

(A) brain metastasis

(B) meningioma

(C) aneurysm

(D) oligodendroglioma

(E) pilocytic astrocytoma

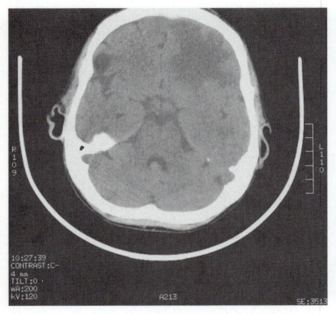

FIG. 10a

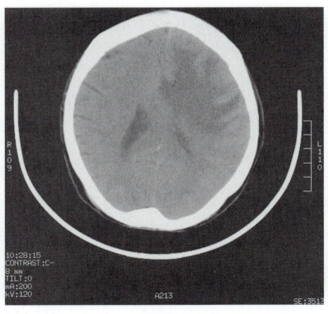

FIG. 10c

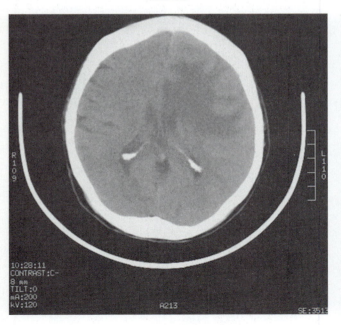

FIG. 10b

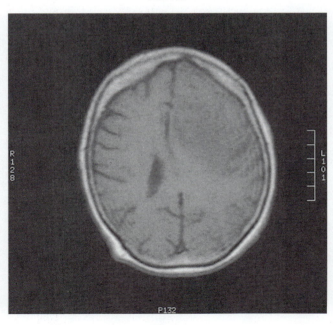

FIG. 10d

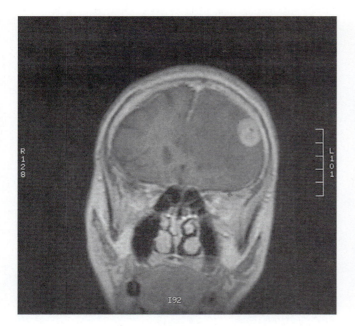

FIG. 10e

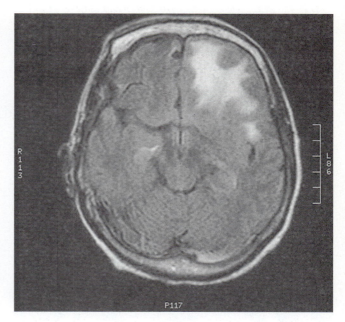

FIG. 10g

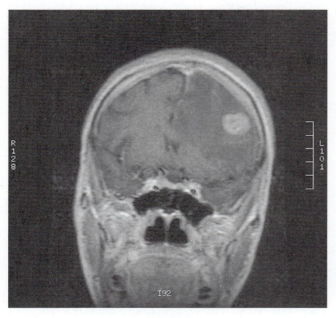

FIG. 10f

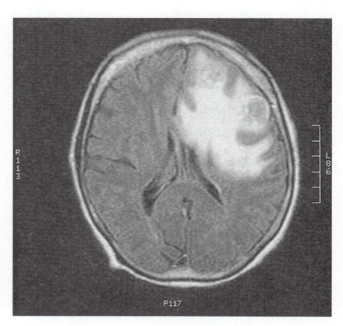

FIG. 10h

11. This is the imaging study of a 20-year-old woman with new onset of acute headache, sub-acute fever, and new onset seizures. The most likely diagnosis is

(A) normal head MRI
(B) viral meningitis
(C) left anterior cerebral artery stroke
(D) superior sagittal sinus thrombosis
(E) cortical dyplasia

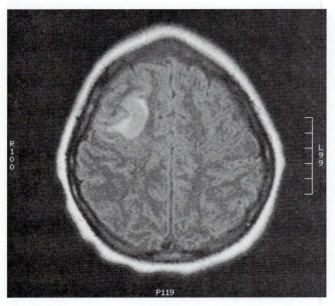

FIG. 11a

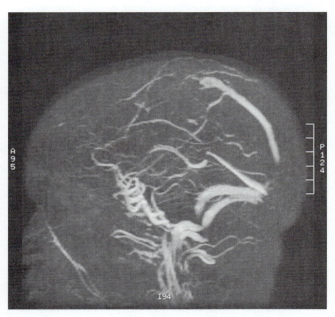

FIG. 11c

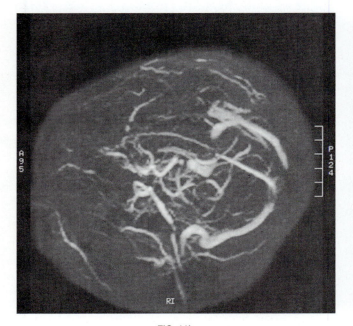

FIG. 11b

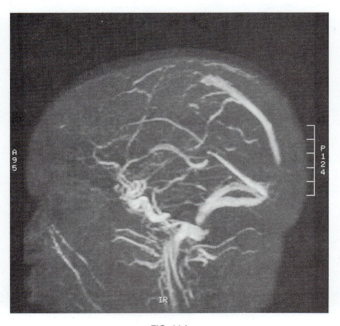

FIG. 11d

Answers and Explanations

1. **(B)** This is an unenhanced CT scan of the head. It shows a large area of hypodensity within the left medial frontal lobe. There is a similar region of hypodensity within the right medial frontal region, which is smaller in size. These findings are typical of evolving infarcts within the territory of the left and right anterior cerebral arteries (ACA). There is no mass or midline shift. The basal cisterns are intact. The ventricles are normal in size and shape.

   Infarction in the ACA distribution is uncommon and bilateral infarction is rare. ACA infarctions are cortical or subcortical and are caused by embolism. The clinical spectrum of unilateral infarction in the ACA territory is broad and may include disinhibition and hemiparesis predominant in the leg. Bilateral infarction in the ACA territories causes a profound neurological syndrome, highlighted by akinetic mutism and poor recovery. *(Minagar and Noble, 886)*

2. **(D)** These are multiple axial images of the brain MRI, with and without contrast. There is a left cerebellar mass with low signal intensity on T1-weighted images demonstrating minimal enhancement. This mass causes compression of the fourth ventricle. There is also increased signal intensity in the subependymal region consistent with transependymal resorption of cerebrospinal fluid. The lateral and third ventricles are dilated. These findings are consistent with obstructive hydrocephalus.

   This profile is suggestive of a metastatic tumor. Most brain metastases that present with an unknown primary tumor suffer from lung cancer. A more extensive search for the primary tumor does not appear to improve overall survival. The search for a primary tumor should focus on tumors that are sensitive to systemic treatment. Magnetic resonance imaging (MRI) is superior to computed tomography (CT) for detection of metastatic disease. *(Van den Bent, 717–723)*

3. **(C)** MRI examination of the brain parenchyma demonstrates a right cerebellar lesion with a fluid level, a surrounding edema, and minimal gadolinium enhancement. There is a lesion with a left posterior temporal fluid level and a surrounding edema as well as mass-effect upon the posterior horn of the left lateral ventricle. There are multiple intracranial lesions demonstrating fluid levels and hemorrhagic components consistent with hemorrhagic metastasis.

   Cerebral metastases from melanoma, renal cell carcinoma, thyroid carcinoma, and choriocarcinoma have a propensity to bleed. Although metastases from breast and lung cancer are less prone to bleed, a cerebral hemorrhagic metastasis is still more likely to originate from lung or breast cancer because these are the most frequently occurring malignancies. A single cerebral hemorrhagic mass should lead one to suspect a primary brain tumor such as glioblastoma multiforme. *(Grossman and Yousen, 79–82)*

4. **(B)** This image shows a 2-cm nonenhancing suprasellar mass. It is rounded, with regular borders, and signal characteristics similar to cerebrospinal fluid. These characteristics are consistent with an arachnoid cyst.

   Arachnoid cysts are usually a congenital malformation derived from the meninx primitiva. Their most common location is the middle cranial fossa. Less commonly, they may be seen in the cerebral convexities, the basal cisterns, and the retrocerebellar region. They result from a splitting of normal arachnoid membranes by congenital aberrations of increased CSF pulsatile flow. They constitute 1% of all intracranial space-occupying lesions. On MRI scan, an arachnoid cyst follows the intensity of the cerebrospinal fluid with low signal intensity on T1-weighted images and a high signal intensity on T2-weighted images. The major differential diagnosis with arachnoid cyst is epidermoid cyst. The latter may show an internal matrix on T1-weighted non-enhanced MRI, and hyperintense signal compared to cerebrospinal fluid on FLAIR images. *(Grossman and Yousem, 247–249; Pollice et al., 764–765)*

5. **(D)** This is a magnetic resonance study with T1-weighted image, T2-weighted image, FLAIR, and diffusion weighted images. There are areas of abnormal signal present on the FLAIR weighted images in the pons; the left inferior pons is particularly bright on the diffusion-weighted images. The abnormal signals on the FLAIR and T2-weighted images in the periventricular deep white matter, which are not seen on diffusion, correspond to small vessel ischemic changes. The ventricular system is normal in size and is midline. The subarachnoid spaces are unremarkable. These findings are compatible with the diagnosis of acute left pontine ischemic stroke.

    Clinical symptoms of pontine stroke are variable and depend on the location and extension of the ischemic damage. In a ventral pontine infarct, motor symptoms vary from mild hemiparesis in a small ventrolateral pontine infarction, to contralateral hemiplegia with dysarthria and ataxia in a ventromedial infarction. Tegmental pontine lesions may cause sensory disturbances and ipsilateral cranial nerve dysfunction, such as facial palsy. Basilar artery branch disease is more commonly associated with pontine stroke than cardioembolism or large arteries stenosis. Large ventral infarcts carry the worst prognosis. *(Bassetti et al., 165–175)*

6. **(B)** This is a head MRI study with T1- and T2-weighted images, including sagittal and coronal sections. It shows a large (4.0 × 2.5 cm) pituitary sellar mass, with suprasellar extension and bowing into the sphenoid sinus that has intermediate signal on T1 and T2. The mass protrudes ventrally into the sphenoid sinus and superiorly compresses the optic chiasm. There is no evidence of chronic hemorrhage or methemoglobin. This lesion is most consistent with pituitary macroadenoma. MRI of the sellar and parasellar regions is the imaging study of choice for the diagnosis of pituitary adenoma. The size of the pituitary gland is variable and depends on the age and sex of the patient. The maximum height allowed for the pituitary gland is 12 mm in women in late pregnancy and postpartum, 10 mm in women of child bearing, 8 mm in men and postmenopausal women, and 6 mm in children. Microadenomas are more common than macroadenomas; their MRI detection rate varies from 65% to 90%. MRI signs of microadenomas may include hypointensity on T1-weighted sequences, focal enlargement of the gland, and sella floor thinning or erosion. In case of macroadenomas, head MRI may show sellar enlargement in 94% to 100% of cases. It may also show a lobulated pituitary margin. MRI of the pituitary gland is a useful tool in defining the extent of a pituitary mass to the cavernous sinus, and in following the effect of medical treatment on the size of the macroadenoma. *(Anderson et al., 703–721)*

7. **(B)** Magnetic resonance image of the brain shows decrease in sulcation over the temporal, frontal, and right occipital lobes consistent with the diagnosis of lissencephaly. The ventricular system is in the midline. There is dilatation of both lateral ventricles; the right lateral ventricle is significantly more dilated than the left. Especially dilated are the occipital horns of both lateral ventricles. Lissencephaly is divided into two types based on histological criteria, extent of damage, and clinical features. In both types, the brain appears smooth on gross inspection. In lissencephaly type 1, the neocortex has 4 poorly organized layers instead of 6 well-organized layers. In type 2 lissencephaly, the cortex is unlayered, with a cobblestone surface and thickened meninges. The clinical spectrum of lissencephaly is heterogeneous and may include seizures, motor delay, hypotonia, and mental retardation. *(Porter et al., 361–365)*

8. **(C)** Figure 8a is a head CT upper left image without contrast. It shows a lesion approximately 1.2 cm in diameter of hyperdensity along the region of the genu of the right internal capsule. This represents hemorrhage. There is no subarachnoid hemorrhage and no associated mass lesion. The rest of the imaging study is head MRI images that include T1, proton density, gradient echo images, and T2-weighted images. Gradient-echo images demonstrate multiple foci of markedly decreased signal. These are consistent with hemosiderin staining, likely related to multiple cavernous hemangiomas. Cavernous hemangioma is a benign vascular lesion that may occur at any site within the central nervous system. It is formed by ectatic, endothelial, lined channels without mural muscular or elastic fibers and without any neuronal elements. It does not have a direct high-pressure arterial supply or distinct venous drainage, which distinguish cavernous hemangioma from arteriovenous malformation. It is characterized, on T2-weighted MRI, by a reticulated core of mixed signal representing blood various state of degradation surrounded by a hypointense halo due to hemosiderin. *(Moran et al., 561–568)*

9. **(B)** This imaging study shows a contrast-enhancing lesion within the right basal ganglion with significant vasogenic edema and mass-effect on the surrounding structures, with compression of the anterior horn of the right lateral ventricle and midline shift. These findings are suggestive of either toxoplasmosis or lymphoma and less likely PLM. These three diagnoses are particularly increased in frequency in AIDS, whereas bacterial abscess, glioblastoma multiforme, and bacterial metastasis are not. Primary central nervous system lymphoma (PCNSL) accounts for 1% to 1.5% of all primary brain tumors. It is a common complication for HIV patients and occurs in as many as 20% of patients. The most common presenting signs of PCNSL are altered level of consciousness, focal neurological deficits, and seizures. Radiological signs of PCNSL may include a homogeneous enhancing lesion on CT scan in the central gray matter, corpus callosum, or ring-enhancing lesion. Head MRI is more sensitive than CT scan for detecting CNS lymphoma. Most lesions are located close to the ependymal or meningeal areas. The main differential diagnosis of PCNSL in HIV patient is CNS toxoplasmosis and progressive multifocal leukoencephalopathy. Lesions in CNS toxoplasmosis may have the tendency to have more multiple enhancing lesions of smaller size than PCNSL on CT scan. PET or SPECT scanning can help confirm the diagnosis. Biopsy is now rarely performed. *(Ciacci et al., 213–221)*

10. **(A)** The head CT scan of this patient shows a large region of hypoattenuation within the anterior left frontal region, suggesting the presence of edema with mass effect on the lateral ventricle and a shift of the midline. MRI examination of the brain shows, within the superior left frontal lobe, inhomogeneously enhancing lesions with edema and mass-effect as well as minimal midline shift. These findings are suggestive of brain metastasis.

   Brain metastasis is the most common cause of intracranial mass in adults. It is an important cause of morbidity and mortality in cancer patients. They are found at autopsy in approximately 25% of patients who die of cancer. Metastases are often multiple; however, in 30% to 50% of cases they may be a solitary lesion on brain imaging. Cancers of the lung, breast, skin, kidney, and thyroid frequently metastasize to the brain. Most patients that present with a brain metastasis of unknown origin suffer from lung cancer. The typical location of brain metastasis is the gray-white matter junction because tumor cells lodge in the small caliber vessels in this location. Head MRI with contrast is the imaging technique of choice in detecting brain tumors. It is more sensitive than head CT scan with contrast in detecting brain metastasis. Metastatic brain lesion typically has an enhanced, rounded, and circumscribed mass surrounded by a disproportionate vasogenic edema, which is manifested by an increased signal on T2-weighted images. *(Van den Bent, 717–723)*

11. **(D)** The FLAIR head MRI of this patient shows a serpiginous right frontal hyperintensity signal. MR venography reveals cut-off of the anterior half of the superior sagittal sinus. These findings suggest a right frontal lobe infarction secondary

to superior sagittal venous thrombosis. Cerebral venous thrombosis (CVT) is commonly under-diagnosed, causing a delay in recognizing this entity, which may lead to devastating disability, and even death. The clinical spectrum of the disease includes seizures, focal neurological signs, headache, and papilledema related to increased intracranial pressure. Computed axial tomography (especially without contrast) as well as conventional T1- and T2-weighted MRI images have a low sensitivity for diagnosing CVT. Alteration in blood flow and hemoglobin degradation in cerebral venous thrombosis may produce signal changes in conventional MRI imaging that may suggest the diagnosis; however, these changes are often subtle. MR venography (MRV) and echo-planar T2 imaging are becoming the techniques of choice to establish the diagnosis of CVT and should be performed when there is a high index of suspicion of the disease. *(Selim et al., 1021–1026)*

REFERENCES

Anderson, JR. Antoun, N. Burnet, N. Chatterjee, K. Edwards, O. Pickard, JD. Sarkies, N. Neurology of the pituitary gland. *J Neurol Neurosurg Psychiatr.* 1999;66:703–721.

Atlas SW, Grossman RI, Gomri M et al. Hemorrhagic intracranial malignant neoplasms: spin-echo MR imaging. *Radiology.* 1987;164:71–77.

Bassetti C, Bogousslavsky J, Barth, A, Regli F. Isolated infarcts of the pons. *Neurology.* 1996;46:165–175.

Ciacci JD. Tellez C. VonRoenn J. Levy RM. Lymphoma of the central nervous system in AIDS. *Sem Neurol.* 1999;19:213–221.

Grossman RI, Yousem DM. *Neuroradiology: The Requisites.* St. Louis: Mosby; 2002.

Minagar A, David NJ. Bilateral infarction in the territory of the anterior cerebral arteries. *Neurology.* 1999;52:886–888.

Moran NF, Fish DR, Kitchen N, Shorvon S, Kendall BE, Stevens JM. Supratentorial cavernous haemangiomas and epilepsy: *J Neurol Neurosurg Psychiatr.* 1999;66:561–568.

Pollice PA, Bhatti NI, Niparko JK. Imaging quiz case 1. Posterior fossa arachnoid cyst. *Arch Otolaryngol Head Neck Surg.* 1997;123:762, 764–765.

Porter BE, Brooks-Kayal, A, Golden JA. Disorders of cortical development and epilepsy. *Arch Neurol.* 2002;59:361–365.

Selim M, Fink J, Linfante I, Kumar S, Schlaug G, Caplan LR. Diagnosis of cerebral venous thrombosis with echo-planar T2*-weighted magnetic resonance imaging. *Arch Neurol.* 2002;59:1021–1026.

Van den Bent MJ. The diagnosis and management of brain metastases. *Curr Opin Neurol.* 2001;14:717–723.

CHAPTER 17

Psychiatry
Questions

1. The highest rate of completed suicide among adult males is at the age of

   (A) 20 years
   (B) 35 years
   (C) 55 years
   (D) 65 years
   (E) 75 years

2. The peak of a panic attack is reached within

   (A) 6 hours
   (B) 3 hours
   (C) 1 hour
   (D) 20 seconds
   (E) 10 minutes

3. At what age does an infant drink from a cup, walk, and say dada/mama nonspecifically?

   (A) Four months
   (B) Six months
   (C) Eight months
   (D) Ten months
   (E) Twelve months

4. Autonomy versus shame and the doubt stage of Erikson's epigenetic model of development correspond to which stage of Freud's psychosexual model of development?

   (A) Oral phase
   (B) Anal phase
   (C) Phallic phase
   (D) Latency phase
   (E) Adolescence phase

5. A 6-year-old boy was brought to the outpatient clinic by his mother because of easy distractibility and poor school performance. The mother states that for the past 12 months, her son experienced difficulty engaging in quiet leisure activities, talked excessively, and interrupted others frequently. In school, he was reported to avoid activities that require mental effort, to have poor concentration, and to be easily distractible. What is the most likely diagnosis?

   (A) Oppositional defiant disorder
   (B) Bipolar disorder
   (C) Obsessive compulsive disorder
   (D) Conduct disorder
   (E) Attention deficit hyperactivity disorder

6. Which of the following medications is contraindicated in the management of acute agitation in an 84-year-old man with a history of normal pressure hydrocephalus and coronary artery disease with arrhythmia?

   (A) Midazolam
   (B) Haloperidol
   (C) Droperidol
   (D) Morphine sulfate
   (E) Lorazepam

7. The positive reinforcement of alcohol is mediated by

   (A) activation of glutamate receptors
   (B) activation of GABA A receptors
   (C) decreased norepinephrine activity in the brain
   (D) inhibition of dopamine release
   (E) opioid release inhibition

8. A 30-year-old alcoholic man was admitted to the emergency room because he was found by his neighbors to be acting agitated and confused. Which of the following is more suggestive of delirium tremens rather than acute alcoholic hallucination?

   (A) Mild tremor
   (B) Auditory hallucination
   (C) 20 days' duration
   (D) Dilated pupils with slow reaction to light
   (E) Clear sensorium

9. What is the mechanism of action of disulfiram?

   (A) Inhibition of intestinal absorption of alcohol
   (B) Inhibition of liver transport of alcohol
   (C) Inhibition of alcohol dehydrogenase
   (D) Inhibition of aldehyde dehydrogenase
   (E) Increased renal excretion of alcohol

10. Which of the following questions is NOT a part of the CAGE questionnaire?

   (A) Have you gotten into physical fights when drinking?
   (B) Have you ever felt you should cut down on your drinking?
   (C) Have people annoyed you by criticizing your drinking?
   (D) Have you ever felt bad or guilty about your drinking?
   (E) Have you ever had a drink first thing in the morning to steady your nerves or to get rid of a hangover?

11. The craving for alcohol is reduced by

   (A) lorazepam
   (B) naltrexone
   (C) disulfiram
   (D) diazepam
   (E) amitriptyline

12. In the central nervous system, cocaine acts by

   (A) blocking D1 dopamine receptors
   (B) inhibiting acetylcholine esterase in the central nervous system

   (C) mediating its rewarding effect through dopamine cells in the ventral tegmentum area that projects to the basal ganglia
   (D) increasing the reuptake of norepinephrine
   (E) activating GABA receptors

13. Epidemiological studies have shown that in schizophrenia

   (A) women tend to have earlier age of onset of the disease and poorer outcome than men
   (B) urban poor population has a lower incidence of the disease
   (C) the majority of cases occurring after the age of 40 are men
   (D) at-risk children have a normal scholastic test
   (E) children who have been abused have an earlier age of onset and a poorer outcome

14. Major depression is characterized by loss of interest or pleasure for more than

   (A) 2 years
   (B) 6 months
   (C) 3 months
   (D) 6 weeks
   (E) 2 weeks

15. Which of the following statements about major depression is TRUE?

   (A) The lifetime prevalence rates for adult men range from 3% to 9%.
   (B) Relapse after a single episode is about 50%.
   (C) Thirty precent of individuals with a single episode of major depression develop bipolar disorder.
   (D) An average age of onset of unipolar major depression is 50 years.
   (E) Full recovery from major depression occurs in 25% of patients by 6 months.

16. A good correlation between the blood level and the clinical effect of an antidepressant is seen with

(A) imipramine

(B) fluoxetine

(C) paroxetine

(D) trazodone

(E) phenelzine

17. Which of the following is NOT a cardinal feature of mania?

(A) Insomnia

(B) Distractibility

(C) Low self-esteem

(D) Flight of ideas

(E) Thoughtlessness

18. The treatment of choice of rapid cycling bipolar disorder is

(A) lithium

(B) valproic acid

(C) carbamazepine

(D) clonazepam

(E) haloperidol

19. Posttraumatic stress disorder spares the

(A) thalamus

(B) prefrontal cortex

(C) red nucleus

(D) hippocampus

(E) amygdala

Questions 20 through 24

Link the following.

(A) Somatization disorder

(B) Hypochondriasis

(C) Both

(D) Neither

20. Fear of having a serious illness despite adequate medical evaluation

21. "La belle indifference"

22. Depression may be a comorbid condition

23. Family history of substance abuse

24. Delusion is a common feature

25. Factitious disorder is differentiated from malingering by which one of the following characteristics?

(A) The production of physical signs is under voluntary control.

(B) The absence of secondary gain.

(C) The presence of a serious organic disorder as a comorbid factor.

(D) The primary motivation of the patient is to assume the sick role.

(E) The patient may intentionally produce symptoms of another person who is under his care.

26. Which of the following anatomical structures is responsible for the genesis of rapid eye movement sleep?

(A) Ascending reticular activating system

(B) Thalamus

(C) Red nucleus

(D) Putamen

(E) Nucleus coeruleus (Locus ceruleus)

27. Restless leg syndrome may be exacerbated by using

(A) fluoxetine

(B) L dopa

(C) bromocriptine

(D) clonazepam

(E) pergolide

28. Neuroleptic malignant syndrome results from

(A) anaphylactic reaction to a neuroleptic medication

(B) depletion of synatic dopamine stores in the CNS

(C) blockade of central dopamine receptors

(D) central dopamine receptor hypersensitivity to neuroleptics

(E) inhibition of serotonin reuptake in the CNS

Questions 29 through 32
Link each of the following biological or genetic markers to the appropriate psychiatric disorder.

    (A) Short arm of chromosome 4
    (B) X chromosome
    (C) 5 hydroxyindoleacetic acid
    (D) A1 allele of D2 receptors

29. Tourette syndrome

30. Infantile autism

31. Huntington disease

32. Suicidal behavior

Questions 33 through 38
Link each of the following antipsychotic agents to its corresponding side effect.

    (A) Thioridazine
    (B) Haloperidol
    (C) Clozapine
    (D) Risperidone
    (E) Olanzapine
    (F) Quetiapine

33. Agranulocytosis

34. Akathisia

35. QT interval prolongation and risk of arrhythmia

36. Thyroid dysfunction

37. Orthostatic hypotension

38. Elevation of hepatic transaminase

39. Grand mal seizure is the most prominent side effect of

    (A) bupropion
    (B) phenelzine
    (C) fluoxetine
    (D) amitriptyline
    (E) venlafaxine

40. Delirium with abnormal EEG and abnormal renal function is seen at a minimal lithium range level of

    (A) 1.2 to 1.5 meq meq/L
    (B) 1.6 to 1.9 meq/L
    (C) 2.0 to 2.5 meq/L
    (D) 2.6 to 3 meq/L
    (E) above 3 meq/L

41. Stimulant drugs appear to be more effective in the treatment of which of the following symptoms of narcolepsy?

    (A) Sleep paralysis
    (B) Sleep attacks
    (C) Cataplexy
    (D) Hypnagogic hallucination
    (E) Restless nighttime sleep

42. The lithium level increases with the co-administration of

    (A) theophylline
    (B) mannitol
    (C) sodium chloride
    (D) acetazolamide
    (E) captopril

43. Drug-induced hypertension may be seen with the use of

    (A) venlafaxine
    (B) imipramine
    (C) clozapine
    (D) nortriptyline
    (E) risperidone

44. A 30-year-old woman was evaluated over a 5 year period for various symptoms including headaches, arthralgia, and pain in the abdomen, chest, and pelvis. An extensive workup as an outpatient in different subspecialty clinics (neurology, cardiology, gastroenterolgy, rheumatology, pulmonary, gynecology, and urology) has been negative. The patient reports a chaotic lifestyle because of her condition despite the absence of an organic abnormality. What is the most likely diagnosis?

(A) Somatization disorder

(B) Dysmorphic disorder

(C) Factitious disorder

(D) Malingering

(E) Conversion disorder

45. Weight gain is LEAST likely to be caused by the long term use of

(A) clozapine

(B) piperidine

(C) haloperidol

(D) molindone

(E) risperidone

46. A 10-year-old boy was brought to a psychiatric clinic by his mother because of marked impairment in his social interaction. He has no friends and does not make eye contact. He is unable to identify objects of interest to other people and exhibits stereotyped and repetitive hand and finger flapping. He has normal language and cognitive development. Neurological examination is normal. What is the most likely diagnosis?

(A) Asperger's disorder

(B) Autism

(C) Pervasive development disorder not otherwise specified

(D) Schizoid personality disorder

(E) Rett syndrome

47. With kleptomaniacs,

(A) objects are stolen for their financial value

(B) thievery is pleasurable

(C) there is antisocial behavior

(D) there is a decreasing sense of tension immediately before the theft

(E) after the theft, there is anger and vengeance

48. Priapism is a serious side effect of

(A) haloperidol

(B) lorazepam

(C) trazodone

(D) risperidone

(E) valproic acid

49. The next step in the treatment of a child who has attention deficit hyperactive disorder and who fails to respond to methylphenidate is to use

(A) bupropion

(B) clonidine

(C) magnesium pemoline

(D) dextroamphetamine

(E) guafenosine

50. A 20-year-old woman with no past medical history consults a physician because of recurrent abdominal pain, nausea, vomiting, and weakness in the lower extremities. She also reports paranoid ideation and auditory hallucination. What is the most likely diagnosis?

(A) Hepatic encephalopathy

(B) Acute intermittent porphyria

(C) Niacin deficiency

(D) Thiamine deficiency

(E) Cobalamin deficiency

51. What is the substance most likely to provoke an acute panic attack in a patient suffering from a panic disorder?

(A) Carbon dioxide inhalation

(B) Dopamine

(C) Lactate

(D) Caffeine

(E) Yohimbine

52. Which of the following medications is most appropriate for an 80-year-old man with major depression and history of glaucoma, orthostatic hypotension, and urinary hesitation?

(A) Nortriptyline

(B) Amitriptyline

(C) Trimipramine

(D) Doxepin

(E) Imipramine

53. Which of the following symptoms is the earliest indication of lithium intoxication?

    (A) Impaired consciousness
    (B) Myoclonus
    (C) Seizures
    (D) Coarse tremor
    (E) Acute renal failure

54. Which of the following is NOT a sign of lithium toxicity?

    (A) Dry mouth
    (B) Seizure
    (C) Constipation
    (D) Delirium
    (E) Polyuria

55. Neurotoxicity of lithium may increase with the co-administration of which of the following drugs?

    (A) Sodium bicarbonate
    (B) Caffeine
    (C) Mannitol
    (D) Acetazolamide
    (E) Amlodipine

Questions 56 through 59
Link each of the following side effects to the drug most likely to cause it.

    (A) Agranulocytosis
    (B) Hepatoxicity
    (C) Cardiac conduction disturbance
    (D) Hypothyroidism

56. Clozapine

57. Lithium

58. Pemoline

59. Imipramine

60. In which stage of pregnancy do major pharmacokinetic changes of lithium metabolism occur?

    (A) First trimester
    (B) Second trimester

    (C) Third trimester
    (D) At delivery
    (E) Postpartum and during breast-feeding

61. Functional neuroimaging of patients with attention-deficit hyperactivity disorder shows decreased activity in which region of the brain?

    (A) The prefrontal cortex
    (B) The temporal lobe
    (C) The parietal lobe
    (D) The thalamus
    (E) The amygdala

62. Irreversible pigmentation of the retina is seen as a side effect with the chronic use of

    (A) chlorpromazine
    (B) thioridazine
    (C) lithium
    (D) risperidone
    (E) valproic acid

63. Which of the following is TRUE about the effect of chronic alcohol consumption on sleep?

    (A) Decreased REM sleep
    (B) Increased stage IV sleep
    (C) Decreased sleep fragmentation
    (D) Increased sleep latency

Questions 64 through 70
Link each of the following abused substances to the most appropriate signs of acute intoxication.

    (A) Alcohol
    (B) Cocaine
    (C) Heroin
    (D) Cannabis
    (E) Phencyclidine
    (F) LSD (Lysergic acid diethylamide)
    (G) Caffeine

64. Impairment in attention or memory, slurred speech, euphoria, and pupillary vasoconstriction

65. Anxiety, depression, paranoid ideation, subjective intensification of perceptions, hallucinations, tachycardia, and sweating

66. Dysarthria, ataxia, muscle rigidity, decreased response to pain, vertical nystagmus, and labile affect

67. Impaired judgment, slurred speech, incoordination, unsteady gait, and nystagmus

68. Euphoria, tachycardia, elevated blood pressure, pupillary dilatation, and seizure

69. Excitement, restlessness, tachycardia, muscle twitching, insomnia, and diuresis

70. Euphoria, conjunctival injection, increased appetite, tachycardia, and impaired judgment

Questions 71 through 75
Link each of the following abused substances to the most appropriate signs of withdrawal.

   (A) Alcohol
   (B) Cocaine
   (C) Heroin
   (D) Nicotine
   (E) Caffeine

71. Insomnia, transient visual, tactile or auditory hallucination, and autonomic hyperactivity

72. Dysphoric mood, fatigue, vivid unpleasant dreams, and increased appetite

73. Headache, nausea, vomiting, marked fatigue and depression

74. Dysphoric mood, nausea, vomiting, muscle aches, pupillary dilation, piloerection, and sweating

75. Depressed mood, insomnia, decreased heart rate, and increased appetite

76. Electroconvulsive therapy is least likely to be successful in which of the following diseases?

   (A) Major depression
   (B) Acute schizophrenia
   (C) Acute manic episodes
   (D) Chronic schizophrenia
   (E) Obsessive-compulsive disorder

77. The CAGE questionnaire is used in case of

   (A) catatonic schizophrenia
   (B) Pick disease
   (C) mental retardation
   (D) bipolar disorder
   (E) alcohol abuse

78. Alprazolam's half life increases with the co-administration of

   (A) fluoxetine
   (B) fluvoxamine
   (C) paroxetine
   (D) sertraline
   (E) clozaril

Answers and Explanations

1. **(E)** Suicide, the eighth leading cause of death in the United States, accounts for more than 30,000 deaths per year. The suicide rate in men (18.7 suicides per 100,000 men in 1998) is more than 4 times that in women (4.4 suicides per 100,000 women in 1998). In females, suicide rates remain relatively constant beginning in the midteens. In males, suicide rates are stable from the late teenage years until the late 70s, when the rate increases substantially to 41 suicides per 100,000 persons annually in men 75 to 84 years of age. *(Mann, 302–311)*

2. **(E)** Panic disorder is a syndrome characterized by unexpected and unprovoked attacks of anxiety that produce both cognitive and physical symptoms. The lifetime prevalence of panic disorder in the general population is 1.6%. The disorder has a unimodal distribution, peaking in the third decade of life. Panic disorder affects more females than males. The major distinguishing feature of panic disorder is the combination of cognitive and physical symptoms. Onset is rapid, peaking within 10 minutes, and the attack lasts about 60 minutes. The typical patient has 2 to 4 attacks per week, often accompanied by anticipatory anxiety. A patient who sustains 4 panic attacks in 4 weeks or 1 or more attacks followed by 4 weeks of continuous anticipatory anxiety may be said to have panic disorder. *(Zun, 92–96)*

3. **(E)** At the age of 12 months, an infant with normal psychomotor development can drink from a cup, walk, and say dada/mama non-specifically. *(Stern et al., 25)*

4. **(B)** Erikson's formulations were based on the concept that epigenetic development occurs in sequential, clearly defined stages, and that each stage must be satisfactorily resolved for development to proceed smoothly. If successful resolution of a particular stage does not occur, all subsequent stages reflect the failure in the form of physical, cognitive, social, or emotional maladjustment. Erikson described 8 stages of the life cycle:

   Stage 1 corresponds to trust versus mistrust.
   Stage 2 corresponds to autonomy versus shame and doubt.
   Stage 3 corresponds to initiative versus guilt.
   Stage 4 corresponds to industry versus inferiority.
   Stage 5 corresponds to ego identity versus role confusion.
   Stage 6 corresponds to intimacy versus isolation.
   Stage 7 corresponds to generativity versus stagnation.
   Stage 8 corresponds to ego integrity versus despair.

Stage 2 is the autonomy versus shame and doubt (about 1 to 3 years) stage and corresponds to the anal phase of Freud's psychosexual model of development. Autonomy concerns children's sense of mastery over themselves and over their drives and impulses. For Erikson, it is the time for children either to retain feces (holding in) or to eliminate feces (letting go); both behaviors have an effect on the mother. Children in the second and third years of life learn to walk alone, to feed themselves, to control the anal sphincter, and to talk. Muscular maturation sets the tone for this stage of development. When parents permit children to function with some autonomy and are supportive without being overprotective, toddlers gain self-confidence and feel that they can control themselves and their world. But if toddlers are punished for being autonomous or are overcontrolled, they feel angry and ashamed. If parents show approval when children show self-control, children's self-esteem is enhanced, and a sense of pride develops. *(Kaplan and Sadock, 214–215, 233–239)*

5. **(E)** The patient in this vignette has symptoms of inattention (he was reported to avoid activities that require mental effort, to have poor concentration, and to be easily distractible), hyperactivity (had difficulty engaging in leisure activity quietly), and impulsivity (grabbed things and interrupted others frequently). These symptoms are highly suggestive of attention deficit hyperactivity disorder.

Attention deficit hyperactivity disorder (ADHD) is characterized by poor ability to attend to a task, motor overactivity, and impulsivity. Oppositional and aggressive behaviors are often seen in conjunction with ADHD. The cause of ADHD is unknown. Genetic factors as well as other factors affecting brain development during prenatal and early postnatal life are most likely responsible. An association of the dopamine receptor D4 gene with a refined phenotype of ADHD has been demonstrated. Growing evidence shows that children with ADHD differ from normal children on neuroimaging measures of brain structure and function. In particular, a prefrontal-striatal-thalamocortical circuit has been implicated. ADHD-afflicted children display various behaviors indicative of problems with attention, hyperactivity, and impulsivity.

According to DSM-IV, inattentiveness is manifested when a child often or constantly (1) makes careless mistakes, failing to give close attention; (2) has difficulty sustaining attention; (3) does not seem to listen; (4) does not follow through on tasks; (5) has difficulty getting organized; (6) dislikes or avoids sustained mental effort; (7) loses things; (8) is easily distracted; and (9) is forgetful. Hyperactivity is evidenced when a child often or constantly

(1) fidgets; (2) is out of his or her seat; (3) runs and climbs excessively; (4) has difficulty playing quietly; (5) is always on the go as though driven by a motor; and (6) talks excessively. Impulsivity is reflected in a child who often or constantly (1) blurts out answers; (2) has difficulty awaiting his or her turn; and (3) interrupts or intrudes on others.

Diagnosis of ADHD requires the presence of at least 6 manifestations from the inattentiveness cluster, the hyperactivity/impulsivity cluster, or both. Children whose symptoms are predominantly from 1 cluster are said to be primarily inattentive or hyperactive/impulsive. Clinical diagnosis requires that the symptoms be evident before age 7 years and be constant for at least 6 months. *(Behrman, 107–110)*

6. **(B)** High doses of haloperidol have been associated with prolongation of cardiac conduction. Patients with a previous history of dilated ventricles, arrhythmia, or alcohol abuse have an increased risk of developing torsade de point. *(Stern et al., 392)*

7. **(B)** Addictive behavior associated with alcoholism is characterized by compulsive preoccupation with obtaining alcohol, loss of control over consumption, and development of tolerance and dependence, as well as impaired social and occupational functioning. Like other addictive disorders, alcoholism is characterized by chronic vulnerability to relapse after cessation of drinking. To understand the factors that compel some individuals to drink excessively, alcohol research has focused on the identification of brain mechanisms that support the reinforcing actions of alcohol and the progression of changes in neural function induced by chronic ethanol consumption that lead to the development of dependence. More recently, increasing attention has been directed toward the understanding of neurobiological and environmental factors in susceptibility torelapse.

Ethanol interacts with dopamine function in the mesolimbic "reward" pathway by activating the dopaminergic neurons of the ventral tegmental area (VTA). Ethanol increases the firing of VTA DA neurons through direct excitation. The activation of GABA A receptors which open chloride channels inducing a primary central nervous system depressant effect as well as the inhibition of glutamate NMDA receptors are the positive reinforcement of alcohol effect. Other factors involved in the positive reinforcement of alcohol include interaction with serotonin systems and the release of opioid peptides. *(Stern et al., 73–74; Weiss and Porrino, 3332–3337)*

8. **(D)** Both delirium tremens and acute alcoholic hallucinosis occur during the withdrawal period in an alcoholic dependent patient. Acute alcoholic hallucinosis may start without a drop in blood alcohol concentration, and without delirium, tremor, or autonomic hyperactivity. Hallucinations are usually auditory and paranoid and may last more than 10 days. In delirium tremens, the patient is confused, with prominent tremor and psychomotor activity, disturbed vital signs, autonomic dysfunction with dilated pupils, and a slow reaction to light. Hallucinations are usually of the visual type. There is difficulty sustaining attention, disorganized thinking, and perceptual disturbances. The duration of symptoms is between 3 to 10 days whereas in acute alcoholic hallucinosis symptom duration is between 5 to 30 days. *(Stern et al., 75)*

9. **(D)** Disulfiram is an alcohol-sensitizing agent that alters the response of the body to alcohol, making its ingestion unpleasant or toxic. It inhibits aldehyde dehydrogenase, the enzyme that catalyzes the oxidation of acetaldehyde, causing blood acetaldehyde levels to increase. The disulfiram-ethanol reaction (DER) varies inversely with the dose of disulfiram and the volume of alcohol consumed. The most common symptoms of the DER are warmness and flushed skin, especially in the upper chest and face, tachycardia, palpitations, and decreased blood pressure. Nausea, vomiting, shortness of breath, sweating, dizziness, blurred vision, and confusion may also occur. In addition to its effects on aldehyde dehydrogenase, disulfiram inhibits a variety of other enzymes, including dopamine beta-hydroxylase. Thus, in addition to the toxicity of the DER caused by the accumulation of acetaldehyde, adverse effects of disulfiram or its metabolites can occur as a result of multiple drug interactions. *(Kranzler et al., 401–423)*

10. **(A)** The CAGE test has a quick and reliable tool to assess alcohol abuse. It has four simple questions:

    "C": Have you ever felt you should cut down on your drinking?
    "A" Have people annoyed you by criticizing your drinking?
    "G" Have you ever felt bad or guilty about your drinking?
    "E" Have you ever had a drink first thing in the morning to steady your nerves or to get rid of a hangover?

    A yes answer is scored 1 and a no answer is scored 0. A score of 2 or more is considered clinically significant. *(Mayfield et al., 1121–1123)*

11. **(B)** Naltrexone is a pure competitive antagonist principally of m, but also of k and d, opioid receptors in the central nervous system. The effect of naltrexone on alcohol craving is not well understood but presumably involves antagonism of endogenous opioid agonists, which may be released on alcohol ingestion and which may contribute to the subjective high. It aids in achieving the goal of abstinence by preventing relapse and decreasing alcohol consumption. *(Kaplan and Sadock, 1064–1067)*

12. **(C)** Cocaine acts by blocking reuptake of neurotransmitters (norepinephrine, dopamine, and serotonin) at the synaptic junctions, resulting in increased neurotransmitter concentrations. Because norepinephrine is the primary neurotransmitter of the sympathetic nervous system, sympathetic stimulation results and leads to vasoconstriction, tachycardia, mydriasis, and hyperthermia. Central nervous system stimulation may appear as increased alertness, energy, talkativeness, repetitive behavior, diminished appetite, and increased libido. Psychological stimulation by cocaine produces an intense euphoria that is often compared to orgasm. Pleasure and reward sensations in the brain have been correlated with increased neurotransmission in the mesolimbic or mesocortical

dopaminergic tracts (or both). Cocaine increases the functional release of dopamine, which activates the ventral tegmental-nucleus accumbens pathway, which seems to be a major component of the brain reward system. Activation of this pathway is essential for the reinforcing actions of psychomotor stimulants. *(Warner, 226–235; Withers et al., 63–78)*

13. **(E)** The prevalence of schizophrenia varies by region in the United States. Its incidence appears to be higher among the urban poor areas. Males manifest the illness between the age of 18 and 25 years whereas females manifest the illness between the age of 26 and 45 years. Twenty percent of cases of schizophrenia occur after the age of 40 years; most are women. Children at risk of schizophrenia have a lower scholastic test score, abnormal affect, and thought disorder early in infancy. Those who are abused have an earlier onset and a poorer course. *(Stern et al., 99)*

14. **(E)** Major depression is a cluster of psychological and physical symptoms that persist for 2 or more weeks and that interfere with a person's ability to function or enjoy life. *(Kaplan and Sadock, 534)*

15. **(B)** The National Comorbidity Survey carried out a structured psychiatric interview of a representative sample of the general population and reported a lifetime rate of major depression of 21.3% in women and 12.7% in men producing a female-to-male ratio of 1.0 to 1.7. A gender difference was found beginning in early adolescence and persisting through the mid-50s. Although this increased tendency for depression in women reflects a long-term trend, over the short term, an increase has also been seen in the rate of depression among young women. The highest rate occurs in adult women aged more than 44 years. Major depression is a recurrent illness; the risk of relapse after one episode is about 50%, whereas it is greater than 80% after 3 episodes. The average lifetime number is 4. The average age of onset of unipolar depression is 29 years. Five to ten percent of individuals with a single episode of major depression will eventually develop bipolar disease whereas 50% of cases of major depression will have full

recovery by 6 months. *(Brown, 241–268; Stern et al., 104–105)*

16. **(A)** Blood level can be obtained for all antidepressant drugs. But not all of them have shown a correlation between the therapeutic effect and the blood level. In 1985, a task force examined the present status of studies investigating the relationship between blood plasma concentrations of tricyclic antidepressants and clinical outcome. It discussed some of the discrepancies that have developed among various antidepressant drugs and evaluates the clinical implications of the current status of blood level monitoring. The task force concluded that plasma level measurements of imipramine, desmethylimipramine, and nortriptyline are unequivocally clinically useful in certain situations. For imipramine, the percentage of favorable responses correlates with plasma levels in a linear manner between 200 and 250 ng/mL, but some patients may respond at a lower level. At levels that exceed 250 ng/mL, there is no improved favorable response, and side effects increase. *(Task Force, 155–162)*

17. **(C)** The diagnosis of manic episodes is established by the presence of irritability or euphoria associated with 3 (euphoria) or 4 (irritability) of the 7 cardinal symptoms of mania. The cardinal symptoms of mania are distractibility, insomnia, grandiosity, flight of ideas, increased activities, pressured speech, and thoughtlessness. *(Stern et al., 116)*

18. **(B)** Divalproex sodium (valproic acid with sodium valproate) was approved by the FDA for the treatment of acute mania in 1995. A therapeutic blood-level window of 45 to 125 mug/mL has been demonstrated to correlate with antimanic response. Valproate might have better efficacy than lithium in the treatment of mixed manic states, rapid cycling mania or other complex, comorbid forms of bipolar disorder, and could synergize with lithium to prevent relapses. Valproate can also be useful in the treatment of AIDS-related mania. *(Goldberg, 211–231)*

19. **(C)** The neurobiology of posttraumatic stress disorder (PTSD) involves the thalamus as a relay

of information about a threat to the prefrontal cortex and amygdala. The hippocampus was found to be affected in adults with PTSD and appears to be related to increased exposure to excitatory amino acids and glucocorticoids. The amygdala plays a key role in consolidating the emotional significance of events. In fact, Vietnam combat veterans with PTSD showed left amygdala activation on SPECT study in response to exposure to combat sound, whereas combat veterans without PTSD and noncombatant controls did not exibit amygdala activation. *(Newport and Nemeroff, 211–218)*

20. **(B)**

21. **(D)**

22. **(C)**

23. **(A)**

24. **(D)**

Explanations 20 through 24

Somatization disorder is characterized by the recurrence of multiple somatic complaints not accounted for by medical findings. It is a chronic condition with female predominance. Hypochondriasis is also a chronic condition characterized by a fear or belief that one has a serious illness despite adequate medical evaluation. Its prevalence is 4% to 9% of medical outpatients with equal incidence between men and women. Major depression is a comorbid condition of both somatization disorder and hypochondriasis. Family history of somatization disorder, antisocial disorder, and substance abuse are reported in somatization disorder whereas a history of illness in family members is reported in hypochondriasis. La belle indifference is an associated feature of conversion disorder, where symptoms do not conform to anatomic pathways. Delusion is not a common feature of either somatization disorder or hypochondriasis. Delusional disorder may be a comorbid condition in body dysmorphic disorder. *(Stern et al., 144–146)*

25. **(B)** Absence of secondary gain is the main feature that differentiates factitious disorder from malingering. In factitious disorder, the patient intentionally produces physical or psychological signs or symptoms that are under voluntary control and are not explained by any other underlying physical or mental disorder. The primary motivation of the behavior is to assume the sick role. There is no secondary gain such as economic benefit or avoidance of legal responsibilities. In malingering, the patient has an obvious recognizable secondary gain in producing their signs and symptoms such as avoiding work or prosecution, or obtaining financial gain. *(Stern et al., 147–150)*

26. **(E)** Hobson proposed the most currently acceptable neuroanatomic model for wakefulness and sleep where rapid eye movement is proposed to arise from the activation of the nucleus ceruleus and the gigantocellular tegmental field, whereas wakefulness is maintained by the ascending reticular activating system. *(Hobson, 1990, 371–382; Hobson, 1975, 369–403; Stern et al., 76)*

27. **(A)** Serotonin reuptake inhibitors such as fluoxetine may exacerbate symptoms of restless leg syndrome whereas medications such as benzodiazepines, levodopa, quinine, opioids, propranolol, and carbamazepine (Tegretol) have some benefit. *(Stern et al., 178)*

28. **(C)** Neuroleptic malignant syndrome is an uncommon but potentially fatal idiosyncratic reaction characterized by the development of altered consciousness, hyperthermia, autonomic dysfunction, and muscular rigidity on exposure to neuroleptic (and probably other psychotropic) medications. The pathophysiology of neuroleptic malignant syndrome (NMS) is poorly understood. The postulated mechanism involves blockade of central dopamine receptors in the basal ganglia, the hypothalamus, and peripherally in postganglionic sympathetic neurons and smooth muscle. The known plasticity of the mesostriatal-mesolimbic dopaminergic system is important in protecting the brain against severe biopsychosocial stressors by means of an appropriately timed receptor down-regulation.

In most people, this homeostatic mechanism is sufficient to protect against psychosis; neuroleptics may help further decrease dopamine receptor sensitivity when the native mechanisms are insufficient. For some patients, however, this further reduction in general dopaminergic tone will result in NMS. As a corollary, it was suggested that the primary mesolimbic hyperdopaminergia might induce a homeostatic response, via GABAergic feedback from the nucleus accumbens, consisting of down-regulation of dopamine receptors in the mesostriatum and hypothalamus. Such a response would then result in a reduction in local dopaminergic tone sufficient to produce lethal catatonia, despite the fact that such mesolimbic hyperdopaminergia would simultaneously cause psychosis. *(Longhurst, 537–538)*

29. **(D)**

30. **(B)**

31. **(A)**

32. **(C)**

Explanations 29 through 32

The prevalence of the D2A1 allele in a range of impulsive, compulsive, addictive disorders ranged from 42.3% to 54.5%. An indication of the importance of the dopamine D2 receptor in Tourette syndrome comes from SPECT studies of monozygotic twins discordant for tic severity. Differences in the D2 receptor density in the head of the caudate nucleus predicted differences in phenotypic severity with a high correlation coefficient, suggesting that striatal dopamine D2 receptor density accounted for 98% of the variance of tic severity. Dopamine is a stress-responsive neurotransmitter. Some studies, using single-photon-emission computed tomography or PET, show increased density of the presynaptic dopamine transporter and the postsynaptic D2 dopamine receptor in Tourette syndrome. These studies suggest that there is abnormal regulation of dopamine release and uptake in this disease.

Fragile X syndrome is primarily a disorder of neurodevelopment, although other organ systems are also involved. In addition to mental retardation, the mutation also predisposes affected individuals to a variety of psychiatric syndromes. A substantial number of males with the fragile X mutation have autism. In one study, nearly 100% have one or more behaviors commonly observed in autism, such as hand flapping and biting, poor eye contact, or tactile defensiveness.

Huntington's disease has an autosomal dominant transmission. Its gene is located on the short arm of chromosome 4.

Platelet 5-HT$_{2A}$ receptors have been found to be increased in proportion to the lethality of the suicide attempt in depressed subjects. Approximately two-thirds of studies comparing subjects who have attempted suicide versus nonattempters show that those who have attempted suicide have low levels of CSF 5-HIAA. One of the factors that is correlated with a low CSF 5-HIAA level is the medical severity of the attempt. CSF 5-HIAA is low in serious suicide attempters, even when the presence of a psychiatric illness (e.g., major depression) is controlled for, and the patients are studied in a drug-free, controlled environment. *(Comings, 50–83; Margolis et al., 1019–1031; Oquendo, 11–25; Weeks, 401–408)*

33. **(C)**

34. **(B)**

35. **(A)**

36. **(F)**

37. **(D)**

38. **(E)**

Explanations 33 through 38

Thioridazine is a D2 dopamine antagonist of low potency. Central nervous system side effects include drowsiness that may be encountered on occasion, especially where large doses are given early in treatment. Generally, this effect tends to subside with continued therapy or a reduction in dosage. Pseudoparkinsonism and other extrapyramidal symptoms may occur but are infrequent. Nocturnal confusion, hyperactivity, lethargy, psychotic reactions, restlessness, and headache have been reported but are extremely rare. Adverse cardiovascular reactions are the most serious side effects and include a dose-related prolongation of the QTc interval, which is associated with the ability to cause torsade de pointes-type arrhythmias, a potentially fatal polymorphic ventricular tachycardia, and sudden death. Autonomic nervous system side effects of thioridazine include dryness of mouth, blurred vision, constipation, nausea, vomiting, diarrhea, and urinary retention.

Haloperidol is a neuoleptic of high potency. Extrapyramidal syndrome (EPS) during its administration has been reported frequently, often during the first few days of treatment. EPS can be categorized generally as having Parkinson-like symptoms, akathisia, or dystonia (including opisthotonos and oculogyric crisis). While all can occur at relatively low doses, they occur more frequently and with greater severity at higher doses. The symptoms may be controlled with dose reductions or administration of antiparkinson drugs such as benztropine.

Clozapine is classified as an "atypical" antipsychotic drug because its profile of binding to dopamine receptors and its effects on various dopamine-mediated behaviors differ from those exhibited by more typical antipsychotic drug products. In particular, although clozapine does interfere with the binding of dopamine at D1, D2, D3, and D5 receptors, and has a high affinity for the D4 receptor, it does not induce catalepsy. This evidence, consistent with the view that clozapine is preferentially more active at limbic than at striatal dopamine receptors, may explain the relative lack of clozapine-induced extrapyramidal side effects. Clozapine also acts as an antagonist at adrenergic, cholinergic, histaminergic, and serotonergic receptors. The incidence of clozapine-induced agranulocytosis is about 1.3% at 1 year, based on the occurrence of 15 U.S. cases out of 1743 patients in the pre-marketing period. This reaction could prove fatal if not detected early and therapy interrupted. The incidence rates of agranulocytosis based upon a weekly monitoring schedule rose steeply during the first 2 months of therapy, peaking in the third month. Among clozapine patients who continued the drug beyond the third month, the weekly incidence of agranulocytosis fell to a substantial degree, so that by the sixth month the weekly incidence of agranulocytosis was reduced to 3 per 1000 person-years. After 6 months, the weekly incidence of agranulocytosis declines still further; however, it never reaches zero.

Risperidone is an antipsychotic agent belonging to the benzisoxazole derivatives. The mechanism of action of risperidone, as with other antipsychotic drugs, is unknown. However, it has been proposed that this drug's antipsychotic activity is mediated through a combination of dopamine type 2 (D2) and serotonin type 2 ($5HT_2$) antagonism. Antagonism at receptors other than D2 and $5HT_2$ may explain some of the other effects of risperidone. It may induce orthostatic hypotension associated with dizziness, tachycardia, and in some patients, syncope, especially during the initial dose-titration period, probably reflecting its alpha-adrenergic antagonistic properties. Syncope was reported in 0.2% of risperidone-treated patients in phase 2 and phase 3 studies.

Olanzapine is an antipsychotropic agent that belongs to the thienobenzodiazepine class. Olanzapine is a selective monoaminergic antagonist with high affinity binding to the following receptors: serotonin $5HT_{2(A)2C}$, dopamine D1-D4, muscarinic M_{1-5}, histamine H_1, and adrenergic _1 receptors. In placebo-controlled studies, clinically significant ALT (SGPT) elevations ($\geq$3 times the upper limit of the normal range) were observed in 2% of patients exposed to olanzapine compared to none of the placebo patients. Periodic assessment of transaminases is recommended in patients with significant hepatic disease.

Quetiapine fumarate is an antagonist at multiple neurotransmitter receptors in the brain: serotonin $5HT_{1A}$ and $5HT_2$, dopamine D1 and D2, histamine H_1 and adrenergic _1 and _2 receptors. Clinical trials with quetiapine fumarate demonstrated a dose-related decrease in total and free thyroxin (T4) of approximately 20% at the higher end of the therapeutic dose range, which was maximal in the first 2-4 weeks of treatment and maintained without adaptation or progression during more chronic therapy. Generally, these changes were of no clinical significance and TSH was unchanged in most patients, and levels of TBG were unchanged. In nearly all cases, cessation of quetiapine fumarate treatment was associated with a reversal of the effects on total and free T4, irrespective of the duration of treatment. *(Enna and Coyle, 34–42)*

39. **(A)** Bupropion is associated with grand mal seizures in approximately 0.4% (4/1000) of patients treated at doses up to 450 mg/day. This incidence of seizures may exceed that of other marketed antidepressants by as much as 4-fold. This relative risk is only an approximate estimate because of the lack of direct comparative studies. The estimated seizure incidence for Bupropion increases almost 10-fold between 450 and 600 mg/day, which is twice the usually required daily dose (300 mg). *(Enna and Coyle, 107)*

40. **(C)** Lithium adverse reactions may be encountered at serum levels below 1.5 mEq/L. Mild to moderate adverse reactions may occur at levels from 1.5–2.5 mEq/L, and moderate to severe reactions may be seen at levels of 2.0 mEq/L and above. Fine hand tremor, polyuria, and mild thirst may occur during initial therapy for the acute manic phase, and may persist throughout treatment. Transient and mild nausea and general discomfort may also appear during the first few days of lithium administration. Diarrhea, vomiting, drowsiness, muscular weakness, and lack of coordination may be early signs of lithium intoxication, and can occur at lithium levels below 2.0 mEq/L. At a level between 2 and 2.5 mEq/L moderate to severe signs of toxicity may appear such as delirium, abnormal EEG, abnormal renal function cardiac arrhythmia, and risk of coma. At a level above 2.5 mEq/L, signs of severe intoxication may appear that include acute renal failure seizure and death. Treatment is by dialysis. *(Enna and Coyle, 125–128; Kaplan and Sadock, 1050)*

41. **(B)** Stimulants appear most effective against daytime somnolence and sleep attacks associated with narcolepsy; they are less beneficial for catalepsy. *(Stern et al., 177–178)*

42. **(E)** The lithium level decreases with the co-administration of mannitol, urea, theophylline and aminophyline, sodium chloride, acetazolamide, and sodium bicarbonate. It increases with the co-administration of ACE inhibitors, thiazide diuretics and nonsteroidal antiinflammatory drugs. *(Stern et al., 385)*

43. **(A)** Venlafaxine is an effective antidepressant drug that acts by nonselective inhibition of the reuptake of 3 biogenic amines: serotonin, norepinephrine, and dopamine. An increase in blood pressure was seen in clinical trials in patients treated with venlafaxine. This occurred most often with doses above 200 mg venlafaxine per day and seems to be dose dependent. *(Stern et al., 356)*

44. **(A)** The patient in this vignette has recurrent multiple chronic somatic complaints that started at the age of 25 years. This objective pathology is found despite evaluations; she also has a chaotic lifestyle. This is most suggestive of somatization disorder; the patient has a chronic condition without identifiable secondary gain. Dysmorphic disorder is unlikely, since the patient did not report an imagined ugliness. Conversion disorder is unlikely, because her condition is not self-limited. The absence of secondary gain makes the diagnosis of malingering unlikely. The absence of voluntary control of the symptoms makes the diagnosis of factitious disorder unlikely. *(Stern et al., 139–140)*

45. **(D)** A common adverse effect of treatment with dopamine receptor antagonists is weight gain, which can be significant in some cases. Molindone and, perhaps, loxapine are not associated with the symptom and may be indicated in patients for whom weight gain is a serious health hazard or a reason for noncompliance. *(Kaplan and Sadock, 1030)*

46. **(A)** Asperger's disorder is characterized by a severe, sustained impairment in social interaction

and restricted, repetitive patterns of behavior, interests, and activities. Unlike autistic disorder, in Asperger's disorder there are no significant delays in language, cognitive development, or age-appropriate self-help skills. The cause of Asperger's disorder is unknown, but family studies suggest a possible relation to autistic disorder. The similarity of Asperger's disorder to autistic disorder leads to genetic, metabolic, infectious, and perinatal hypotheses. The clinical features include at least 2 of the following indications of qualitative social impairment: markedly abnormal nonverbal communicative gestures, the failure to develop peer relationships, the lack of social or emotional reciprocity, and an impaired ability to express pleasure in other people's happiness. *(Kaplan and Sadock, 1190–1191)*

47. **(B)** The essential feature of kleptomania is a recurrent failure to resist impulses to steal objects not needed for personal use or for monetary value. The objects taken are often given away, returned surreptitiously, or kept and hidden. People with kleptomania usually have the money to pay for the objects they impulsively steal. Like other impulse-control disorders, kleptomania is characterized by mounting tension before the act, followed by gratification and lessening of tension with or without guilt, remorse, or depression during the act. The stealing is not planned and does not involve others, but is the goal of the patient with kleptomania. Although the thefts do not occur when immediate arrest is probable, people with kleptomania do not always consider their chances of being apprehended, even though repeated arrests lead to pain and humiliation. These people may feel guilt and anxiety after the theft, but they do not feel anger or vengeance. Furthermore, when the stolen object is itself the goal, the diagnosis is not kleptomania; in kleptomania only the act of stealing is the goal. *(Kaplan and Sadock, 763–764)*

48. **(C)** Trazodone is associated with the rare occurrence of priapism, the symptom of prolonged erection in the absence of sexual stimuli. That symptom appears to result from the α2-adrenergic antagonism of trazodone. *(Kaplan and Sadock, 1098–1100)*

49. **(D)** Dextroamphetamine is usually the second line of pharmacological treatment when methylphenidate is not effective. Pemoline has the advantage of a longer half-life and thereby allows less frequent dosing and round-the-clock effects, but there have been some recent reports of serious liver failure in-patients being treated with pemoline. *(Kaplan and Sadock, 1198)*

50. **(B)** The most likely diagnosis in this vignette is acute intermittent porphyria. It is a disorder of heme biosynthesis, which results in excessive accumulation of porphyrin. It is characterized by the triad of symptoms: acute abdominal pain, motor polyneuropathy, and psychosis. Acute intermittent porphyria is an autosomal dominant disorder that affects more women than men; its onset is between ages 20 and 50. The psychiatric symptoms include anxiety, insomnia, lability of mood, depression, and psychosis. Some studies have found that between 0.2% and 0.5% of chronic psychiatric patients may have undiagnosed porphyria. Barbiturates precipitate or aggravate the attacks of acute porphyria, and the use of barbiturates for any reason is absolutely contraindicated in a person with acute intermittent porphyria and in anyone who has a relative with the disease. Niacin deficiency is unlikely to be the diagnosis. The neuropsychiatric symptoms of pellagra include apathy, irritability, insomnia, depression, and delirium; the medical symptoms include dermatitis, peripheral neuropathy, and diarrhea.

Thiamine deficiency is unlikely, because there is no history of ethanol abuse, and no signs of or psychiatric symptoms such as apathy, depression, irritability, nervousness, and poor concentration. The presence of a clear sensorium and the associated clinical and psychiatric symptoms argue against the diagnoses of hepatic encephalopathy and cobalamin deficiency, respectively. *(Kaplan and Sadock, 362–363)*

51. **(C)** Up to 72% of patients with panic disorder have a panic attack when administered an intravenous injection of sodium lactate. Therefore, lactate provocation is used to confirm a diagnosis of panic disorder. Hyperventilation, another known trigger of panic attacks in predisposed persons, is not as sensitive as lactate provocation

in inducing panic attacks. Carbon dioxide (CO_2) inhalation also precipitates panic attacks in those so predisposed. *(Kaplan and Sadock, 262)*

52. **(A)** Amitriptyline, imipramine, trimipramine, and doxepin have the most anticholinergic side effects of the tricyclic antidepressants. Amoxapine, nortriptyline, and maprotiline are less anticholinergic; and desipramine may be the least anticholinergic. Anticholinergic effects include dry mouth, constipation, blurred vision, and urinary retention. Narrow-angle glaucoma can also be aggravated by anticholinergic drugs, and the precipitation of glaucoma requires emergency treatment with a miotic agent. Severe anticholinergic effects can lead to a CNS anticholinergic syndrome with confusion and delirium, especially if tricyclic and tetracyclic drugs are administered with antipsychotics or anticholinergic drugs. The most common autonomic effect of tricyclic antidepressant medications, partly because of alpha1-adrenergic blockade, is orthostatic hypotension, which can result in falls and injuries in affected patients. Nortriptyline may be the drug least likely to cause the problem, and some patients respond to fludrocortisone (Florinef), 0.05 mg twice a day. Other possible autonomic effects are profuse sweating, palpitations, and increased blood pressure. *(Kaplan and Sadock, 1104)*

53. **(D)** The early signs and symptoms of lithium toxicity include coarse tremor, dysarthria, and ataxia; the later signs and symptoms include impaired consciousness, muscular fasciculations, myoclonus, seizures, and coma. The higher the lithium levels (and the longer they have been elevated), the worse the symptoms of lithium toxicity. *(Kaplan and Sadock, 1050)*

54. **(C)** Diarrhea, vomiting, drowsiness, muscular weakness and lack of coordination may be early signs of lithium intoxication, and can occur at lithium levels below 2.0 mEq/L. At higher levels, ataxia, giddiness, tinnitus, blurred vision and a large output of dilute urine may be seen. Serum lithium levels above 3.0 mEq/L may produce a complex clinical picture, involving multiple organs and organ systems. Serum lithium levels should not be permitted to exceed 2.0 mEq/L

during the acute treatment phase. *(Enna and Coyle, 125–127)*

55. **(E)** Concurrent use of calcium channel blocking agents with lithium may increase the risk of neurotoxicity in the form of ataxia, tremors, nausea, vomiting, diarrhea, and tinnitus. Caution should be used when lithium and diuretics are used concomitantly because diuretic-induced sodium loss may reduce the renal clearance of lithium and increase serum lithium levels with risk of lithium toxicity. Patients receiving such combined therapy should have serum lithium levels monitored closely and the lithium dosage adjusted if necessary. Lithium levels should be closely monitored when patients initiate or discontinue nonsteroidal antiinflammatory drug (NSAID) use. Concurrent use of metronidazole with lithium may provoke lithium toxicity due to reduced renal clearance. There is evidence that angiotensin-converting enzyme inhibitors, such as enalapril and captopril, may substantially increase steady-state plasma lithium levels, sometimes resulting in lithium toxicity. When such combinations are used, lithium dosage may need to be decreased, and plasma lithium levels should be measured more frequently. The concomitant administration of lithium with selective serotonin reuptake inhibitors should be undertaken with caution as this combination has been reported to result in symptoms such as diarrhea, confusion, tremor, dizziness, and agitation. The following drugs can lower serum lithium concentrations by increasing urinary lithium excretion: acetazolamide, urea, xanthine preparations, and alkalinizing agents such as sodium bicarbonate. *(Enna and Coyle, 127; Stern et al., 366–367)*

56. **(A)**

57. **(D)**

58. **(B)**

59. **(C)**

Explanations 56 through 59

Hepatotoxicity has been reported with the use of pemoline. Agranulocytosis has been estimated to occur in association with clozapine use at a cumulative incidence at 1 year of approximately 1.3% of patients. Its incidence rate based upon a weekly monitoring schedule rose steeply during the first 2 months of therapy, peaking in the third month. Lithium use has been associated with the formation of euthyroid goiter, hypothyroidism accompanied by lower T3 and T4. Imipramine use may be associated with cardiovascular side effects such as arrhythmias, heart block, ECG changes, orthostatic hypotension, hypertension, tachycardia, palpitation, and myocardial infarction. *(Enna and Coyle, 38, 126; Kaplan and Sadock, 566–569, 953)*

60. **(D)** The maternal lithium level must be monitored closely during pregnancy and especially after delivery because of the significant change in renal function with massive fluid shift that occurs over that time period. Lithium should be discontinued shortly before delivery, and the drug should be restarted after an assessment of the usually high risk of postpartum mood disorder and the mother's desire to breast-feed her infant. *(Kaplan and Sadock, 1051)*

61. **(A)** Functional neuroimaging studies of people with attention deficit hyperactivity disorder (ADHD) have either been normal or have shown decreased volume of the right prefrontal cortex and the right globus pallidus. In addition, whereas normally the right caudate nucleus is larger than the left caudate nucleus, people with ADHD may have caudate nuclei of equal size. These findings suggest dysfunction of the right prefrontal-striatal pathway for control of attention. *(Kaplan and Sadock, 1194)*

62. **(B)** Thioridazine is associated with irreversible pigmentation of the retina when given in dosages of more than 800 mg a day. An early symptom of this effect can sometimes be nocturnal confusion related to difficulty with night vision. The pigmentation is similar to that seen in retinitis pigmentosa; it can progress even after the thioridazine is stopped and can finally result in blindness. In contrast, chlorpromazine is associated with benign pigmentation of the eyes. Most patients who show the deposits are those who have ingested 1 to 3 kg of chlorpromazine throughout their lives. *(Kaplan and Sadock, 1030)*

63. **(A)** Although alcohol consumed in the evening usually results in an increased ease of falling asleep (decreased sleep latency), alcohol also has adverse effects on sleep architecture. Specifically, alcohol use is associated with decreased rapid eye movement sleep (REM or dream sleep), decreased deep sleep (stage 4), and increased sleep fragmentation, with more and longer episodes of awakening. *(Kaplan and Sadock, 396)*

64. **(C)**

65. **(F)**

66. **(E)**

67. **(A)**

68. **(B)**

69. **(G)**

70. **(D)**

Explanations 64 through 70

The CNS effects of acute alcohol intoxication depend on the blood level of alcohol. Signs of intoxication include loss of inhibition, slurred speech, staggering gait, euphoria, nystagmus, motor incoordination, confusion, stupor, and coma with high levels of alcohol in the blood.

Signs of cocaine intoxication include vasoconstriction, increased heart rate and blood pressure, chest pain, pupillary dilation, muscle weakness, respiratory depression, euphoria, increased energy, anxiety, and increased risk of psychosis.

Acute heroin intoxication results in an initial euphoria followed by apathy, dysphoria, psychomotor agitation, or retardation. Other signs include pupillary constriction, slurred speech, impaired attention or memory, and drowsiness or coma depending on the severity of the heroin overdose.

Acute cannabis intoxication results in clinically significant maladaptive behavioral or psychological changes such as impaired motor coordination, euphoria, anxiety, sensation of slowed time, and impaired judgment. Other symptoms of cannabis intoxication include conjunctival injection, increased appetite, dry mouth, and tachycardia.

Symptoms of phencyclidine intoxication include clinically significant maladaptive behavioral changes such as belligerence, assaultiveness, impulsiveness, unpredictability, vertical or horizontal nystagmus, hypertension or tachycardia, numbness or diminished responsiveness to pain, ataxia, dysarthria and muscle rigidity, hyperacusis. Seizure and coma may occur in case of severe intoxication.

LSD intoxication is characterized by marked behavioral abnormalities such as marked anxiety or depression, ideas of reference, fear of losing one's mind, paranoid ideation, and impaired judgment. Perceptual changes may occur in a state of full wakefulness and alertness: the patient may express a subjective intensification of perceptions, depersonalization, derealization, illusions, and hallucination. Other physical signs of LSD intoxication include pupillary dilation, tachycardia, blurred vision, incoordination, and sweating.

Caffeine overdose results in restlessness, nervousness, excitement, insomnia, flushed face, diuresis, gastrointestinal disturbance, and muscle twitching. *(Kaplan and Sadock, 379–383; Stern et al., 73, 85, 89)*

71. **(A)**

72. **(B)**

73. **(E)**

74. **(C)**

75. **(D)**

Explanations 71 through 75

Alcohol withdrawal signs are divided into minor and major symptoms. Minor symptoms start 8 to 9 hours after the last drink. The patient may have insomnia, sweating, hallucinations, and seizures. Major symptoms occur 48 to 96 hours after the last drink. The patient may have increased psychomotor activity, tremor, hallucinations, profound disorientation, and increased autonomic activity.

Cocaine withdrawal involves a dysphoric mood, fatigue, vivid and unpleasant dreams, insomnia or hypersomnia, increased appetite, and agitation or psychomotor retardation.

Heroin withdrawal is characterized by a dysphoric mood, nausea or vomiting, muscle aches, lacrimation, pupillary dilation, fever diarrhea, piloerection, and sweating.

Signs of nicotine withdrawal include dysphoric or depressed mood, insomnia, irritability, frustration, or anger, anxiety, difficulty concentrating, restlessness, decreased heart rate, and increased appetite or weight gain. These symptoms are associated with significant distress or impairment in social functioning.

Abrupt cessation of caffeine use, or reduction in the amount of caffeine used causes headache associated with marked fatigue and anxiety, possible depression, and nausea or vomiting, as well as clinically significant distress and impaired social functioning. *(Kaplan and Sadock, 379–383; Stern et al., 75, 85, 89)*

76. **(D)** Catatonia, mania, major depression, and acute exacerbation of schizophrenia are well-established indications of electroconvulsive therapy (ECT). Other indications of electroconvulsive therapy with less evidence of its effectiveness include Parkinson disease, obsessive-compulsive disorder, neuroleptic malignant syndrome, and intractable epilepsy. ECT is only effective in the treatment for acute symptoms of schizophrenia, not those of chronic schizophrenia. *(Kaplan and Sadock, 1116–1118; Stern et al., 360)*

77. **(E)** Four clinical interview questions, the CAGE questions, have proved useful in helping to make a diagnosis of alcoholism. The questions focus on Cutting Down, Annoyance by Criticism, Guilty Feeling, and Eye-Openers. The acronym "CAGE" helps the physician recall the questions:

"C": Have you ever felt you should cut down on your drinking?

"A" Have people annoyed you by criticizing your drinking?

"G" Have you ever felt bad or guilty about your drinking?

"E" Have you ever had a drink first thing in the morning to steady your nerves or to get rid of a hangover? *(Ewing, 1905–1907)*

78. **(B)** Among the SSRIs, fluvoxamine appears to present the greatest risk of drug–drug interactions. Fluvoxamine is metabolized by CYP 3A4. Fluvoxamine may increase the half-lives of alprazolam and diazepam and should not be coadministered with these agents. Fluvoxamine may increase theophylline concentrations 3-fold and warfarin concentrations 2-fold, with important clinical consequences. Fluvoxamine raises concentrations and may increase the activity of clozapine, carbamazepine, methadone, propranolol, and diltiazem. *(Kaplan and Sadock, 1090)*

REFERENCES

American Psychiatric Association. *Diagnostic and Statistical Manual of Mental Disorders*, 4th ed. Washington, DC; American Psychiatric Association:1994.

Behrman RE. *Nelson Textbook of Pediatrics.* 16th ed. Philadelphia, PA: WB Saunders;2000.

Brown CS. Depression and anxiety disorders. *Obstet Gynecol Clin North Am.* 2001;28:241–268.

Comings DE. Clinical and molecular genetics of ADHD and Tourette syndrome. Two related polygenic disorders. *Ann NY Acad Sci.* 2001;931:50–83.

Coyle JT, Enna SJ, eds. *Pharmacological Management of Neurological and Psychiatric Disorders.* New York: McGraw-Hill;1998.

Ewing JA. Detecting alcoholism-the CAGE questionnaire. *JAMA* 1984;252:1905–1907

Goldberg JF. New drugs in psychiatry. *Emerg Med Clin North Am.* 2000;18:211–231.

Hobson JA. Sleep and dreaming. *J Neurosci.* 1990;10: 371–382.

Hobson JA. The sleep-dream cycle: A neurobiological rhythm. *Pathobiol Annu.* 1975:5:369–403.

Kaplan BJ, Sadocks VA. *Synopsis of Psychiatry.* 8th ed. Baltimore, MA: Lippincott, Williams & Wilkins;1997.

Kranzler HR, Amin H, Modesto-Lowe V, Oncken C. Pharmacologic treatments for drug and alcohol dependence. *Psychiatr Clin North Am.* 1999;22:401–423.

Longhurst JG. Neuroleptic malignant syndrome. *J Psychiatr.* 1995;166:537–538.

Margolis RL, McInnis MG, Rosenblatt A, Ross CA. Trinucleotide repeat expansion and neuropsychiatric disease. *Arch Gen Psychiatry.* 1999:56:1019–1031.

Mann JJ. A current perspective of suicide and attempted suicide. *Ann Intern Med.* 2002;136:302–311.

Mayfield D, McLeod G, Hall P. The CAGE questionnaire: validation of a new alcoholism screening instrument. *Am J Psychiatry.* 1974;131:1121–1123.

Newport DJ, Nemeroff CB. Neurobiology of posttraumatic stress disorder. *Curr Opin Neurobiol.* 2000;10:211–218.

Oquendo MA The biology of impulsivity and suicidality. *Psychiatr Clin North Am.* 2000;23:11–25.

Stern TA, Herman JB. *Psychiatry Update and Board Preparation.* New York: McGraw-Hill;2000.

Task Force on the Use of Laboratory Tests in Psychiatry. Tricyclic antidepressants-blood level measurements and clinical outcome: an APA Task Force report. *Am J Psychiatry.* 1985;142:155–162.

Warner EA. Cocaine abuse. *Ann Intern Med.* 1993;119: 226–235.

Weeks RA, Turjanski N, Brooks DJ. Tourette's syndrome: a disorder of cingulate and orbitofrontal function? *QJM.* 1996;89:401–408.

Weiss F. Porrino LJ. Behavioral neurobiology of alcohol addiction: recent advances and challenges. *J Neurosci.* 2002;22:3332–3337.

Withers NW, Pulvirenti L, Koob GF, Gillin JC. Cocaine abuse and dependence. *J Clin Psychopharmacol.* 1995;15: 63–78.

Zun LS. Panic disorder: diagnosis and treatment in emergency medicine. *Ann Emerg Med.* 1997;30:92–96.

Index

Page numbers followed by italic *f* or *t* indicate figures or tables, respectively.